Anesthesiology: A Comprehensive Guide

Anesthesiology: A Comprehensive Guide

Editor: Quentin Hardy

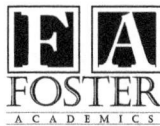

FA
FOSTER
ACADEMICS

www.fosteracademics.com

www.fosteracademics.com

FA
FOSTER
ACADEMICS

Cataloging-in-Publication Data

Anesthesiology : a comprehensive guide / edited by Quentin Hardy.
     p. cm.
Includes bibliographical references and index.
ISBN 978-1-63242-824-0
1. Anesthesiology. 2. Anesthesia--Guidebooks. 3. Surgery. I. Hardy, Quentin.
RD82.2 .A54 2019
617.96--dc23

Foster Academics,
118-35 Queens Blvd., Suite 400,
Forest Hills, NY 11375, USA

ISBN 978-1-63242-824-0 (Hardback)

Contents

Preface

This book has been a concerted effort by a group of academicians, researchers and scientists, who have contributed their research works for the realization of the book. This book has materialized in the wake of emerging advancements and innovations in this field. Therefore, the need of the hour was to compile all the required researches and disseminate the knowledge to a broad spectrum of people comprising of students, researchers and specialists of the field.

Anesthesia is an induced state of temporary and controlled loss of awareness and sensation. It includes paralysis or muscle relaxation, prevention and relief from pain, and unconsciousness. It allows the painless performance of medical procedures, which could cause intolerable pain in an unanesthetized patient. It can be administered such that it leads to a total lack of sensation, or to partial loss of sensation, or inhibit anxiety and the creation of long-term memories. Safe anesthesia administration requires a holistic understanding of the effects of anesthetic drugs, organ support techniques, hemodynamic monitoring, advanced airway management and diagnostic techniques. The practice of anesthesia is known as anesthesiology. This book discusses the fundamentals as well as modern approaches of anesthesiology. It presents researches and studies performed by experts across the globe. The extensive content of this book provides the readers with a thorough understanding of the subject.

At the end of the preface, I would like to thank the authors for their brilliant chapters and the publisher for guiding us all-through the making of the book till its final stage. Also, I would like to thank my family for providing the support and encouragement throughout my academic career and research projects.

Editor

Successful Ultrasound-Guided Femoral Nerve Blockade and Catheterization in a Patient with Von Willebrand Disease

Youmna E. DiStefano and Michael D. Lazar

Department of Anesthesiology, New York Medical College, Valhalla, NY 10595, USA

Correspondence should be addressed to Youmna E. DiStefano; abihaidary@wcmc.com

Academic Editor: Mario Dauri

Peripheral nerve blockade (PNB) is superior to neuraxial anesthesia and/or opioid therapy for perioperative analgesia in total knee replacement (TKR). Evidence on the safety of PNB in patients with coagulopathy is lacking. We describe the first documented account of continuous femoral PNB for perioperative analgesia in a patient with Von Willebrand Disease (vWD). Given her history of opioid tolerance and after an informative discussion, a continuous femoral PNB was planned for in this 34-year-old female undergoing TKR. A Humate-P intravenous infusion was started and the patient was positioned supinely. Using sterile technique with ultrasound guidance, a Contiplex 18 Gauge Tuohy needle was advanced in plane through the fascia iliaca towards the femoral nerve. A nerve catheter was threaded through the needle and secured without complications. Postoperatively, a levobupivacaine femoral catheter infusion was maintained, and twice daily Humate-P intravenous infusions were administered for 48 hours; enoxaparin thromboprophylaxis was initiated thereafter. The patient was discharged uneventfully on postoperative day 4. Given documentation of delayed, unheralded bleeding from PNB in coagulopathic patients, we recommend individualized PNB in vWD patients. Multidisciplinary team involvement is required to guide factor supplementation and thromboprophylaxis, as is close follow-up to elicit signs of bleeding throughout the delayed postoperative period.

1. Introduction

Von Willebrand disease (vWD) is the most common inherited bleeding disorder. Despite advances in the molecular diagnosis and treatment of this disease, the literature remains scarce as to the perioperative management of vWD patients undergoing orthopedic and other types of surgery. In particular, joint replacement surgery is amenable to various regional anesthetic techniques, including neuraxial anesthesia, lumbar plexus blockade, and peripheral nerve blockade (PNB). Evidence has established the superiority of PNB to neuraxial anesthesia and/or opioid therapy in total knee replacement (TKR) patients [1–3] and in orthopedic surgery patients on thromboprophylaxis (ppx) [4]. While PNB among other modalities has been associated with superior pain scores and a more favorable side effect profile, its use in patients with inherited or acquired coagulopathy may carry potentially catastrophic hemorrhagic complications. Certainly, the available evidence regarding the safety of PNB in coagulopathic patients is insufficient to date. To our knowledge, this case study is the first documented account of a continuous femoral nerve catheter insertion for intra- and postoperative pain control in a patient with Von Willebrand disease.

2. Case Report

The patient presented has granted us permission to publish this report. She is a 34-year-old female diagnosed with type 1 vWD associated with a hypercoagulable state, as evidenced by superficial thrombophlebitis and 3 spontaneous abortions in the past. She had a long history of debilitating left knee chondromalacia patellae secondary to a slip and fall injury at age 15; this progressed to advanced patellofemoral arthrosis, resulting in significantly decreased ambulatory capacity and constant knee pain refractory to large doses of nonsteroidal anti-inflammatory medications and Percocet. The patient had failed physical therapy, multiple intra-articular steroid injections, multiple arthroscopic debridements, and tibial tubercle osteotomy with lateral retinacular release; she was thus scheduled to undergo a left TKR. Her medical history was otherwise significant for mild intermittent asthma, and her surgical history was notable for inferior vena cava filter placement, left wrist ganglion cyst excision, 3 dilatation and curettage procedures, and a Caesarean section complicated by severe intraoperative hemorrhage requiring massive transfusion with packed red blood cells, fresh frozen plasma, and factor VIII concentrate. Her height and weight were 170 cm and 70 kg, respectively. She was treated with Singulair, albuterol, nonsteroidal anti-inflammatory medications, and Percocet; she also had an allergy to penicillin.

During the preanesthetic evaluation, the patient expressed an interest in a femoral nerve block for postoperative pain control, given her history of opioid tolerance and in light of a self-review of the pertinent literature. The risks and benefits of PNB and general endotracheal anesthesia (GETA) were discussed with the patient, with particular reference to her coagulopathy and the risk of bleeding complications from regional anesthesia. The anesthetic plan consisted of intravenous (IV) infusion of Humate-P in compliance with the hematologist's recommendations and it was dosed using body weight and baseline plasma vWF ristocetin cofactor activity. This was to be followed by ultrasound-guided continuous left femoral nerve blockade and GETA.

In the operating room, the patient was positioned supinely and standard American Society of Anesthesiologists monitors were applied. The patient was premedicated with midazolam 2 mg IV and fentanyl 50 mcg IV; the block site was prepared with chlorhexidine and draped in a sterile fashion. An IV infusion of 1876 units of Humate-P was initiated prior to the start of the block. With the ultrasound transducer sterilely covered and positioned transversely over the left inguinal crease, the femoral artery and femoral nerve were identified. Using a Contiplex 18 Gauge Tuohy continuous nerve block tray, the site was locally infiltrated with 6 mL of 2% lidocaine with 1:100,000 epinephrine. The needle was positioned in plane and advanced medially toward the femoral nerve. Once adequate local anesthetic spread was visualized, the nerve catheter was threaded through the needle and advanced 4 cm past the needle tip. A total of 20 mL of 0.5% levobupivacaine and 10 mL of 2% lidocaine with 1:100,000 epinephrine was injected during the procedure. The catheter was secured at the skin with a Tegaderm dressing and reinforced with adhesive tape. There were no signs of vascular trauma, nerve injury, or bleeding throughout the block procedure.

This was followed by standard induction of general anesthesia, endotracheal intubation, and maintenance with inhalational anesthetic.

Intraoperatively, a left lower extremity tourniquet was applied at a pressure of 250 psi for 76 minutes. Towards the end of the operation, 10 mL of 0.5% levobupivacaine was injected through the femoral catheter. Total surgical time was 79 minutes and blood loss was approximately 50 mL. The patient emerged from anesthesia and was extubated uneventfully. She made no complaints and was transferred to the postanesthesia care unit, where a femoral catheter infusion of 0.2% levobupivacaine at 12 mL per hour was started and

maintained for 2 days postoperatively. This was supplemented through postoperative day (POD) 1 with hydromorphone patient-controlled analgesia; the patient required a total of 7.6 mg of hydromorphone during the 24-hour succeeding surgery. As per recommendations from the consulting hematology team, the patient also received 1600 units of Humate-P every 12 hours for 48 hours postoperatively. After the 4th and last dose of Humate-P was administered (i.e., on the night of POD 2), ppx was initiated with enoxaparin 30 mg subcutaneously daily. The femoral nerve catheter was removed intact on POD 2. The patient's postoperative course was uncomplicated and she was discharged from the hospital on POD 4.

3. Discussion

The need for orthopedic surgery among vWD patients is not uncommon, especially considering the risk of development of disabling arthropathy from repeated bleeding into the involved joints. Our patient was suffering from patellofemoral arthrosis unrelated to her coagulopathy. At any rate, surgical intervention in vWD patients is missing evidence-based standards for safe, quality perioperative management.

According to a meta-analysis of 504 TKRs, PNB is associated with equivalent analgesia, significantly lower rates of hypotension and urinary retention, and higher patient satisfaction as compared to neuraxial blocks [2]. Moreover, while epidural and spinal hematomas carry an alarmingly high risk of permanent neurologic disability, hematomas resulting from PNB tend to develop in more compliant spaces and are theoretically less likely to cause catastrophic nerve impingement [5]. This consideration, however, is by no means definitive and certainly cannot be assumed in states of inherited or acquired coagulopathy as in vWD cases.

Table 1 summarizes the available literature on the outcomes of femoral nerve blockade in patients on ppx and/or at above-standard bleeding risk [6–11]. Two case reports [10, 11] involved temporary lower extremity motor impairment, and one prospective series [9] detailed a case of retroperitoneal hematoma associated with permanent quadriceps femoris denervation. The concerned patient was reportedly self-administering 1 g of aspirin daily pre- and postoperatively, unbeknownst to her caregivers [9]. Importantly, the signs of PNB-associated bleeding described in the literature (Table 1) were not apparent until later in the postoperative period, between POD 2 [9] and POD 10 [11]. It also remains unclear whether or not the bleeding was associated with initiation of ppx therapy versus vascular puncture or delayed intravascular migration of femoral nerve catheters. The unheralded, delayed presentation of PNB-related hemorrhage could account for the higher rate of neurologic complications as a result of the insidious accumulation of blood at the blockade site; this is in contrast to such procedures as transfemoral cardiac catheterization, which, although performed on anticoagulated patients by definition, are marked by a higher incidence of acute blood loss and vascular complications. Lower postprocedure vigilance and surveillance for bleeding could also be incriminated in the insidious yet catastrophic

TABLE 1: Available literature on outcomes of femoral nerve blockade in patients on thromboprophylaxis and/or at above-standard bleeding risk.

Author	Study type	Nb. of blocks	Type of block	ppx or bleeding risk	Complication(s) from femoral block
Chelly and Schilling [6]	Retrospective cohort	1790	Continuous femoral	10% aspirin ppx 20% LMWH ppx 10% fondaparinux ppx 60% warfarin ppx	0
Vanarase et al. [7]	Retrospective cohort	21	Single-shot femoral or sciatic or both	2 vWD patients 13 hemophilia patients	0
Sripada et al. [8]	Case report	2	Single-shot femoral and sciatic	2 hemophilia patients	0
Wiegel et al. [9]	Retrospective cohort	628	Continuous femoral	Not specified	36 vascular punctures 1 retroperitoneal hematoma causing permanent nerve injury*
Bickler et al. [10]	Case report	2	Continuous femoral and sciatic	LMWH ppx	1 swelling & discoloration at block site with temporary lower extremity motor impairment 1 delayed oozing at catheter site
Rodríguez et al. [11]	Case report	1	Single-shot femoral and sciatic	Factor XI deficiency, LMWH ppx	Perineural hematoma with temporary lower extremity paralysis

*Nerve injury was evidenced by complete quadriceps femoris denervation. The concerned patient was reportedly self-administering 1 g of aspirin daily pre- and postoperatively, unbeknownst to her caregivers.
Nb. indicates number; ppx, thromboprophylaxis; LMWH, low molecular weight heparin.

neurologic outcomes of PNB-related hemorrhage, which is in stark contrast to the close patient observation and femoral compression performed immediately after cardiac catheterization.

Perioperative supplementation of vWD patients with Von Willebrand factor/factor VIII (vWF/FVIII) concentrates is commonly recommended by hematologists to mitigate the risk of massive or uncontrolled bleeding. Humate-P is a human plasma-derived vWF/FVIII concentrate with an extensive, three-decade track record of no thrombosis and no cases of viral transmission [12, 13]. It is recommended for surgical prophylaxis and spontaneous bleeding treatment in all types of vWD and in vWD cases that are refractory to desmopressin. As per recommendations from the patient's hematologist, she received a Humate-P preoperative dose of 1876 units, followed by postoperative maintenance doses of 1600 units every 12 hours. These correspond to Humate-P surgical prophylaxis doses, which are calculated based on a formula integrating body weight and baseline plasma vWF ristocetin cofactor activity [14].

The 1st dose of prophylactic enoxaparin was administered to our patient after 48 hours of supplementation with Humate-P, at which point it was felt by the hematology team that the combination of postoperative time and loaded Humate-P dose was favorable for adequate hemostasis. According to the American Academy of Orthopaedic Surgeons (AAOP) guidelines, ppx after total hip or knee replacement procedures in patients at elevated risk for both pulmonary embolism and major bleeding (as in our case subject) should consist of aspirin 325 mg twice daily, or warfarin (with a goal international normalized ratio (INR)

less than or equal to 2.0), or none, in addition to the use of mechanical prophylaxis [15]. The latest ASRA consensus report, however, acknowledges important shortcomings in the current literature on ppx indications. These include failure to ensure adequate case mix balance between patients at risk of thrombosis and patients at risk for major bleeding, the deliberate exclusion of patients with preexisting coagulopathy, and the use of surrogate endpoints instead of the prescribed primary outcomes (i.e., symptomatic deep venous thrombosis and pulmonary embolism) [5].

Until authoritative evidence is generated to guide perioperative anesthetic care in patients with bleeding disorders, we recommend that vWD patients engage in an informed and educated decision regarding their plan of analgesia. Regional anesthetic techniques must be considered on a case-by-case basis, with careful weighing of the inherent risks and benefits. Multidisciplinary involvement by experts in hematology, surgery, anesthesiology, and nursing is required as is adherence to timely clotting factor supplementation and appropriate ppx. Standard PNB techniques using advanced technology, such as ultrasound guidance, are likely advantageous. Additionally, PNB sites and catheters must be carefully inspected and symptoms elicited for signs of bleeding throughout the postoperative period extending several days after surgery.

Disclosure

This work was presented at the 13th Annual ASRA Pain Medicine Meeting in San Francisco, CA.

References

[1] F. J. Singelyn, M. Deyaert, D. Joris, E. Pendeville, and J. M. Gouverneur, "Effects of intravenous patient-controlled analgesia with morphine, continuous epidural analgesia, and continuous three-in-one block on postoperative pain and knee rehabilitation after unilateral total knee arthroplasty," *Anesthesia and Analgesia*, vol. 87, no. 1, pp. 88–92, 1998.

[2] S. J. Fowler, J. Symons, S. Sabato, and P. S. Myles, "Epidural analgesia compared with peripheral nerve blockade after major knee surgery: a systematic review and meta-analysis of randomized trials," *British Journal of Anaesthesia*, vol. 100, no. 2, pp. 154–164, 2008.

[3] J. E. Paul, A. Arya, L. Hurlburt et al., "Femoral nerve block improves analgesia outcomes after total knee arthroplasty: a meta-analysis of randomized controlled trials," *Anesthesiology*, vol. 113, no. 5, pp. 1144–1162, 2010.

[4] C. Hantler, G. J. Despotis, R. Sinha, and J. E. Chelly, "Guidelines and alternatives for neuraxial anesthesia and venous thromboembolism prophylaxis in major orthopedic surgery," *The Journal of Arthroplasty*, vol. 19, no. 8, pp. 1004–1016, 2004.

[5] T. T. Horlocker, D. J. Wedel, J. C. Rowlingson et al., "Regional Anesthesia in the patient receiving antithrombotic or thrombolytic therapy; American Society of Regional Anesthesia and Pain Medicine evidence-based guidelines (Third Edition)," *Regional Anesthesia and Pain Medicine*, vol. 35, no. 1, pp. 64–101, 2010.

[6] J. E. Chelly and D. Schilling, "Thromboprophylaxis and peripheral nerve blocks in patients undergoing joint arthroplasty," *Journal of Arthroplasty*, vol. 23, no. 3, pp. 350–354, 2008.

[7] M. Y. Vanarase, H. Pandit, Y. W. M. Kimstra, C. A. F. Dodd, and M. T. Popat, "Pain relief after knee replacement in patients with a bleeding disorder," *Haemophilia*, vol. 13, no. 4, pp. 395–397, 2007.

[8] R. Sripada, J. J. Reyes, and R. Sun, "Peripheral nerve blocks for intraoperative management in patients with hemophilia A," *Journal of Clinical Anesthesia*, vol. 21, no. 2, pp. 120–123, 2009.

[9] M. Wiegel, U. Gottschaldt, R. Hennebach, T. Hirschberg, and A. Reske, "Complications and adverse effects associated with continuous peripheral nerve blocks in orthopedic patients," *Anesthesia and Analgesia*, vol. 104, no. 6, pp. 1578–1582, 2007.

[10] P. Bickler, J. Brandes, M. Lee, K. Bozic, B. Chesbro, and J. Claassen, "Bleeding complications from femoral and sciatic nerve catheters in patients receiving low molecular weight heparin," *Anesthesia and Analgesia*, vol. 103, no. 4, pp. 1036–1037, 2006.

[11] J. Rodríguez, M. Taboada, F. García, M. Bermúdez, M. Amor, and J. Alvarez, "Intraneural hematoma after nerve stimulation-guided femoral block in a patient with factor XI deficiency: case report," *Journal of Clinical Anesthesia*, vol. 23, no. 3, pp. 234–237, 2011.

[12] G. Auerswald and W. Kreuz, "Haemate P/Humate-P for the treatment of von Willebrand disease: considerations for use and clinical experience," *Haemophilia*, vol. 14, supplement 5, pp. 39–46, 2008.

[13] E. Berntorp, W. Archey, G. Auerswald et al., "A systematic overview of the first pasteurised VWF/FVIII medicinal product, Haemate P/Humate-P: history and clinical performance," *European Journal of Haematology*, vol. 80, supplement 70, pp. 3–35, 2008.

[14] CSL Behring GmbH, *Humate-P Antihemophilic Factor/Von Willebrand Factor Complex (Human): Prescribing Information*, CSL Behring GmbH, 2013, http://labeling.cslbehring.com/PI/US/Humate-P/EN/Humate-P-Prescribing-Information.pdf.

[15] American Academy of Orthopaedic Surgeons, accessed in November 5, 2014, http://www.aaos.org/guidelines.pdf.

In Vitro Contracture Test Results and Anaesthetic Management of a Patient with Emery-Dreifuss Muscular Dystrophy for Cardiac Transplantation

Frank Schuster,[1] **Carsten Wessig,**[2] **Christoph Schimmer,**[3] **Stephan Johannsen,**[1] **Marc Lazarus,**[1] **Ivan Aleksic,**[3] **Rainer Leyh,**[3] **and Norbert Roewer**[1]

[1] *Department of Anaesthesia and Critical Care, University of Wuerzburg, 97080 Wuerzburg, Germany*
[2] *Department of Neurology, University of Wuerzburg, 97080 Wuerzburg, Germany*
[3] *Department of Cardiothoracic and Thoracic Vascular Surgery, University of Wuerzburg, 97080 Wuerzburg, Germany*

Correspondence should be addressed to Frank Schuster, schuster_f@klinik.uni-wuerzburg.de

Academic Editors: S. Faenza, R. S. Gomez, A. Han, and E. A. Vandermeersch

Emery-Dreifuss muscular dystrophy (EDMD) is a hereditary neuromuscular disorder characterized by slowly progressive muscle weakness, early contractures, and dilated cardiomyopathy. We reported an uneventful general anaesthesia using total intravenous anaesthesia (TIVA) for cardiac transplantation in a 19-year-old woman suffering from EDMD. In vitro contracture test results of two pectoralis major muscle bundles of the patient suggest that exposition to triggering agents does not induce a pathological sarcoplasmic calcium release in the lamin A/C phenotype. However, due to the lack of evidence in the literature, we would recommend TIVA for patients with EDMD if general anaesthesia is required.

1. Introduction

Emery-Dreifuss muscular dystrophy (EDMD), initially considered a benign form of Duchenne or Becker muscular dystrophy, is a hereditary neuromuscular disorder characterized by slowly progressive muscle weakness at the outset with humeroperoneal distribution and early contractures of elbow joints, Achilles tendons, and posterior-cervical muscles. EDMD either presents as an *X-linked disorder* due to a mutation in the emerin gene on chromosome Xq28 or as an *autosomal dominant* form, associated with an aberration of lamin A/C proteins on chromosome 1q11-23 [1]. Emerin and lamin A/C are located in the inner nuclear membrane of different cell types, including skeletal und cardiac muscle fibers. The incidence of autosomal dominant EDMD varies from 1 to 3 : 100.000, while the prevalence of the X-linked recessive form is assumed with 1 in 100.000 males [2]. Cardiac disease occurring by adulthood is a predominant feature of EDMD comprising conduction defects and arrhythmias. Implantation of a pacemaker is recommended if sinus or AV node disease develops [3, 4].

Heart transplantations due to dilated cardiomyopathy and heart failure are rare, but may increase as patients with a pacemaker or cardioverter/defibrillator may have longer survival [5].

2. Case Report

After obtaining written informed consent of a 19-year-old woman with a lamin A/C associated EDMD scheduled for high urgent cardiac transplantation we reviewed the specific anaesthetic management of this case and presented histological findings of skeletal and heart muscle and results of in vitro contracture-testing.

Beside minor weakness of anterior cervical muscles and proximal upper limbs preoperative neurologic examination was unremarkable. After surviving a sudden cardiac arrest in 2005 an implantable cardioverter defibrillator (ICD) had been inserted. During the last 3 years, she had frequently been hospitalized because of congestive heart failure. Cardiac evaluation revealed an ongoing progression towards dilated

TABLE 1: Metabolic parameters at different points of time during cardiac transplantation.

	F_iO_2	pH	PCO_2 [mmHg]	PO_2 [mmHg]	Base excess	Laktate [mmol/L]	Creatinkinase [U/L] reference value: <170 U/L	Myoglobin [μg/L] reference value: 25–58 μg/L	Temp. °C
Initial	0.21	7.5	34	62	3.4	0.8	53	30	37.2
Reperfusion	1.0	7.25	44	235	−7.7	8.4	53	56	36.3
After weaning from CPB (central venous)	1.0	7.29	47	59	−7.6	9.5	729	830	36.9
Admission on ICU	0.4	7.32	46	156	−1.9	—	1357	1283	36.3
1 postoperative day	0.35	7.41	48	122	5.8	—	1292	1005	—

cardiomyopathy despite maximum medical therapy. Perioperative echocardiography showed left ventricular and atrial dilatation, an ejection fraction of 22%, moderate tricuspid regurgitation, and an increased systolic pulmonary arterial pressure of 71 mmHg. ECG showed a regular sinus rhythm with incomplete right bundle branch block. After a 3-month waiting period, orthotopic bicaval cardiac transplantation was carried out. Prior to arrival at the operating room, the anaesthetic workstation (Dräger Primus, Germany) was prepared according to our standardized procedure for patients with known malignant hyperthermia susceptibility or muscular disorders: Vapors were removed, carbon dioxide absorbent, fresh gas hose, and breathing circuit were exchanged and the system was flushed with a fresh gas flow of 18 L/min for at least 25 min. Prior to surgery, arterial, central venous, and pulmonary artery catheters for hemodynamic monitoring were inserted under local anaesthesia. Preoperative arterial blood gases (ABG) and metabolic parameters were unremarkable (Table 1). Due to the known muscle dystrophy a total intravenous anaesthesia (TIVA) supplemented with nondepolarising muscle relaxants was carried out. Following 5 min of preoxygenation anaesthesia was induced with 1 μg/kg sufentanil, 2 mg/kg propofol and maintained with continuous propofol (5 mg/kg/h) and sufentanil (1 μg/kg/h) infusion. Rocuronium (0,6 mg/kg) was given to facilitate oral airway intubation and ventilation was adjusted to ABG using low tidal volumes (4–6 mL/kg). Anticoagulation with heparin (500 UI/kg) was monitored by activated clotting time (ACT) in 20 min intervals to maintain ACT > 500 seconds. Tranexamic acid was administered as loading dose of 15 mg/kg within 15 min followed by continuous infusion of 2 mg/kg for 6 hours. During induction of anaesthesia vital signs remained stable. After aortic and bicaval cannulation, cardiopulmonary bypass (CPB) was initiated and cardiac transplantation was performed as described by Shumway and colleagues [6]. Reperfusion phase was prolonged due to reduced donor organ function with an estimated ejection fraction of 30%. Hence, an intra-aortic balloon pump counterpulsation was inserted via the left femoral artery. Afterwards, the patient was weaned from CPB on epinephrine (0.07 μg/kg/min), norepinephrine (0.25 μg/kg/min), enoximone (0.17 mg/kg/h), and inhaled nitric oxide (25 ppm). At this time, a lactic acidosis was noticed, most likely caused by a prolonged episode of low

cardiac output (Table 1). Towards sternal closure hemodynamic instability with sudden rise of pulmonal arterial pressure to 60/24 mmHg occurred. The sternum was reopened and inhaled nitric oxide concentration was increased to 34 ppm. Subsequently the patient could be transferred to the ICU in stable condition with an open chest. On the first postoperative day the patient went to the operating room for definite sternal closure and was extubated on the third day after cardiac transplantation. Neurological status after extubation was unaltered to initial findings and the patient was discharged from hospital 30 days after transplantation.

2.1. In Vitro Contracture Test and Histological Findings. With prior informed consent of the patient, two bundles of the pectoralis major muscle were excised during the operative procedure. According to the guidelines of the European Malignant Hyperthermia Group an in vitro contracture test was carried out and the muscle bundles were incubated with increasing concentrations of caffeine (0.5; 1; 1.5; 2; 3; 4; 32 mM), respectively, halothane (0.11; 0.22; 0.44; 0.66 mM) [7]. Neither caffeine nor halothane induced significant muscular contractures at the threshold concentrations. There was no evidence of pathologic sarcoplasmic calcium release in response to malignant hyperthermia triggering agents in this patient. Histology of pectoralis major muscle showed mild myopathic changes with slightly increased variation in fiber size, some atrophic fibers, internal nuclei and slight increase of intramuscular fibrous tissue (Figure 1(a)). In the ventricular myocardium many atrophic cardiomyocytes and an increase of connective tissue were detected (Figure 1(b)).

3. Discussion

Due to lack of evidence in the current literature, the choice of the best anaesthetic management for patients with muscular dystrophies remains controversial. Several case reports documented the safe application of inhalational agents in patients with Duchenne and Becker type muscular dystrophy [8]. On the other hand, rhabdomyolysis, hyperkalemia and intraoperative or postoperative cardiac arrest occurred in affected patients independently of the use or absence of volatile anesthetics and/or the depolarising

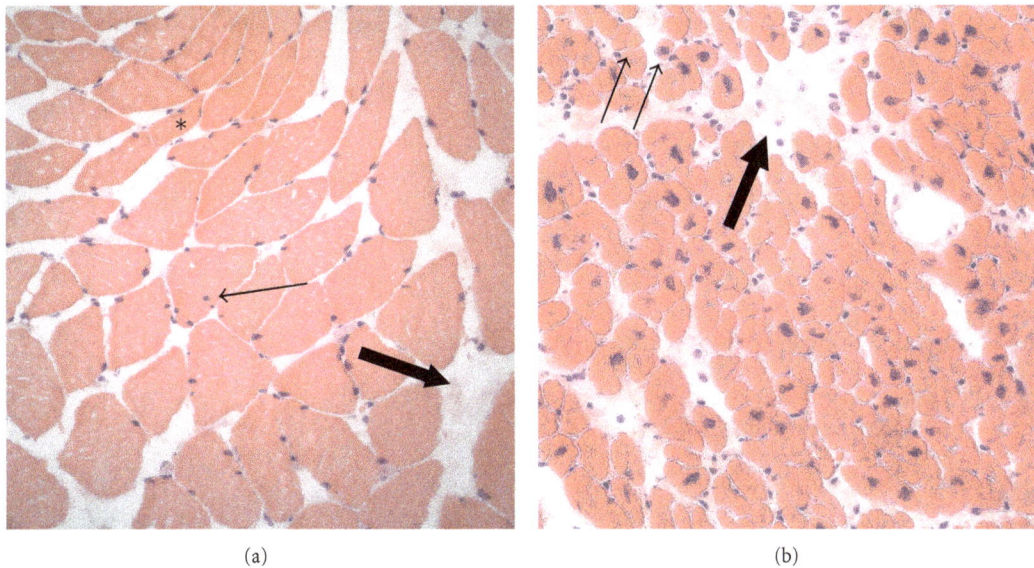

(a)   (b)

FIGURE 1: Histology (hematoxylin-eosin staining) of pectoralis major muscle (a) and heart muscle (b). In the pectorals major, mild myopathic changes with hypotrophic fibers (asterisk), some internal nuclei (small arrow), and an increase of fibrous tissue (large arrow) are seen. In the myocardium, there are some atrophic cardiomyocytes (small arrows) and a mild increase in connective tissue.

muscle relaxant succinylcholine [9]. Explicit recommendations or even guidelines concerning the anaesthetic practice for patients with EDMD are not available. While spinal or epidural anaesthesia were applied without any difficulty for orthopaedic surgery [10–12] and caesarean sections [13, 14], only two cases of uneventful general anaesthesia in EDMD patients using enflurane and succinylcholine [11], or TIVA [15] were described. In contrast to Duchenne and Becker muscular dystrophy, caused by a mutation of the muscle-stabilizing protein dystrophin, EDMD is associated with an aberration of the inner nuclear membrane proteins emerin or lamin A/C. As emerin and lamin A/C are suspected being responsible for the fixation and stabilization of the myonuclei during muscular contraction, alterations of these nuclear membrane proteins may cause defective cellular signalling in response to mechanical stimulations [16]. However, the impact on sarcoplasmic calcium release remains cloudy [17]. The missing muscular response to caffeine and halothane in the performed in vitro contracture test may be a hint that exposition to triggering agents does not lead to a dysfunction of calcium homeostasis in the lamin A/C phenotype. However, we should be cautious transferring in vitro results to in vivo conditions and drawing conclusions based on this single investigation. For safety reasons and in absence of significant publications on anaesthesia in patients with EDMD we decided to use TIVA in our patient. During and after anaesthesia no signs of hypermetabolism or rhabdomyolysis were observed. The lactic acidosis during reperfusion and after weaning from CPB was most likely a result of the initially reduced cardiac output of the transplanted organ, while the increase of serum creatine kinase and myoglobin were comparable to other major surgical procedures [18].

Interestingly, the extent of cardiac involvement does not correlate with the degree of skeletal muscle symptoms. Progressive cardiomyopathy without peripheral muscular symptoms similar to our patient has been previously reported for lamin A/C phenotypes [19]. In affected patients ECG abnormalities, for example, low amplitude P waves, prolonged PQ interval and atrial fibrillation or flutter may occur. These changes may proceed to atrial and ventricular conduction blocks, possibly resulting in complete heart block and necessitating temporary or permanent cardiac pacing. During the course of the disease cardiomyopathy leading to congestive heart failure may develop [4]. In patients with significant cardiomyopathy myocardial depressant agents should be avoided and cardiac pacing must be readily available at any time in the perioperative period.

Early appearance of skeletal muscle contractures before onset of muscular weakness is unique to EDMD. Involvement of posterior-cervical muscles may significantly reduce possible neck flexion and complicate endotracheal intubation, even with a normal Mallampati score [15]. If in doubt awake fiberoptic intubation should be preferred to secure the airway. Furthermore, lumbar paravertebral muscle contractures may hamper the application of spinal or epidural anaesthesia [13].

In summary, we reported an uneventful general anaesthesia using TIVA for cardiac transplantation in a 19-year-old woman suffering from EDMD. The in vitro contracture test results of the patient suggest that exposition to triggering agents does not induce a pathological sarcoplasmic calcium release in the lamin A/C phenotype. However, due to the lack of evidence in the literature, the authors would recommend TIVA for patients with EDMD if general anaesthesia is required.

Funding

This study was supported by departmental funding only.

References

[1] M. Puckelwartz and E. M. McNally, "Emery-Dreifuss muscular dystrophy," *Handbook of Clinical Neurology*, vol. 101, pp. 155–166, 2011.

[2] G. Lattanzi, S. Benedetti, and E. Bertini, "Laminopathies: many diseases, one gene. Report of the first Italian Meeting Course on Laminopathies," *Acta Myologica*, vol. 30, no. 2, pp. 138–143, 2011.

[3] J. Finsterer and C. Stöllberger, "Primary myopathies and the heart," *Scandinavian Cardiovascular Journal*, vol. 42, no. 1, pp. 9–24, 2008.

[4] M. C. E. Hermans, Y. M. Pinto, I. S. J. Merkies, C. E. M. de Die-Smulders, H. J. G. M. Crijns, and C. G. Faber, "Hereditary muscular dystrophies and the heart," *Neuromuscular Disorders*, vol. 20, no. 8, pp. 479–492, 2010.

[5] G. Boriani, M. Gallina, L. Merlini et al., "Clinical relevance of atrial fibrillation/flutter, stroke, pacemaker implant, and heart failure in Emery-Dreifuss muscular dystrophy: a long-term longitudinal study," *Stroke*, vol. 34, no. 4, pp. 901–908, 2003.

[6] N. E. Shumway, R. R. Lower, and R. C. Stofer, "Transplantation of the heart," *Advances in surgery*, vol. 2, pp. 265–284, 1966.

[7] F. R. Ellis, P. J. Halsall, and H. Ording, "A protocol for the investigation of malignant hyperpyrexia (MH) susceptibility. The European malignant hyperpyrexia group," *British Journal of Anaesthesia*, vol. 56, no. 11, pp. 1267–1269, 1984.

[8] J. J. Driessen, "Neuromuscular and mitochondrial disorders: what is relevant to the anaesthesiologist?" *Current Opinion in Anaesthesiology*, vol. 21, no. 3, pp. 350–355, 2008.

[9] H. Gurnaney, A. Brown, and R. S. Litman, "Malignant hyperthermia and muscular dystrophies," *Anesthesia and Analgesia*, vol. 109, no. 4, pp. 1043–1048, 2009.

[10] D. Shende and R. Agarwal, "Anaesthetic management of a patient with Emery-Dreifuss muscular dystrophy," *Anaesthesia and Intensive Care*, vol. 30, no. 3, pp. 372–375, 2002.

[11] V. Jensen, "The anaesthetic management of a patient with Emery-Dreifuss muscular dystrophy," *Canadian Journal of Anaesthesia*, vol. 43, no. 9, pp. 968–971, 1996.

[12] P. Morrison and R. H. Jago, "Emery-Dreifuss muscular dystrophy," *Anaesthesia*, vol. 46, no. 1, pp. 33–35, 1991.

[13] O. M. O. Kim and D. Elliott, "Elective caesarean section for a woman with Emery-Dreifuss muscular dystrophy," *Anaesthesia and Intensive Care*, vol. 38, no. 4, pp. 744–747, 2010.

[14] M. Sariego, A. Bustos, A. Guerola, I. Romero, and A. García-Baquero, "Anesthesia for cesarean section in a patient with Emery-Dreifuss muscular dystrophy," *Revista Espanola de Anestesiologia y Reanimacion*, vol. 43, no. 8, pp. 288–290, 1996.

[15] R. J. Aldwinckle and A. S. Carr, "The anesthetic management of a patient with Emery-Dreifuss muscular dystrophy for orthopedic surgery," *Canadian Journal of Anesthesia*, vol. 49, no. 5, pp. 467–470, 2002.

[16] J. Lammerding, J. Hsiao, P. C. Schulze, S. Kozlov, C. L. Stewart, and R. T. Lee, "Abnormal nuclear shape and impaired mechanotransduction in emerin-deficient cells," *Journal of Cell Biology*, vol. 170, no. 5, pp. 781–791, 2005.

[17] F. Chevessier, S. Bauché-Godard, J. P. Leroy et al., "The origin of tubular aggregates in human myopathies," *Journal of Pathology*, vol. 207, no. 3, pp. 313–323, 2005.

[18] A. S. Laurence, "Serum myoglobin and creatine kinase following surgery," *British Journal of Anaesthesia*, vol. 84, no. 6, pp. 763–766, 2000.

[19] D. Fatkin, C. Macrae, T. Sasaki et al., "Missense mutations in the rod domain of the lamin A/C gene as causes of dilated cardiomyopathy and conduction-system disease," *New England Journal of Medicine*, vol. 341, no. 23, pp. 1715–1724, 1999.

Asystole after Orthotopic Lung Transplantation: Examining the Interaction of Cardiac Denervation and Dexmedetomidine

Christopher Allen-John Webb,[1] Paul David Weyker,[1] and Brigid Colleen Flynn[1, 2]

[1] Columbia University College of Physicians and Surgeons, Columbia University Medical Center, New York, NY 10032, USA
[2] Division of Critical Care, Department of Anesthesiology, Columbia University Medical Center,
 622 West 168th Street PH 5-505, New York, NY 10032, USA

Correspondence should be addressed to Brigid Colleen Flynn, bf2184@columbia.edu

Academic Editors: M. J. C. Carmona, M. R. Chakravarthy, and E. A. Vandermeersch

Dexmedetomidine is an α_2-receptor agonist commonly used for sedation and analgesia in ICU patients. Dexmedetomidine is known to provide sympatholysis and also to have direct atrioventricular and sinoatrial node inhibitory effects. In rare instances, orthotopic lung transplantation has been associated with disruption of autonomic innervation of the heart. The combination of this autonomic disruption and dexmedetomidine may be associated with severe bradycardia and/or asystole. Since orthotopic lung transplant patients with parasympathetic denervation will not respond with increased heart rate to anticholinergic therapy, bradyarrhythmias must be recognized and promptly treated with direct acting beta agonists to avoid asystolic cardiac events.

1. Introduction

Bradycardia and asystole in the cardiothoracic intensive care unit (CTICU) setting can be due to a broad range of etiologies. Certain patients may be more predisposed to bradyarrhythmias and/or asystole due to a combination of factors such as the surgical procedure, medications being administered, and preexisting patient comorbidities. We report a case of severe bradycardia leading to asystole after a bilateral orthotopic lung transplantation (OLT) in a patient receiving dexmedetomidine sedation. We consider the possibility that cardiac sympathetic denervation secondary to the OLT in conjunction with atrial-ventricular node conduction delay caused by the dexmedetomidine may have led to the asystolic event.

2. Case Description

A 55-year-old woman with sarcoidosis was admitted to the CTICU after receiving a bilateral OLT involving significant tracheal dissection. On postoperative day 1, sedation was weaned, and she was communicating appropriately while intubated and desired to have an epidural catheter placed for pain control prior to extubation. Timing of the epidural for patients on anticoagulation was in accordance with the American Society of Regional Anesthesia and Pain Medicine guidelines [1]. Two hours prior to the procedure, the patient was started on a dexmedetomidine infusion at 0.5 micrograms/kilogram/hour for anxiolysis during the procedure. Since bradycardia is oftentimes associated with large boluses and high-dose infusions of dexmedetomidine, we decided to start the infusion at a lower dose two hours prior to procedure. She remained spontaneously breathing, comfortable, and cooperative. Her hemodynamics remained unchanged during the initiation of the dexmedetomidine infusion.

With her assistance and the endotracheal tube remaining in place, she was placed in a sitting position for epidural placement, and 50 micrograms of intravenous fentanyl was given for additional analgesia. Hemodynamic and respiratory stability was maintained with a sinus rhythm of 95 beats per minute, blood pressure of 130/63 mmHg, and SpO$_2$ of 95% and was consistent with her vitals prior to initiating the dexmedetomidine infusion. After obtaining the sitting position, her sinus rhythm deteriorated to bradycardia of 30 beats per minute, and she subsequently became hypotensive.

She became agitated, ceased following commands, and became unresponsive. The dexmedetomidine infusion was immediately stopped, and one milligram of intravenous atropine was administered for the bradycardia with no effect. The bradycardia continued to decline and deteriorated to an asystolic event confirmed by arterial pressure monitoring, and cardiopulmonary resuscitation (CPR) was initiated. After 3–5 minutes of CPR, an additional 1-milligram bolus of intravenous atropine was administered along with a 1-milligram bolus of intravenous epinephrine, resulting in a heart rate of 130 beats per minute and a systolic blood pressure of 220 mmHg, which rapidly decreased to 130 mmHg. Her hemodynamic profile remained stable, and the epidural placement was aborted. Transesophageal echocardiogram (TEE) failed to show any signs of a pulmonary embolus.

Differential diagnosis for the asystolic arrest included myocardial infarction, pulmonary embolism (PE), relative hypovolemia, a vasovagal event, the Bezold-Jarisch reflex, cardiac sarcoidosis, and direct atrial-ventricular conduction inhibition by dexmedetomidine. Our patient had increased troponin levels; however, these were difficult to interpret due to the CPR efforts and the previous day's lung transplantation operation. Her electrocardiogram remained in sinus rhythm after the resuscitation with no ST abnormalities, and her TEE was unchanged from her baseline, arguing against a saddle embolus or myocardial infarction as the cause of the arrest. While patients with systemic inflammatory diseases are at risk for developing a deep venous thrombosis, this patient was on prophylactic subcutaneous heparin. Cardiac sarcoidosis was also considered; however, this was less likely given that during the preoperative evaluation she denied any previous history of arrhythmias or knowledge of cardiac sarcoidosis. In terms of relative hypovolemia, our patient's fluid balance was negative; however, she was maintaining adequate perfusion pressures with sufficient urine output. Additionally, her ICU bed had previously been positioned in the semirecumbent position with no hemodynamic instability. Unfortunately, she never regained consciousness following the arrest. Computed tomography (CT) of her head and electroencephalogram (EEG) did not demonstrate pathology explaining her comatose state, and she did not meet the criteria for brain death. She remained unresponsive and expired almost a month later from massive gastrointestinal bleeding. On postmortem autopsy, several small pulmonary infarcts consistent with pulmonary emboli were noted. However, the significance and timing of these infarcts could not be established with certainty.

3. Discussion

Dexmedetomidine, a D-enantiomer of medetomidine, is a highly selective agonist of G-protein-coupled α_2-adrenergic receptors. These receptors are further categorized into three main subtypes which exist in the periphery (α_{2A}), brain, and spinal cord (α_{2B}, α_{2C}) [2, 3]. Dexmedetomidine is a useful sedative/analgesic commonly used in the ICU for several reasons. It has been shown to decrease time on the ventilator [4], decrease length of ICU stay [3], decrease anxiety, and

have opioid-sparing effects due to its analgesic properties [5, 6]. Particularly, in postthoracotomy patients, it has been shown that intravenous dexmedetomidine, in addition to a thoracic epidural bupivicaine infusion, decreases opioid requirements and may decrease the potential for respiratory depression [6]. A significant advantage of dexmedetomidine is its potential attenuation of delirium in ICU patients [6]. This delirium-sparing effect may be due to action on α_2 receptors in the locus ceruleus producing a sedative state similar to physiologic sleep. Lastly, dexmedetomidine is especially beneficial for postsurgical patients in that it preserves the respiratory drive, provides sympatholysis and decreases the inflammatory response [7].

The most common side effects during dexmedetomidine infusion are hypotension and bradycardia [3]. According to the manufacturers of Precedex (Hospira, Inc., Lake Forest, IL), 14% of patients experience bradycardia defined as a heart rate < 40 bpm or >30% decrease from baseline. Other authors have reported an incidence of bradycardia of up to 42% [4]. Bradycardia seen with dexmedetomidine is likely due to sympatholysis in addition to direct inhibitory effects on the sinoatrial (SA) and atrial-ventricular (AV) nodes [8]. This bradycardia usually resolves with cessation of the infusion or treatment with an anticholinergic agent. We believe that dexmedetomidine-induced SA and AV nodal depression proved refractory to anticholinergic medication (atropine) owing to cardiac denervation occurring at the time of lung transplantation.

It is known that during heart transplantation, both sympathetic and parasympathetic denervation occur leading to an increase in basal heart rate as the heart rate and electrical activity of the transplanted heart become entirely dependent on the intrinsic electrical system of the heart rather than relying on the neurological input from the recipient. The milieu of the denervated heart is complicated by the fact that while separation of sympathetic and parasympathetic occurs centrally, there is evidence that postganglionic fibers remain functional in these patients [9]. In other words, following cardiac transplantation, the sinus node becomes decentralized rather than totally denervated [10]. Surgical decentralization of the sinus node may be associated with supersensitivity to catecholamine stimulation [10], because α and β receptors are still present on the heart. The decentralized heart will continue to respond to directly acting catecholamine agents, such as epinephrine, isoproterenol, and dobutamine [11]. However, due to interruption of parasympathetic tone, the heart is not responsive to anticholinergic agents.

However, there is less knowledge of cardiac decentralization following lung transplantation. The operative dissection, especially that surrounding the trachea, likely leads to interruption of sympathetic and parasympathetic pathways to the heart [12]. This was illustrated in a study by Schaefers et al. which demonstrated that lung transplant recipients displayed abnormal responses to carotid sinus massage and Valsalva maneuvers [12]. In fact, half of the patients studied had no response to atropine, similar to what was observed in our patient. Following OLT, it is thought that reinnervation may occur at around 12 months.

While atrial arrhythmias following lung transplantation can occur during the immediate postoperative period, bradycardia is less defined in the literature. Atrial arrhythmias following lung transplantation are commonly due to inflammation or edema at the pulmonary vein left atrial anastomoses [13]. The arrhythmias occur early during the postoperative period and decrease over time [13].

Previous case reports have emerged citing dexmedetomidine as a contributing source of bradycardia followed by asystole in various settings [14–16]. In these reports and in our patient, it is likely that a combination of factors contributed to the asystolic arrest. While the use of concomitant sedatives with sympatholytic properties, that is, fentanyl, may have augmented the bradycardia and/or asystole associated with dexmedetomidine, it is likely that cardiac sympathetic decentralization following OLT placed our patient at significant risk for an asystolic event especially when sedated with dexmedetomidine. To our knowledge, only one other case report has described dexmedetomidine-induced asystole in a patient status after double lung transplant [16]. However, the transient bradycardia and asystole in that patient are confounded by the presence of pulmonary hypertension and a preexisting vagal response to coughing which led to hypoxemia [16]. Additionally, treatment with atropine or glycopyrrolate was not required in this patient. Our case is unique given that our patient demonstrated a refractory response to atropine and required epinephrine for management of the asystolic arrest.

Clinicians must be aware of the possibility of cardiac chronotropic alterations following OLT, similar to that following heart transplantation. Acknowledging the valuable and beneficiary role that dexmedetomidine plays in the management of OLT patients, we would suggest that heightened vigilance and prompt recognition of dysrhythmias when using dexmedetomidine in these patients may prevent a life-threatening event.

Authors' Contributions

C. A.-J. Webb, P. D. Weyker, and B. C. Flynn helped write the paper, all authors approved the final paper.

Disclosure

Written consent could not be obtained from the patient since she is currently deceased. No current contact information for next of kin could be obtained. Since she is currently deceased, she does not qualify as a human subject according to the definition set forth by the Institutional Review Board (IRB) of Columbia University Medical Center. As such, the paper did not qualify for IRB review.

Acknowledgment

The authors would like to thank Joshua S. Mincer, M.D. and Ph.D., for reviewing the paper.

References

[1] T. T. Horlocker, D. J. Wedel, J. C. Rowlingson et al., "Regional Anesthesia in the patient receiving antithrombotic or thrombolytic therapy; American Society of Regional Anesthesia and Pain Medicine evidence-based guidelines (Third Edition)," *Regional Anesthesia and Pain Medicine*, vol. 35, no. 1, pp. 64–101, 2010.

[2] A. Paris and P. H. Tonner, "Dexmedetomidine in anaesthesia," *Current Opinion in Anaesthesiology*, vol. 18, no. 4, pp. 412–418, 2005.

[3] J. A. Tan and K. M. Ho, "Use of dexmedetomidine as a sedative and analgesic agent in critically ill adult patients: a meta-analysis," *Intensive Care Medicine*, vol. 36, no. 6, pp. 926–939, 2010.

[4] R. R. Riker, Y. Shehabi, P. M. Bokesch et al., "Dexmedetomidine vs midazolam for sedation of critically Ill patients A randomized trial," *Journal of the American Medical Association*, vol. 301, no. 5, pp. 489–499, 2009.

[5] T. Z. Guo, J. Y. Jiang, A. E. Buttermann, and M. Maze, "Dexmedetomidine injection into the locus ceruleus produces antinociception," *Anesthesiology*, vol. 84, no. 4, pp. 873–881, 1996.

[6] S. Wahlander, R. J. Frumento, G. Wagener et al., "A prospective, double-blind, randomized, placebo-controlled study of dexmedetomidine as an adjunct to epidural analgesia after thoracic surgery," *Journal of Cardiothoracic and Vascular Anesthesia*, vol. 19, no. 5, pp. 630–635, 2005.

[7] J. Mantz, J. Josserand, and S. Hamada, "Dexmedetomidine: new insights," *European Journal of Anaesthesiology*, vol. 28, no. 1, pp. 3–6, 2011.

[8] G. B. Hammer, D. R. Drover, H. Cao et al., "The effects of dexmedetomidine on cardiac electrophysiology in children," *Anesthesia and Analgesia*, vol. 106, no. 1, pp. 79–83, 2008.

[9] U. Nellessen, T. C. Lee, T. A. Fischell et al., "Effects of acetylcholine on epicardial coronary arteries after cardiac transplantation without angiographic evidence of fixed graft narrowing," *American Journal of Cardiology*, vol. 62, no. 16, pp. 1093–1097, 1988.

[10] J. S. Strobel, A. E. Epstein, R. C. Bourge, J. K. Kirklin, and G. N. Kay, "Nonpharmacologic validation of the intrinsic heart rate in cardiac transplant recipients," *Journal of Interventional Cardiac Electrophysiology*, vol. 3, no. 1, pp. 15–18, 1999.

[11] S. Akhtar, *Ischemic Heart Disease*, Churchill Livingstone, Philadelphia, Pa, USA, 5th edition, 2008.

[12] H. J. Schaefers, M. B. Waxman, G. A. Patterson et al., "Cardiac innervation after double lung transplantation," *Journal of Thoracic and Cardiovascular Surgery*, vol. 99, no. 1, pp. 22–29, 1990.

[13] T. W. Lim, C. H. Koay, R. McCall, V. A. See, D. L. Ross, and S. P. Thomas, "Atrial arrhythmias after single-ring isolation of the posterior left atrium and pulmonary veins for atrial fibrillation: mechanisms and management," *Circulation Arrhythmia and Electrophysiology*, vol. 1, no. 2, pp. 120–126, 2008.

[14] E. Ingersoll-Weng, G. R. Manecke, and P. A. Thistlethwaite, "Dexmedetomidine and cardiac arrest," *Anesthesiology*, vol. 100, no. 3, pp. 738–739, 2004.

[15] A. N. Shah, J. Koneru, A. Nicoara, L. B. Goldfeder, K. Thomas, and F. A. Ehlert, "Dexmedetomidine related cardiac arrest in a patient with permanent pacemaker; a cautionary tale," *Pacing and Clinical Electrophysiology*, vol. 30, no. 9, pp. 1158–1160, 2007.

Triad of Idiopathic Thrombocytopenic Purpura, Preeclampsia, and HELLP Syndrome in a Parturient: A Rare Confrontation to the Anesthetist

Tanu Mehta, Geeta P. Parikh, and Veena R. Shah

Department of Anaesthesia and Critical Care, Smt. K. M. Mehta and Smt. G. R. Doshi Institute of Kidney Diseases and Research Center, Dr. H. L. Trivedi Institute of Transplantation Sciences, Civil Hospital Campus, Asarwa, Ahmedabad, Gujarat 380016, India

Correspondence should be addressed to Tanu Mehta; tanu.khushi@yahoo.com

Academic Editor: Eugene A. Vandermeersch

Idiopathic thrombocytopenic purpura (ITP) with HELLP represents a rare complication that requires combined care of obstetrician, anesthesiologist, hematologist, and neonatologist. At 37-week gestation a 35-year-old parturient (G2A1P0) a known case of chronic ITP presented with severe pregnancy induced hypertension (PIH), thrombocytopenia, and elevated liver enzymes. We describe successful anesthetic management of this patient who was taken for emergency caesarean section.

1. Introduction

The concomitance of chronic ITP, preeclampsia-eclampsia syndrome, and HELLP syndrome in a parturient is not very well described in literature. In January 2010, Ben et al. did a bibliographical search in PubMed and Cochrane database of systematic reviews and no similar cases were reported [1]. We describe the anesthetic management of a patient of chronic ITP who develops preeclampsia syndrome with HELLP syndrome.

2. Case Report

A 35-year-old parturient (G2A1P0) at 37 weeks of gestation presented at emergency department with severe preeclampsia. An urgent lower segment caesarean section (LSCS) was planned by the obstetric team and anaesthesia consultation was sought for it. Her antenatal history revealed that she was a patient of chronic ITP which was diagnosed 1 year back when she developed menorrhagia after diagnostic hysterolaparoscopy. She had thrombocytopenia and her bone marrow biopsy revealed normocellular marrow with megakaryocytes. She received methylprednisolone (20 mg/day) for 6 months which was later tapered down. She was on regular antenatal care (ANC) and did not receive any treatment during pregnancy as she had mild thrombocytopenia and her platelets remained around $100–150 \times 10^9$/L. In her last ANC which was 5 days prior to admission her platelets were normal and BP was 130/80 mm of Hg. On admission she had c/o headache and blurring of vision with severe epigastric pain and vomiting. Her BP was 210/110 mm Hg and was treated with sublingual depin 10 mg and loading dose of Inj. $MgSO_4$ followed by 5 gm IM in each buttock alternately. Inj. dexona 2 mg IV was given. Since her liver enzymes were elevated (SGPT 422 IU/L, SGOT 765 IU/L, S. Bilirubin total 3.6, direct 2.4, and indirect 1.2) HELLP syndrome was suspected. CBC showed normal S. creatinine (0.7) and electrolytes (Na, K, Ca, and Mg). Her Hb was 9 gms%. Platelet count was 60×10^9/L, LDH was 958 IU/L, and INR was normal. Blood products including platelet concentrates were kept available. She was transported to the OT with a wedge under right hip. Premedication included IV ranitidine (150 mg) and metoclopramide (10 mg). Following adequate preoxygenation with 100% O_2, induction of anesthesia was achieved with thiopentone sodium 300 mg (5 mg/kg). Aided with Sellicks manoeuvre, tracheal intubation was done with Portex Cuffed Endotracheal Tube number 7.0 after adequate relaxation with succinylcholine (2 mg/kg). Anesthesia was maintained with sevoflurane before and nitrous oxide after the delivery of baby and bolus doses of atracurium were given as muscle relaxant. IV fentanyl 100 μg was given after the baby was delivered. Intraoperative monitoring included temperature, pulse, BP, SpO$_2$, ECG, and etCO$_2$. A healthy female child was delivered 16 minutes after incision and APGAR scores were 7 and 9 at 1 and 5 minutes, respectively. Five minutes after baby delivery BP went up to 180/100 mm of Hg and NTG infusion was started. Inj. oxytocin 20 U in IV infusion was started and Inj. prostodin 250 mg IM was given immediately after the baby's delivery. Surprisingly there were no problems of haemostasis and the patient received 1.5 litres of crystalloids. She was reversed with neostigmine (2.5 mg) and glycopyrrolate (0.2) and shifted to ICU for postoperative care. IV tramadol (2 mg/kg) was given for postoperative analgesia. In the first two postoperative days platelets went down to 25×10^9/L and LDH increased to 1592 IU/L. From the 3rd postoperative day platelet counts started improving with a decreasing trend of liver enzymes and LDH. The patient was discharged on 9th postoperative day with normal liver enzymes and platelets and LDH was down to 493 IU/L. There was no evidence of neonatal thrombocytopenia.

3. Discussion

ITP is present in 0.01-0.02% of women during pregnancy. The decreased platelet count is due to binding of autoantibodies directed against target antigens on platelets, specifically the glycoprotein IIb-IIIa complex or glycoprotein Ib. These antibodies serve as opsonins accelerating platelet clearance by phagocytic cells in the reticuloendothelial system [2]. Management of a pregnant woman with ITP is based on the assessment of the risk of significant hemorrhage. The platelet count usually falls as pregnancy progresses with the greatest rate of decline occurring in the 3rd trimester [3]. Frequent monitoring of platelet count is required to ensure a safe platelet count at the time of delivery. In our patient platelets remained normal throughout the pregnancy and the first episode of thrombocytopenia was at the time of admission. Severe preeclampsia was diagnosed as the patient had hypertension with epigastric pain (stretching of liver capsule) and headache (sign of cerebral edema) and urine albumin was +2 by dip stick test. Elevated liver enzymes and S. Bilirubin and raised LDH correspond to the diagnosis of HELLP syndrome. As a part of preanaesthetic evaluation strategic planning is essential for anticipating difficulties like hemorrhage in the respiratory tract, aspiration of gastric contents, uncontrolled hypertension, convulsion, and fetal hypoxia and controlling these problems promptly. ITP itself is not an indication for caesarean delivery or general anesthesia. Mode of delivery and anesthesia in a pregnant patient with ITP is based on obstetric indication with avoidance of procedures associated with increased hemorrhagic risk. Maternal anesthesia must be based on safety of the mother. The HELLP syndrome affects 10–20% of women with severe preeclampsia but 15–20% of women do not have antecedent hypertension or proteinuria and symptoms may be absent [4]. However, since our patient was already symptomatic

and signs of haemolysis were present (increased LDH) we decided to give her general anesthesia (GA). In addition to the usual precautions of GA in pregnancy there are special problems that increase the anesthetic risk associated with such concomitant conditions. These include edema of upper airway, severe hypertensive response to laryngoscopy, interaction of magnesium with muscle relaxants, and risk of haemorrhage. Preoperative medication, Sellicks manoeuvre, and rapid sequence induction were used to avoid Mendelson's syndrome. Another therapeutic dilemma was the issue of platelet transfusion. Patients with ITP are generally refractory to platelet transfusion because of platelet alloantibodies. Conventionally a platelet count of $\geq 50 \times 10^9$/L should target transfusion count and unnecessary transfusion of platelet concentrates in the absence of haemostatic failure may stimulate more autoantibodies and worsen maternal thrombocytopenia [2]. Low platelets in our patient were more likely due to HELLP and not ITP as she was in remission; however, we did not transfuse any platelets as her preoperative platelet count was 60×10^9/L and there was no problem with haemostasis. Risk of hemorrhage in respiratory tract due to thrombocytopenia and compromised airway was avoided by treatment with smooth, rapid, and atraumatic intubation with the help of small endotracheal tube, adequate expertise, and better muscle relaxation with succinylcholine. Hypertensive response to laryngoscopy was attenuated with IV lignocaine. Intensive postpartum monitoring is necessary in women with HELLP because laboratory parameters frequently worsen 24–48 hours after delivery with peak rise in LDH and platelet nadir and platelet count begins to rise by 4th day postpartum [5] as was the case in our patient where parameters started improving by day 3. ITP is characterized by a reduced platelet count and increased peripheral destruction of platelets and augmented platelet production was evidenced by increased circulating megathrombocytes and higher number of megakaryocytes in bone marrow. Preeclamptic individuals have similar antiplatelet antibody profiles. The disorder differs in that the neonatal platelet counts are not depressed in preeclampsia whereas in ITP neonatal thrombocytopenia results from placentally transmitted maternal antibody [6]. Therefore platelet count of the neonate should be obtained at delivery to determine the need for immediate therapy. In neonates with thrombocytopenia platelet count is obtained daily because its nadir is frequently seen in 2–5 days after birth. A spontaneous rise of platelet count is usually seen by day 7. There was no evidence of neonatal thrombocytopenia in our patient. Another rare differential diagnosis to HELLP is TTP (thrombotic thrombocytopenic purpura). TTP represents a rare complication mainly in the second trimester and mimics HELLP syndrome in its early stage. Patients with HELLP syndrome completely recover following delivery. In contrast TTP does not usually improve dramatically following delivery or monotherapy with corticosteroids. Also, if LDH to AST ratio exceeds 25 : 1, especially in association with severe haematuria with failure of the platelet count and LDH to respond to therapy, a presumptive diagnosis of TTP can be considered and emergent plasma exchange (PEX) needs to be initiated [6].

However, since the patient improved after caesarean section and LDH to AST ratio was low [7] it further corresponded to a diagnosis of PIH with HELLP in a patient of ITP.

4. Conclusion

In summary, a high level of vigilance and team work is necessary in a parturient with ITP. Medical and expectant management can suddenly change into surgical and anesthetic management if patient develops HELLP syndrome. Establishment of an accurate diagnosis and individualized management is required to obtain best outcome in this clinically diverse condition.

References

[1] S. Ben, F. Rodríguez, C. Severo, and N. Debat, "A case of HELLP syndrome in a patient with immune thrombocytopenic purpura," *Obstetrics and Gynecology International*, vol. 2010, Article ID 692163, 4 pages, 2010.

[2] T. Y. Euliano, M. S. Zumberg, and M. Frölich, "Cesarean section combined with splenectomy in a parturient with immune thrombocytopenic purpura," *Journal of Clinical Anesthesia*, vol. 13, no. 4, pp. 313–318, 2001.

[3] V. Suri, N. Aggarwal, S. Saxena, P. Malhotra, and S. Varma, "Maternal and perinatal outcome in idiopathic thrombocytopenic purpura (ITP) with pregnancy," *Acta Obstetricia et Gynecologica Scandinavica*, vol. 85, no. 12, pp. 1430–1435, 2006.

[4] K. Haram, E. Svendsen, and U. Abildgaard, "The HELLP syndrome: clinical issues and management. A review," *BMC Pregnancy and Childbirth*, vol. 9, article 8, 2009.

[5] T. Gernsheimer, A. H. James, and R. Stasi, "How I treat thrombocytopenia in pregnancy," *Blood*, vol. 121, no. 1, pp. 38–47, 2013.

[6] P. Samuels, E. K. Main, A. Tomaski, M. T. Mennuti, S. G. Gabbe, and D. B. Cines, "Abnormalities in platelet antiglobulin tests in preeclamptic mothers and their neonates," *American Journal of Obstetrics and Gynecology*, vol. 157, no. 1, pp. 109–113, 1987.

[7] S. D. Keiser, K. W. Boyd, J. F. Rehberg et al., "A high LDH to AST ratio helps to differentiate pregnancy-associated thrombotic thrombocytopenic purpura (TTP) from HELLP syndrome," *Journal of Maternal-Fetal and Neonatal Medicine*, vol. 25, no. 7, pp. 1059–1063, 2012.

Unilateral Hypoglossal Nerve Palsy after Use of the Laryngeal Mask Airway Supreme

**Kenichi Takahoko, Hajime Iwasaki, Tomoki Sasakawa,
Akihiro Suzuki, Hideki Matsumoto, and Hiroshi Iwasaki**

*Department of Anesthesiology and Critical Care Medicine, Asahikawa Medical University, Midorigaoka Higashi 2-1-1-1,
Asahikawa, Hokkaido 078-8510, Japan*

Correspondence should be addressed to Kenichi Takahoko; ken-ichi@asahikawa-med.ac.jp

Academic Editor: Pavel Michalek

Purpose. Hypoglossal nerve palsy after use of the laryngeal mask airway (LMA) is an exceptionally rare complication. We present the first case of unilateral hypoglossal nerve palsy after use of the LMA Supreme. *Clinical Features.* A healthy 67-year-old female was scheduled for a hallux valgus correction under general anesthesia combined with femoral and sciatic nerve blocks. A size 4 LMA Supreme was inserted successfully at the first attempt and the cuff was inflated with air at an intracuff pressure of 60 cmH$_2$O using cuff pressure gauge. Anesthesia was maintained with oxygen, nitrous oxide (67%), and sevoflurane under spontaneous breathing. The surgery was uneventful and the duration of anesthesia was two hours. The LMA was removed as the patient woke and there were no immediate postoperative complications. The next morning, the patient complained of dysarthria and dysphasia. These symptoms were considered to be caused by the LMA compressing the nerve against the hyoid bone. Conservative treatment was chosen and the paralysis recovered completely after 5 months. *Conclusion.* Hypoglossal nerve injury may occur despite correct positioning of the LMA under the appropriate intracuff pressure. A follow-up period of at least 6 months should be taken into account for the recovery.

1. Introduction

Hypoglossal nerve injury associated with laryngeal mask airway (LMA) is a rare complication but can cause severe symptoms such as dysarthria and dysphasia. To our knowledge, eight cases of hypoglossal nerve palsy after use of the LMA have previously been reported [1–8]. In all these cases, LMAs which have silicone cuffs (e.g., LMA Classic and LMA ProSeal) were used. LMA Supreme (The Laryngeal Mask Company Ltd., St. Helier, Jersey, UK) is a disposable LMA which has anatomically curved airway and oval-shaped polyvinyl chloride (PVC) cuff. We present the first case of unilateral hypoglossal nerve palsy after use of the LMA Supreme.

2. Case Description

A 67-year-old female (weight 55 kg, height 155 cm) was scheduled for a hallux valgus correction. Her preoperative physical

examination was normal and she had no past medical history (American Society of Anesthesiologists physical status I). No premedication was given. On arrival at the operating room, ultrasound-guided femoral and sciatic nerve blocks were performed under sedation with midazolam 2 mg and fentanyl 0.05 mg. After confirming the effects of blocks, general anesthesia was induced with propofol 3 mg·kg^{-1}. A size 4 LMA Supreme was inserted successfully at the first attempt without difficulty using the standard insertion technique. The cuff was inflated with air at an intracuff pressure of 60 cmH$_2$O using cuff pressure gauge (VBM Medizintechnik, Sulz, Germany). The LMA appeared to be in the correct position because there was gas leakage at a positive pressure of approximately 25 cmH$_2$O and insertion of a gastric tube was smooth. Anesthesia was maintained with sevoflurane 1.5% and nitrous oxide 67% in oxygen under spontaneous breathing. The patient was in the supine position and hemodynamic parameters were stable during the surgery. The surgery was uneventful and the duration of anesthesia

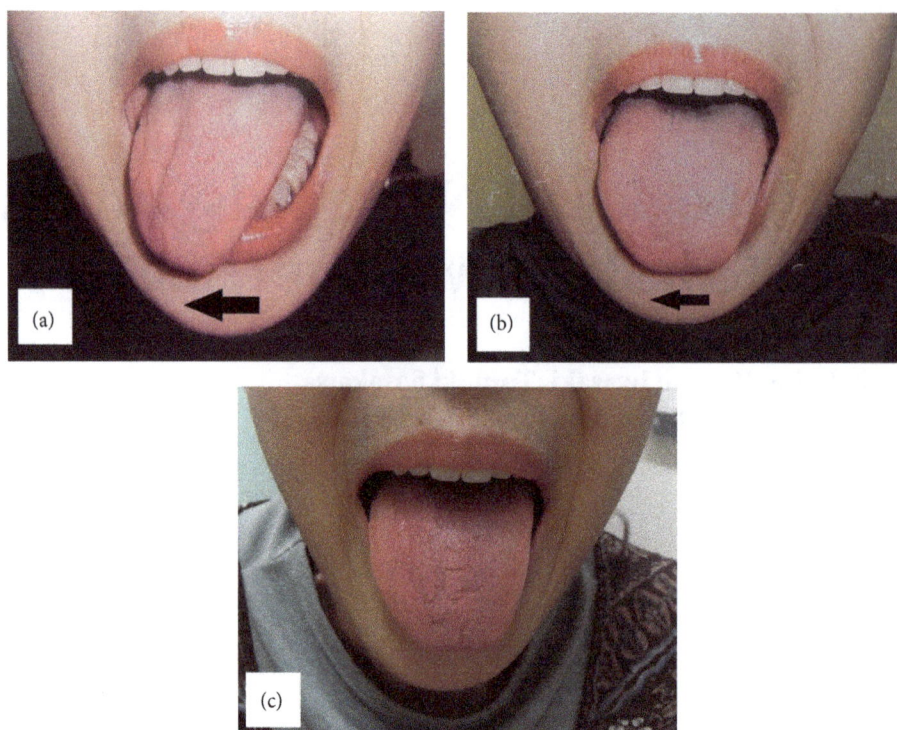

FIGURE 1: (a) Physical examination of the tongue on postoperative day 1. The tongue was deviated to the right side on protrusion demonstrating the right hypoglossal nerve palsy. (b) Physical examination of the tongue three months later. The deviation of the tongue slightly improved. (c) Physical examination of the tongue five months later. The deviation of the tongue disappeared showing a complete recovery of hypoglossal nerve function.

was two hours. The LMA was removed as the patient woke and there were no immediate postoperative complications.

The next morning, the patient complained of difficulty in swallowing and slurred speech. Physical examination showed the deviation of the tongue to the right on protrusion (Figure 1(a)). The gag reflex and global and taste sensations of the tongue were normal. To exclude cerebrovascular diseases or internal carotid artery dissection, CT scan was performed, confirming the absence of abnormalities. These findings revealed isolated right hypoglossal nerve palsy after use of the LMA. In reference to previous reports [1–8], conservative management (including speech therapy and regular assessment) was chosen in the hope of spontaneous recovery. Medical follow-up was performed every 2–4 weeks. Although recovery was slow, the symptoms continued to improve and made a complete recovery after 5 months (Figures 1(b) and 1(c)).

3. Discussion

The LMA is one of the most widely used supraglottic airway devices. Although rare, neural damage such as lingual nerve injury [9], trauma to the recurrent laryngeal nerve [10], or hypoglossal nerve injury may be associated with an insertion of the LMA. On search of the literature, eight cases of hypoglossal nerve injuries associated with LMA have previously been reported [1–8]. One report was with LMA ProSeal [6] and all the others were with LMA Classic

[1–5, 7, 8]. The LMA Supreme is the most recent type of laryngeal mask airway. This disposable device has a curved rigid stem copying the upper airway anatomy and allowing easy insertion and PVC cuff resistant to gas diffusion. As far as we know, neural damage associated with the LMA Supreme is extremely rare and only two cases of lingual nerve injury have been reported to date [11, 12]. We believe our report is the first case of unilateral hypoglossal nerve injury associated with LMA Supreme.

Potential risk factors for hypoglossal nerve injury are use of nitrous oxide, inappropriate size of the LMA, the lateral position, extreme head side rotation, primary illnesses, and difficult insertion of the LMA [13]. In our case, manufacturer's recommended size of the mask was chosen based on the body weight, the patient remained supine during the surgery and had no past medical history, and the mask was inserted successfully at the first attempt. Among the risk factors, only the use of nitrous oxide applied to our case. It is well known that nitrous oxide will diffuse into the LMA cuff and increase the cuff pressure with time during anesthesia [14]. The cuff pressure of LMA Classic and LMA ProSeal has been shown to increase from $60\,cmH_2O$ to over $100\,cmH_2O$ following 30 min of nitrous oxide exposure [14]. However, there are reports that LMAs with PVC cuff are less susceptible to hyperinflation caused by nitrous oxide compared to the ones with silicone cuff [15–17]. Anand et al. reported that intracuff pressure of LMA Supreme remained stable at approximately $60\,cmH_2O$ during an hour of nitrous oxide anesthesia [17].

Moreover, van Zundert et al. suggested that continuous cuff monitoring can be omitted in pediatric LMA with a PVC cuff during nitrous oxide anesthesia [18]. Therefore, excessive cuff pressure due to nitrous oxide anesthesia might not be the main factor which caused the nerve injury in our case.

Our case suggests that a correctly positioned LMA Supreme can occasionally cause a nerve injury. Correct position of the LMA was confirmed by the oropharyngeal leak pressure of approximately 25 cmH$_2$O and easy gastric tube insertion [19]. Oropharyngeal leak pressure is the pressure at which a gas leak occurs around the LMA cuff. Oropharyngeal leak pressure in LMA Supreme at intracuff pressure of 60 cmH$_2$O is reported to be approximately 20 cmH$_2$O, similar to that in our case [20]. By any chance, rigid airway tube might have caused adverse effect. We postulate that the right hypoglossal nerve was compressed between the LMA cuff and the hyoid bone inadvertently during the anesthesia.

Hypoglossal nerve originates from the hypoglossal nerve nucleus in the medulla oblongata and leaves the skull through the hypoglossal canal of the occipital bone. It then descends between the internal carotid artery and the internal jugular vein. At the level of the angle of the mandible it becomes superficial, passes just above the greater horn of the hyoid bone, and enters the floor of the mouth [2]. Thus, a likely site of injury is at the greater horn of the hyoid bone where the inflated cuff of the LMA can compress the nerve against the bone [21]. The complete recovery of hypoglossal nerve injury has been reported to occur within the first 6 months, while there was one case of permanent recurrent nerve palsy after use of the LMA which resulted in no improvement [22]. These data suggest that the nerve function is temporarily impaired due to compression (i.e., neurapraxia). Depending on the extent of the exerted compression, the nerve may be permanently damaged due to collapse of its fibers (i.e., axonotmesis or neurotmesis). When the patient was diagnosed with hypoglossal nerve palsy caused by the LMA, a follow-up period of at least 6 months should be taken into account without invasive surgical procedures because spontaneous recovery is usually expected.

References

[1] K. Nagai, C. Sakuramoto, and F. Goto, "Unilateral hypoglossal nerve paralysis following the use of the laryngeal mask airway," *Anaesthesia*, vol. 49, no. 7, pp. 603–604, 1994.

[2] C. King and M. K. Street, "Twelfth cranial nerve paralysis following use of a laryngeal mask airway," *Anaesthesia*, vol. 49, no. 9, pp. 786–787, 1994.

[3] N. Umapathy, T. G. Eliathamby, and M. S. Timms, "Paralysis of the hypoglossal and pharyngeal branches of the vagus nerve after use of a LMA and ETT," *British Journal of Anaesthesia*, vol. 87, no. 2, p. 322, 2001.

[4] A. Stewart and W. A. Lindsay, "Bilateral hypoglossal nerve injury following the use of the laryngeal mask airway," *Anaesthesia*, vol. 57, no. 3, pp. 264–265, 2002.

[5] M. Sommer, M. Schuldt, U. Runge, S. Gielen-Wijffels, and M. A. E. Marcus, "Bilateral hypoglossal nerve injury following the use of the laryngeal mask without the use of nitrous oxide," *Acta Anaesthesiologica Scandinavica*, vol. 48, no. 3, pp. 377–378, 2004.

[6] P. Trümpelmann and T. Cook, "Unilateral hypoglossal nerve injury following the use of a ProSeal laryngeal mask," *Anaesthesia*, vol. 60, no. 1, pp. 101–102, 2005.

[7] T. S. Lo, "Unilateral hypoglossal nerve palsy following the use of the laryngeal mask airway," *Canadian Journal of Neurological Sciences*, vol. 33, no. 3, pp. 320–321, 2006.

[8] L. Trujillo, D. Anghelescu, and G. Bikhazi, "Unilateral hypoglossal nerve injury caused by a laryngeal mask airway in an infant," *Paediatric Anaesthesia*, vol. 21, no. 6, pp. 708–709, 2011.

[9] N. S. Ahmad and S. M. Yentis, "Laryngeal mask airway and lingual nerve injury," *Anaesthesia*, vol. 51, no. 7, pp. 707–708, 1996.

[10] S. Inomata, T. Nishikawa, A. Suga, and S. Yamashita, "Transient bilateral vocal cord paralysis after insertion of a laryngeal mask airway," *Anesthesiology*, vol. 82, no. 3, pp. 787–788, 1995.

[11] P. Rujirojindakul, C. Prechawai, and E. Watanayomnaporn, "Tongue numbness following laryngeal mask airway Supreme and i-gel insertion: two case reports," *Acta Anaesthesiologica Scandinavica*, vol. 56, no. 9, pp. 1200–1203, 2012.

[12] V. Thiruvenkatarajan, R. M. van Wijk, I. Elhalawani, and A. M. Barnes, "Lingual nerve neuropraxia following use of the Laryngeal Mask Airway Supreme," *Journal of Clinical Anesthesia*, vol. 26, pp. 65–68, 2014.

[13] J. Brimacombe, G. Clarke, and C. Keller, "Lingual nerve injury associated with the ProSeal laryngeal mask airway: a case report and review of the literature," *British Journal of Anaesthesia*, vol. 95, pp. 420–423, 2005.

[14] A. B. Lumb and M. W. Wrigley, "The effect of nitrous oxide on laryngeal mask cuff pressure. In vitro and in vivo studies," *Anaesthesia*, vol. 47, no. 4, pp. 320–323, 1992.

[15] P. Maino, A. Dullenkopf, V. Bernet, and M. Weiss, "Nitrous oxide diffusion into the cuffs of disposable laryngeal mask airways," *Anaesthesia*, vol. 60, no. 3, pp. 278–282, 2005.

[16] J. Brimacombe, C. Keller, R. Morris, and D. Mecklem, "A comparison of the disposable versus the reusable laryngeal mask airway in paralyzed adult patients," *Anesthesia and Analgesia*, vol. 87, no. 4, pp. 921–924, 1998.

[17] L. K. Anand, M. Singh, D. Kapoor, and N. Goel, "Intracuff pressure comparison between ProSeal and Supreme laryngeal mask airways," *Anaesthesia*, vol. 68, pp. 1202–1203, 2013.

[18] A. van Zundert, K. Fonck, B. Al-Shaikh, and E. P. Mortier, "Comparison of cuff-pressure changes in LMA-Classic and the new Soft Seal laryngeal masks during nitrous oxide anaesthesia in spontaneous breathing patients," *European Journal of Anaesthesiology*, vol. 21, no. 7, pp. 547–552, 2004.

[19] A. I. J. Brain, C. Verghese, and P. J. Strube, "The LMA "ProSeal"— a laryngeal mask with an oesophageal vent," *British Journal of Anaesthesia*, vol. 84, no. 5, pp. 650–654, 2000.

[20] L. Zhang, E. Seet, V. Mehta et al., "Oropharyngeal leak pressure with the laryngeal mask airway Supreme at different intracuff pressures: a randomized controlled trial," *Canadian Journal of Anesthesia*, vol. 58, no. 7, pp. 624–629, 2011.

[21] A. I. Brain, "Course of the hypoglossal nerve in relation to the position of the laryngeal mask airway," *Anaesthesia*, vol. 50, no. 1, pp. 82–83, 1995.

[22] D. Lowinger, B. Benjamin, and L. Gadd, "Recurrent laryngeal nerve injury caused by a laryngeal mask airway," *Anaesthesia and Intensive Care*, vol. 27, no. 2, pp. 202–205, 1999.

A Rare Complication of Tracheal Intubation: Tongue Perforation

Loreto Lollo,[1] Tanya K. Meyer,[2] and Andreas Grabinsky[1]

[1] Department of Anesthesiology & Pain Medicine, Harborview Medical Center, University of Washington, No. 359724,
325 Ninth Avenue, Seattle, WA 98104, USA
[2] Department of Otolaryngology, Harborview Medical Center, University of Washington, 325 Ninth Avenue, Seattle, WA 98104, USA

Correspondence should be addressed to Loreto Lollo, lollomd@uw.edu

Academic Editors: T. Horiguchi, C.-H. Hsing, I.-O. Lee, E. W. Nielsen, and R. Riley

Aim. To describe the subsequent treatment of airway trauma sustained during laryngoscopy and endotracheal intubation. *Methods.* A rare injury occurring during laryngoscopy and endotracheal intubation that resulted in perforation of the tongue by an endotracheal tube and the subsequent management of this unusual complication are discussed. A 65-year-old female with intraparenchymal brain hemorrhage with rapidly progressive neurologic deterioration had the airway secured prior to arrival at the referral institution. The endotracheal tube (ETT) was noted to have pierced through the base of the tongue and entered the trachea, and the patient underwent operative laryngoscopy to inspect the injury and the ETT was replaced by tracheostomy. *Results.* Laryngoscopy demonstrated the ETT to perforate the base of the tongue. The airway was secured with tracheostomy and the ETT was removed. *Conclusions.* A wide variety of complications resulting from direct and video-assisted laryngoscopy and tracheal intubation have been reported. Direct perforation of the tongue with an ETT and ability to ventilate and oxygenate subsequently is a rare injury.

1. Introduction

A wide variety of complications resulting from direct and video-assisted laryngoscopy and tracheal intubation have been reported [1, 2]. Although infrequent these injuries include lacerations of the pharyngeal structures such as the soft palate and palatoglossal fold, as well as the esophagus, which can result in severe hemorrhage that obscures visualization during laryngoscopy for tracheal intubation [3, 4]. These injuries can create a false lumen with potential for catastrophic outcomes such as pneumomediastinum, infection, or even lack of ventilation [5, 6]. Other infrequent injuries have resulted in hoarseness or areas of oropharyngeal numbness attributed to unilateral and bilateral palsies of the recurrent laryngeal and lingual nerves [7, 8]. Arytenoid dislocation and fractures of the thyroid cartilage and tracheal rings have also been described [9–11]. A rare injury occurring during laryngoscopy and endotracheal intubation that resulted in perforation of the tongue by an endotracheal tube, the subsequent management of this unusual complication, is reported.

2. Case Description

A 65-year-old Caucasian female with ASA physical status 2 sustained an intraparenchymal brain hemorrhage with rapidly progressive neurologic deterioration that required the airway to be secured. Tracheal intubation was performed prior to arrival at the admitting referral institution. A chart review of placement of the endotracheal tube (ETT) did not document any difficulty or injury with the procedure.

A chart review after admission documented preanesthetic airway assessment for unrelated surgery seven years prior. She was classified as a Mallampati class 2 airway. Tracheal intubation at that time was hindered by small mouth opening after induction, an anteriorly positioned glottic opening with a grade 2 laryngoscopic view by the Cormack-Lehane criteria, and inability to place an ETT through the glottis without the assistance of a gum elastic bougie.

During the current admission to the intensive care unit, it was noted that the ETT pierced the patient's tongue. Anesthesiology and otolaryngology services were consulted for ETT exchange and evaluation of the tongue injury.

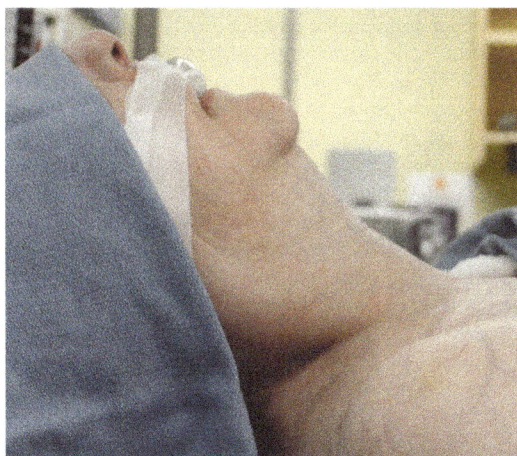

FIGURE 1

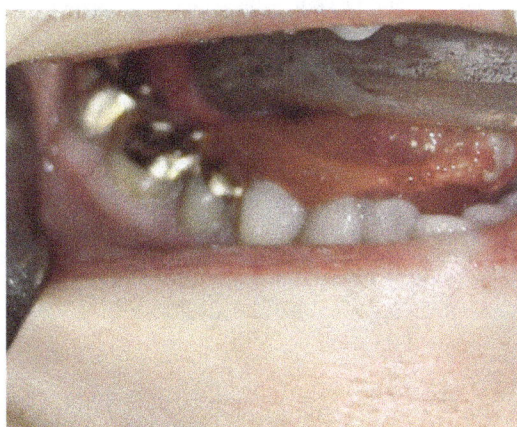

FIGURE 3

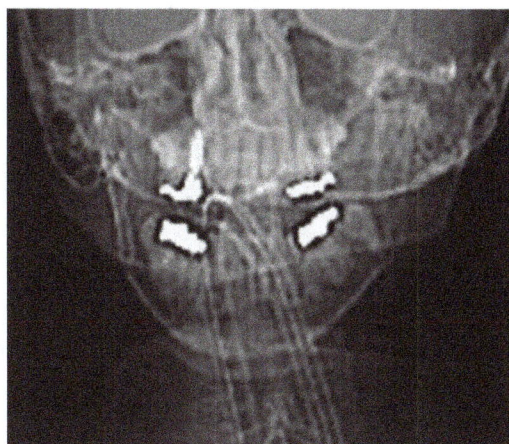

FIGURE 2

Inspection of the oral cavity was restricted by limited mouth opening, a short thyromental distance, and crowded dentition (Figure 1). A 7.0 mm internal diameter ETT on the right side of the oral cavity pierced through the body of the tongue with a 4 mm pedicle of tissue bridging around the ETT. Ecchymosis and edema of the surrounding oropharyngeal tissue made further evaluation difficult but the ETT was in correct position in the trachea (Figure 2). Anteroposterior radiographs of the facial structures demonstrated the ETT to be deviated to the right side of the mandible instead of that in the midline position that the ETT bite block maintains for patients mechanically ventilated with an ETT (Figure 3). Oxygenation and ventilation remained normal at all times during the hospital stay.

The patient's brain injury had resulted in loss of the gag reflex but the cough reflex remained intact. Consent to perform elective tracheostomy followed by operative direct laryngoscopy (DL), removal of the ETT, and repair of injury to the oropharyngeal structures was obtained, and the patient was transferred to the operating room on hospital day 2. DL demonstrated the ETT traversing the floor of the mouth through a laceration at the junction of the floor of the mouth and the posterior tongue on the right side. The

ETT appropriately entered the laryngeal opening (Figure 4). Both the Lindholm and anterior commissure laryngoscopes allowed visualization of the epiglottis, but tilting of the epiglottis to expose the laryngeal inlet or visualization of the laryngeal opening was not possible (Figure 5).

The patient had normal tracheal anatomy, and a standard tracheotomy with placement of a number 4 cuffed Shiley tracheostomy tube was performed. After securing the tracheostomy tube, the ETT was removed and repeat DL revealed no additional injuries. There was no significant bleeding from the tongue or floor of the mouth. The patient had scant drainage of serosanguinous secretions from the laceration site that resolved spontaneously. The patient was placed on palliative care due to the severity of the brain injury and expired on the fifth hospital day.

3. Discussion

Dental injury is the most common complication of DL for tracheal intubation and can result in aesthetic and functional sequelae. Rarely, aspiration of dental fragments can result in pulmonary complications such as pneumonia and atelectasis. Injuries to cartilaginous and neurologic structures of the laryngopharynx during DL and ETT placement are rare but associated with more serious outcomes due to their importance for phonation and airway protection.

Mucosal injuries due to shearing or traction forces applied by the laryngoscope can cause laceration of oropharyngeal tissue. Penetrating injuries can be caused by the ETT, with or without a stylet introducer. Hemorrhage ensuing from an oropharyngeal mucosal laceration may obscure the visual field during laryngoscopy and result in the creation of a false lumen. Inability to ventilate and subcutaneous and mediastinal emphysema may occur if ventilation is attempted with an ETT placed within this false lumen. Delayed sequelae include pain and extension of infection to adjacent structures such as the submental space and mediastinum.

Because this individual had a secure airway with adequate oxygenation and ventilation, the surgical team decided to

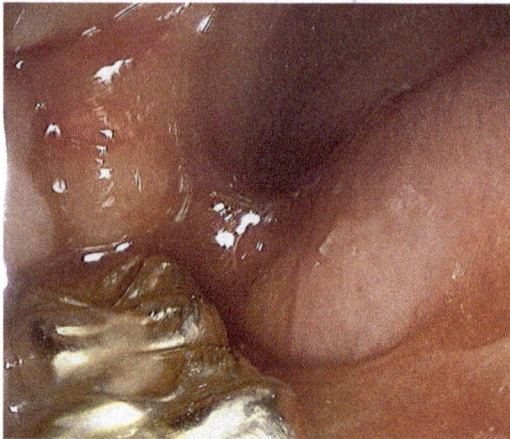

FIGURE 4

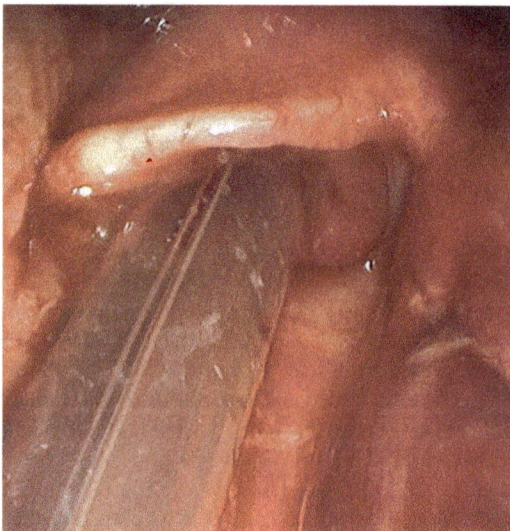

FIGURE 5

perform subsequent manipulations electively in the operating room. This would have allowed for the best possible conditions to control hemorrhage and repair mucosal damage. The presence of the ETT possibly maintained tamponade of hemorrhage from the tongue perforation. Adequate hemostasis was present at the time of removal of the ETT and further operative repair of the tongue laceration was not deemed necessary. Postoperative monitoring of the patient was continued in order to observe any signs of infection resulting from tongue perforation.

References

[1] L. D. Martin, J. M. Mhyre, A. M. Shanks, K. K. Tremper, and S. Kheterpal, "3,423 emergency tracheal intubations at a university hospital: airway outcomes and complications," *Anesthesiology*, vol. 114, no. 1, pp. 42–48, 2011.

[2] M. F. Aziz, D. Healy, S. Kheterpal, R. F. Fu, D. Dillman, and A. M. Brambrink, "Routine clinical practice effectiveness of the glidescope in difficult airway management: an analysis of 2,004 glidescope intubations, complications, and failures from two institutions," *Anesthesiology*, vol. 114, no. 1, pp. 34–41, 2011.

[3] R. M. Cooper, "Complications associated with the use of the GlideScope videolaryngoscope," *Canadian Journal of Anesthesia*, vol. 54, no. 1, pp. 54–57, 2007.

[4] D. S. Bartlett, R. Grace, and S. Newell, "Perforation of and intubation through the palatoglossal fold," *Anaesthesia and Intensive Care*, vol. 37, no. 3, pp. 481–483, 2009.

[5] S. Sejwal, M. Tandon, P. Ganjoo, and A. Sharma, "Pneumomediastinum due to hypopharyngeal injury during orotracheal intubation," *Canadian Journal of Anesthesia*, vol. 54, no. 9, p. 767, 2007.

[6] S. Koscielny and R. Gottschall, "Perforation of the hypopharynx as a rare life-threatening complication of endotracheal intubation," *Anaesthesist*, vol. 55, no. 1, pp. 45–52, 2006.

[7] M. D. Sacks and D. Marsh, "Bilateral recurrent laryngeal nerve neuropraxia following laryngeal mask insertion: a rare cause of serious upper airway morbidity," *Paediatric Anaesthesia*, vol. 10, no. 4, pp. 435–437, 2000.

[8] M. S. Lang and P. D. Waite, "Bilateral lingual nerve injury after laryngoscopy for intubation," *Journal of Oral and Maxillofacial Surgery*, vol. 59, no. 12, pp. 1497–1499, 2001.

[9] V. Tan and S. Seevanayagam, "Arytenoid subluxation after a difficult intubation treated successfully with voice therapy," *Anaesthesia and Intensive Care*, vol. 37, no. 5, pp. 843–846, 2009.

[10] A. P. Reed, "Laryngoscopy complicated by thyroid cartilage fracture," *Anesthesiology*, vol. 113, no. 4, pp. 993–994, 2010.

[11] K. Stannard, J. Wells, and C. Cokis, "Tracheal rupture following endotracheal intubation," *Anaesthesia and Intensive Care*, vol. 31, no. 5, pp. 588–591, 2003.

Successful Treatment of Genitofemoral Neuralgia Using Ultrasound Guided Injection: A Case Report and Short Review of Literature

Harsha Shanthanna

St. Joseph's Hospital, Department of Anesthesiology, McMaster University, Health Sciences Centre 2U1, 1200 Main Street West, Hamilton, ON, Canada L8N 3Z5

Correspondence should be addressed to Harsha Shanthanna; harshamd@gmail.com

Academic Editors: A. Apan, G. Hans, and J. G. Jakobsson

A young male patient developed chronic, severe, and disabling right sided groin pain following resection of his left testicular cancer. Since there is considerable overlap, ultrasound guided, selective diagnostic nerve blocks were done for ilioinguinal, iliohypogastric, and genitofemoral nerves, to determine the involved nerve territory. It was revealed that genitofemoral neuralgia was the likely cause. As a therapeutic procedure, it was injected with local anesthetic and steroid using ultrasound guidance. The initial injection led to pain relief of 3 months. Subsequent blocks reinforced the existing analgesia and were sufficient to allow for maintenance with the use of analgesic medications. This case report describes the successful use of diagnostic selective nerve blocks for the assessment of groin pain, subsequent to which an ultrasound guided therapeutic injection of genitofemoral nerve led to long term pain relief. As a therapeutic procedure, genitofemoral nerve block is done in patients with genitofemoral neuralgia. Ultrasound allows for controlled administration and greatly enhances the technical ability to perform precise localization and injection. There are very few case reports of such a treatment in the published literature. Apart from the case report, we also highlight the relevant anatomy and a brief review of genitofemoral neuralgia and its treatment.

1. Introduction

In 1942, Magee described the condition of pain and paresthesias in the distribution of genitofemoral nerve [1]. He called it as genitofemoral neuralgia (GFN), as it was not widely recognized. It was then reported to be commonly associated with appendicular surgeries. As shown in Figure 1, there is considerable overlap in the areas supplied from inguinal (IL), iliohypogastric (IH), genitofemoral (GF), and lateral cutaneous femoral nerve (LCFN) [2]. These nerves are quiet susceptible to injury following many lower abdominal and pelvic surgeries. Beneš et al. suggest using the term abdominoinguinal pain syndrome, as a common entity [3]. The diagnosis and treatment of these conditions are difficult and challenging. Although the exact incidence of GFN is not known, the incidence of chronic pain after inguinal hernia surgery is quoted around 12%–20% [4]. The inability to distinguish a GFN from ilioinguinal nerve pain can lead to unnecessary nerve exploration surgery and more morbidity [5].

Some have resorted to paravertebral nerve blocks at L1-L2 to alleviate the pain by blocking the common segmental origins [5]. In the following report we describe a patient of severe groin pain who underwent ultrasound guided selective nerve blocks, before being diagnosed and treated as GFN. This report highlights 2 important aspects. Firstly, it reports the unique advantage obtained from ultrasound in performing selective diagnostic nerve blocks around the groin. Secondly, it reports the successful management of GFN using ultrasound guided nerve block. Written permission has been obtained from the patient for this paper.

2. Case Description

A 27-year-old male patient was referred to our pain clinic after having had orchidectomy for a left sided testicular cancer, 2 years earlier. He continued to have a persistent, severe pain in his right groin and scrotal area. The pain was

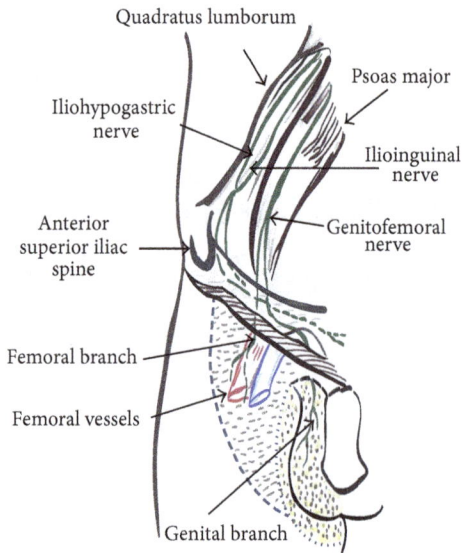

FIGURE 1: Anatomy of nerves around the inguinal region.

continuous and dull with a heavy feeling. He reported the severity to be 8/10, on average. He described this to be a severe, burning, sharp pain, which could make him nauseous and fainting with any physical activity such as running, jumping, sexual intercourse, and physical examination. He also reported significant sensitivity and allodynia. Prior to our consultation, he was investigated with an ultrasound and CT scan on the right side. Since they showed some signs of edema and possible epididymitis, he was treated with antibiotics, without much improvement. He was also tried on nortriptyline 10 mg and (lyrica) pregabalin 150 mg BID, without much improvement. There were no other comorbidities or allergies. He was referred to us for the possibility of inguinal nerve blocks. On examination, he was anxious and quiet worried. His gait and posture were normal. His scrotal examination showed an empty scrotal sac on the left side and a highly sensitive inguinal region and scrotal sac on the right side. There were no signs of infection, swelling, or redness. There were no signs of inguinal or femoral hernia. The maximum tenderness was found to be just at the pubic tubercle and below, extending up to the whole of the right side of scrotum and also slightly over the medial side of thigh. Since the area of the lower abdomen and groin can be supplied by IL, IH, or GF nerve, we decided to perform separate diagnostic blocks to confirm the diagnosis and for a possible treatment. Initially, he underwent an ultrasound guided IL and IH nerve block, by the corresponding author, using 2 mL of 2% lidocaine and 2 mL of 0.25% bupivacaine mixed with 40 mg of depomedrol. The sensory block achieved did not cover the area of his pain. Approximately a month after that we performed an ultrasound guided GF nerve block using 2 mL of 2% lidocaine and 2 mL of 0.25% bupivacaine mixed with 40 mg of depomedrol.

2.1. Description of the Procedure. With patient in supine position, the inguinal area and the area above the femoral vessels were uncovered and wiped with chlorohexidine solution. A high frequency, linear, high resolution probe (GE Ultrasound, LOGIQ e machine) was initially kept perpendicular to the inguinal ligament just above the femoral vessels (Figure 1).

A cephalad movement of the probe identified the iliac artery splitting into femoral and external iliac arteries. This corresponds to the level of the internal inguinal ring [6]. An oval structure lying medial and superficial to the femoral artery is the inguinal canal with its contents. A longitudinal view of the femoral artery is also identified at the same site (Figure 2). The contents of the inguinal canal were identified clearly, with testicular vessels shown laterally and spermatic cord shown medially. We used an in-plane approach to direct the needle towards the spermatic cord to block the genital branch of the GF nerve, using a 50 mm echostim needle (Benlan, Ontario, Canada) (Figure 3). Soon after the block, the patient noticed considerable improvement and tested it by jumping and running, to see if it hurts. The intensity of pain came down to 4/10, and the attacks of sharp pain became infrequent. The initial relief lasted 3 months, and he had a similar effect for the 2nd injection which lasted for 6 months. With an aim to prevent recurrence, he was tried on long acting tramadol 100 mg taken one a day. He underwent a 3rd injection after which his pain relief has continued beyond 12 months. He continues to be fully functional and is able to take part in normal physical activities.

3. Discussion

Our report demonstrates that an ultrasound guided GF nerve block can be an effective treatment for genitofemoral neuralgia. However, it is critical to identify the involved nerve by performing diagnostic nerve blocks of the inguinal nerves, and the GF nerve to rule out their involvement. Similar to the IL nerve, the genitofemoral nerve arises from L1 and L2 (lumbar segments) and forms a part of the lumbar plexus. It predominantly carries sensory fibres, except the cremasteric motor fibres. The nerve lies on the surface of psoas major muscle, crosses the ureter on its descent, and divides into a genital and a femoral branch at a variable point above the inguinal ligament. The femoral component continues along the femoral sheath. The genital branch, also called the external spermatic nerve, gets into the inguinal canal and lies alongside the spermatic cord (round ligament in females). It carries sensory fibres from the lateral and posterior aspect of scrotum (mons pubis and labium majus in females) [7].

Most injuries to the GF nerve occur with hernia repair and pelvic surgeries such as urethral sling [8]. Other causes include blunt trauma, nephrectomy, appendicectomy, and ureterectomy [5]. It is difficult to comment on the exact nature of injury. Bischoff et al. performed a study to see whether intraoperative identification of these nerves, during hernia surgery, makes any difference. Out of 244 patients, GF nerve was identified in 21% of patients, compared to 94% and 97%, respectively, for IL and IH nerves. However intraoperative identification, and hence possibly a much safer technique, did not make a difference on the incidence of chronic pain [9]. The low identification rate is related to

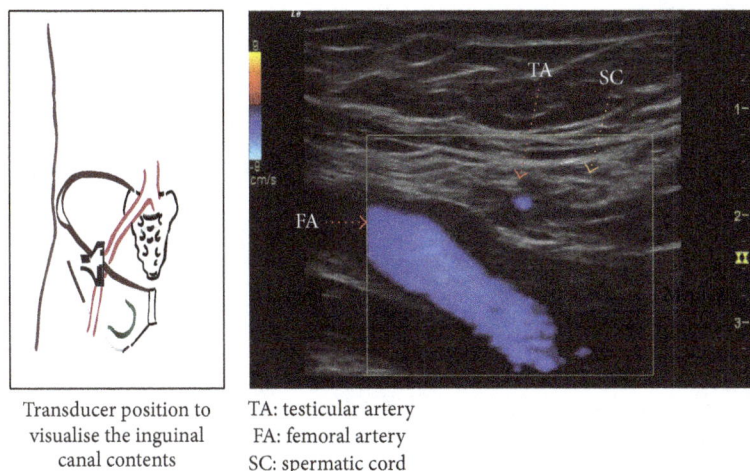

Transducer position to
visualise the inguinal
canal contents

TA: testicular artery
FA: femoral artery
SC: spermatic cord

FIGURE 2: Visualization of structures in the inguinal canal and transducer orientation.

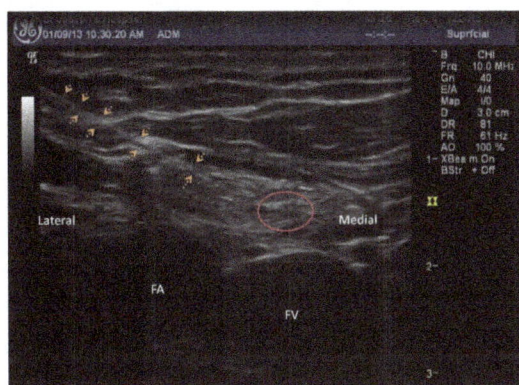

FIGURE 3: Injection into the inguinal canal to block the genitofemoral nerve.

limited dissection, as recommended, near the course of GF nerve which may lie lateral to the external spermatic vein [10]. Laparoscopic hernia surgeries pose similar, if not higher risks. The repair involves placing tacks to secure the mesh from pubic symphysis to anterior superior iliac spine. For one such case, Rho et al. used a fluoroscopic guided injection to successfully treat the condition [11]. It was perhaps easier and safer to do it under ultrasound guidance, which was not as popular at that time. Parris et al. used a CT guided transpsoas approach and ablated the GF nerve, after what seemed to be a successful diagnostic block [12]. The needle was placed, after several attempts, by confirming with electrical stimulation. Unfortunately the patient continued to have persistent pain even after the procedure. Even in this instance an ultrasound guided procedure, near the deep inguinal ring, might have been easier, without the technical difficulties and exposure to radiation. The potential causes of neuropathic pain in these conditions may include inflammation, entrapment, neuroma formation, or deafferentation. Steroid mixed with local anesthetic (LA) solution can block ectopic impulses [13]. Other potential mechanisms include mechanical and anti-inflammatory effect. It must be noted that any such injection must be done preferably at the site of injury or proximal,

to be effective. GF nerve is retroperitoneal until it enters the deep inguinal ring; hence the injury sustained is usually at this level or beyond, and not proximal. The ultrasound guided technique effectively allows for visualisation at this point and can be used for nerve block and pain control. Previously described blind techniques involved injecting 10 mLs of solution just lateral to the pubic tubercle [14]. This can be nonspecific and does not help in differentiating it from the inguinal nerve block. Other options to treatment include operative neurectomy, temporary or permanent neurolysis by using alcohol for phenol, or radiofrequency techniques [15]. Most are invasive and it must be borne in mind that patients can suffer from significant deafferentation pain in a very sensitive area, which itself could be quiet painful.

Through this report, we would like to highlight the need for a differential block, a safe and effective diagnosis, possibly leading to long duration of treatment. All these can be achieved using an ultrasound guided procedure.

Disclosure

Written permission from the patient has been obtained for this report.

References

[1] R. K. Magee, "Genitofemoral Causalgia: (a new syndrome)," *Canadian Medical Association Journal*, vol. 46, no. 4, pp. 326–329, 1942.

[2] M. Rab, J. Ebmer, and A. L. Dellon, "Anatomic variability of the ilioinguinal and genitofemoral nerve: implications for the treatment of groin pain," *Plastic and Reconstructive Surgery*, vol. 108, no. 6, pp. 1618–1623, 2001.

[3] J. Beneš, P. Nádvorník, and J. Doležel, "Abdominoinguinal pain syndrome treated by centrocentral anastomosis," *Acta Neurochirurgica*, vol. 142, no. 8, pp. 887–891, 2000.

[4] E. Aasvang and H. Kehlet, "Surgical management of chronic pain after inguinal hernia repair," *British Journal of Surgery*, vol. 92, no. 7, pp. 795–801, 2005.

[5] B. A. Harms, D. R. DeHaas Jr., and J. R. Starling, "Diagnosis and management of genitofemoral neuralgia," *Archives of Surgery*, vol. 119, no. 3, pp. 339–341, 1984.

[6] P. W. H. Peng and P. S. Tumber, "Ultrasound-guided interventional procedures for patients with chronic pelvic pain— a description of techniques and review of literature," *Pain Physician*, vol. 11, no. 2, pp. 215–224, 2008.

[7] J. R. Starling, B. A. Harms, M. E. Schroeder, and P. L. Eichman, "Diagnosis and treatment of genitofemoral and ilioinguinal entrapment neuralgia," *Surgery*, vol. 102, no. 4, pp. 581–586, 1987.

[8] B. A. Parnell, E. A. Johnson, and D. A. Zolnoun, "Genitofemoral and perineal neuralgia after transobturator midurethral sling," *Obstetrics and Gynecology*, vol. 119, no. 2, pp. 428–431, 2012.

[9] J. M. Bischoff, E. K. Aasvang, H. Kehlet, and M. U. Werner, "Does nerve identification during open inguinal herniorrhaphy reduce the risk of nerve damage and persistent pain?" *Hernia*, vol. 16, no. 5, pp. 573–577, 2012.

[10] S. Alfieri, P. K. Amid, G. Campanelli et al., "International guidelines for prevention and management of post-operative chronic pain following inguinal hernia surgery," *Hernia*, vol. 15, no. 3, pp. 239–249, 2011.

[11] R. H. Rho, T. J. Lamer, and J. T. Fulmer, "Treatment of genitofemoral neuralgia after laparoscopic inguinal herniorrhaphy with fluoroscopically guided tack injection," *Pain Medicine*, vol. 2, no. 3, pp. 230–233, 2001.

[12] D. Parris, N. Fischbein, S. Mackey, and I. Carroll, "A novel CT-guided transpsoas approach to diagnostic genitofemoral nerve block and ablation," *Pain Medicine*, vol. 11, no. 5, pp. 785–789, 2010.

[13] M. Devor, R. Govrin-Lippmann, and P. Raber, "Corticosteroids suppress ectopic neural discharge originating in experimental neuromas," *Pain*, vol. 22, no. 2, pp. 127–137, 1985.

[14] L. Broadman, "Ilioinguinal, iliohypogastric, and genitofemoral nerves," in *Regional Anesthesia. An Atlas of Anatomy and Techniques*, S. G. Gay, Ed., pp. 247–254, Mosby, St. Louis, Mo, USA, 1996.

[15] C. P. Perry, "Laparoscopic treatment of genitofemoral neuralgia," *Journal of the American Association of Gynecologic Laparoscopists*, vol. 4, no. 2, pp. 231–234, 1997.

Myoclonus following a Peripheral Nerve Block

Arlene J. Hudson,[1] **Kevin B. Guthmiller,**[2] **and Marian N. Hyatt**[2]

[1] *Department of Anesthesiology, Uniformed Services University of the Health Sciences, 4301 Jones Bridge Road, Bethesda, MD 20814, USA*
[2] *San Antonio Military Medical Center, 3551 Roger Brooke Drive, San Antonio, TX 78234m, USA*

Correspondence should be addressed to Arlene J. Hudson; arlene.hudson@usuhs.edu

Academic Editors: S. Bele, I.-O. Lee, R. Riley, and C. Seefelder

Myoclonus is an extremely rare perioperative complication following neuraxial anesthesia. It has also been reported to occur due to peripheral nerve lesions. We report a case of self-limiting myoclonus following a routine peripheral nerve block in an otherwise healthy patient.

1. Introduction

A 29-year-old otherwise healthy man presented for an elective left anterior cruciate ligament revision to be performed under a peripheral nerve block. Surgical anesthesia was accomplished with the Labat approach to the sciatic nerve and a live ultrasound guided femoral nerve block. Nerve stimulation was achieved for both nerve blocks at 0.4 mA. On the morning of postoperative day one, the patient developed an involuntary, painless, rhythmic movement of his left lower extremity consistent with spinal myoclonus.

Peripheral nerve blocks are routinely performed for ambulatory orthopedic procedures. Various techniques have been successfully employed including the use of peripheral nerve stimulators as well as ultrasound with excellent efficacy and patient safety. We report a case of myoclonus following a routine peripheral nerve block in an otherwise healthy patient. While myoclonus following neuraxial anesthesia is a rare but recognized phenomenon, myoclonus following a peripheral nerve block has not previously been described.

2. Case Report

A 29-year-old, 90 kilogram, Caucasian man presented for a left anterior cruciate ligament revision. He had previously undergone four uncomplicated left knee procedures all with neuraxial anesthesia. The patient gave consent for regional anesthesia and monitored anesthesia care.

Two blocks for the left lower extremity were performed in a dedicated block area. Oxygen by face mask and routine monitors were applied. Sedation was provided with midazolam (2 mg IV) and fentanyl (100 mcg IV), and the patient remained alert and responsive throughout the procedure. A posterior approach to the sciatic nerve employing Labat's technique was performed. A nerve stimulator was used, and stimulation of the common peroneal segment of the sciatic nerve was achieved at 0.40 mA. Following a positive Raj sign, 30 mL of local anesthetic was injected in a routine fashion using 5 mL aliquots (10 mL of 1.5% mepivacaine with 1 : 400,000 epinephrine, plus 20 mL of 0.5% bupivacaine with 1 : 400,000 epinephrine). The patient was repositioned to the supine, and a femoral block was placed with a technique employing simultaneous live ultrasound (SonoSite MicroMaxx, SonoSite Inc., Bothell, WA; Linear 6–13 MHz) and nerve stimulation. The femoral nerve stimulation was achieved at 0.40 mA. Again, 30 mL of local anesthetic was injected using 5 mL aliquots (0.5% bupivacaine with 1 : 400,000 epinephrine.)

The peripheral nerve blocks provided surgical anesthesia supplemented with dexmedetomidine and fentanyl sedation. The procedure was completed in 3 hours and 51 minutes with a tourniquet time of 125 minutes. The patient recovered overnight in the hospital and received two

Percocet tablets (acetaminophen 325 mg/oxycodone 5 mg) and ketorolac (30 mg IV) for analgesia supplementation. On the morning of postoperative day 1, the patient developed an involuntary, painless, rhythmic movement of his left lower extremity. The patient's left ankle was observed to invert and remain inverted for approximately 1 second before returning to the neutral position. The rhythmic movement exhibited a frequency of 1 every 3 seconds and persisted during sleep as noted by the patient's spouse (see digital video, Supplemental Digital Content 1 in Supplementary Material available online at http://dx.doi.org/10.1155/2013/213472, which is a video of the patient's myoclonus). On exam, full strength and motor function were intact in all muscle groups with the involuntary rhythmic movement being absent during the voluntary motor movement. Residual numbness in the distribution of the femoral nerve was evident, but full sensation was present in the sciatic distribution. Vibratory and position senses were not tested, and cerebellar function was not assessed. A Babinski sign revealed down-going toes bilaterally.

The patient was discharged that morning with instruction for followup with orthopedics as well as the Acute Pain Service. Information pertaining to options for diagnosis was presented, and no immediate consultation was desired by the patient. According to a telephone conversation with the patient, the involuntary rhythmic movement persisted for a total of approximately 6–10 hours followed by spontaneous resolution. No further sequelae were noted.

The authors have obtained written consent from the patient to publish this case report.

3. Discussion

Myoclonus is any brief, involuntary twitching or movement of a muscle or a group of muscles. It is usually caused by muscle contractions (positive myoclonus), but myoclonus also can result from brief lapses of contraction (negative myoclonus). A variety of classification schemes have been developed to categorize myoclonic movements. The "neurophysiologic" classification is a commonly used scheme based on the neuroanatomical origin of electrical discharge and includes the categories cortical, subcortical, spinal, or peripheral myoclonus [1]. In most types of myoclonus, the pathophysiology is unclear although structural lesions, trauma, and abnormalities in neurotransmitter receptors are often present [2]. The neuroanatomical origin of abnormal discharge determines the expressed myoclonic pattern. This may be useful in determining the origin of clinical myoclonus.

Cortical myoclonus arises from the sensorimotor cortex. The transmission of aberrant activity down the corticospinal pathway is characterized by arrhythmic jerks [3]. Subcortical myoclonus originates between the cortex and the spinal cord in the area of the thalamus or brainstem. Subcortical myoclonus is characterized by generalized jerks of the proximal limbs and axial muscles [3].

Spinal myoclonus is typically associated with a lesion in the spinal cord which may cause changes in the afferent signaling from peripheral and supraspinal structures. The duration of the involuntary movements is often longer and more variable than what is seen in cortical or subcortical myoclonus. The movements may be unilateral or bilateral and originate from a spontaneous motor neuron discharge in a single segment of the spinal cord. In one type of spinal myoclonus called segmental spinal myoclonus, the discharge is limited to the level of the lesion and movement is characterized by nonstimulus sensitive rhythmic (0.5–3 Hz) movement. A second type of spinal myoclonus, propriospinal myoclonus, is typified by the propagation of myoclonic jerks along multiple levels of the cord with the myoclonic generator often at the thoracic level. The rhythmic movements are typically slow, bilateral, and usually more extensive than those seen with segmental spinal myoclonus [4, 5].

Lastly, peripheral myoclonus is hypothesized to be caused by lesions of the peripheral nerves that may alter sensory input and induce central reorganization [6]. Peripheral myoclonus is typically not stimulus sensitive and usually results in arrhythmic rapid (200–400 millisecond) jerks. The most commonly encountered peripheral myoclonus is hemifacial spasm.

Our patient exhibited clinical signs suggestive of both spinal and peripheral myoclonus; however, the rhythmic, nonstimulus nature and frequency (0.3–0.5 Hz) of his foot inversion most closely approximates segmental spinal myoclonus. Unfortunately, our patient declined electrophysiological testing, and therefore, our diagnosis is not definitive. Although neuraxial anesthesia has been reported in the literature to cause spinal myoclonus, [7] to our knowledge there are no previous accounts of spinal myoclonus following a regional peripheral nerve block.

Various mechanisms have been suggested as the cause of spinal myoclonus. In general, the loss of inhibitory function of local dorsal horn interneurons, abnormal hyperactivity of local anterior horn cells, and aberrant local axons reexcitation and loss of inhibition from suprasegmental descending pathways have all been suggested as possible etiologies [8]. Given the association of transient spinal myoclonus following neuraxial anesthesia, our patients may have experienced a spread of local anesthetic from the site of injection at the sciatic nerve into the dural sleeves of the nerve roots with migration into the subarachnoid space. This etiology would then be similar to that associated with neuraxial anesthesia and segmental spinal myoclonus. Given the lack of signs suggestive of spinal anesthesia, this explanation appears unlikely.

Peripheral nerve trauma may induce altered sensory inputs and disinhibition of anterior horn neurons via a local sensorimotor integration process. In fact, several cases of spinal myoclonus have been reported in the literature following injury to a peripheral nerve, and some cases have been successfully treated with injections of local anesthetic and botulism toxin. The ensuing success has been attributed to the interruption of abnormal afferent impulse generation [9]. Savrun et al. describe the onset of segmental spinal myoclonus following an ulnar nerve injury [10]. Involuntary movements emerged and intensified over a period of months eventually involving the patient's entire arm. Electromyography confirmed progression to the C5 and C8 nerve roots [10].

Likewise, Assal et al. reported a movement disorder following injury to the cutaneous branch of the deep peroneal nerve with subsequent myoclonus of the first dorsal interosseus muscle [6]. Like our patient, the movements were rhythmic and nonpainful. Proximal local anesthetic injection of the cutaneous branch of the deep peroneal nerve suppressed the myoclonus, suggesting a peripheral origin of the myoclonus with a relay within the spinal cord likely at the L5-S1 level. Shin et al. reported a patient with a known traumatic lesion to the femoral nerve who experienced temporary resolution of the myoclonus with lumbar spinal anesthesia as well as local anesthetic block of the femoral nerve [11], again suggesting a peripheral origin with spinal relay involvement. In all of these cases, however, the movement disorder progressed over a period of months following a permanent peripheral nerve injury. Moreover, other than transient resolution with local anesthetic, in all of these cases the myoclonus persisted.

Ankle inversion, as exhibited by our patient, is accomplished by muscles innervated by branches of the sciatic nerve, specifically the posterior tibial and anterior tibial nerves. The posterior tibial nerve is a branch of the tibial nerve and is comprised of fibers from the L4-5 nerve roots [12]. It innervates muscles which act to invert the ankle while it is in plantarflexion [13]. The anterior tibial nerve is a branch of the deep peroneal nerve and is comprised of fibers from the L5 nerve root. It supplies muscles in the anterior compartment that act to invert the foot while it is in dorsiflexion [12]. Thus, the act of ankle inversion can be accomplished both via anterior or posterior tibial stimulation. Our patient did not appear to be in either excessive plantar or dorsiflexion, and upon examination it was difficult to determine whether the anterior or posterior muscle groups were the primary effectors of ankle movement.

Various techniques for peripheral nerve blocks have been successfully employed including the use of peripheral nerve stimulators as well as ultrasound with excellent efficacy and patient safety. Despite the caution taken with the placement of the two nerve blocks, it is reasonable to consider direct injury or toxicity to the sciatic nerve as the cause of our patient's transient myoclonus. If indeed the sciatic nerve or its branches sustained reversible injury during the regional block, abnormal afferent input generated at the lesion site could have altered the action of local inhibitory spinal interneurons and created a transient involuntary movement disorder.

While myoclonus following neuraxial anesthesia is a recognized phenomenon, albeit exceedingly rare, to our knowledge this case is the first reported myoclonus following a peripheral nerve block.

Acknowledgment

The authors attribute the work to the Department of Anesthesiology at the Walter Reed National Military Medical Center, Bethesda, MD. The views expressed in this article are those of the authors and do not necessarily reflect the official policy or position of the Department of the Navy, Army, Department of Defense, nor the U.S. Government.

References

[1] J. N. Caviness and P. Brown, "Myoclonus: current concepts and recent advances," *Lancet Neurology*, vol. 3, no. 10, pp. 598–607, 2004.

[2] M. R. Pranzatelli and S. R. Snodgrass, "The pharmacology of myoclonus," *Clinical Neuropharmacology*, vol. 8, no. 2, pp. 99–130, 1985.

[3] R. L. Watts and W. C. Koller, *Movement Disorders: Neurologic Principles and Practice*, McGraw-Hill, New York, NY, USA, 2nd edition, 2004.

[4] E. Roze, P. Bounolleau, D. Ducreux et al., "Propriospinal myoclonus revisited: clinical, neurophysiologic, and neuroradiologic findings," *Neurology*, vol. 72, no. 15, pp. 1301–1309, 2009.

[5] W. G. Bradley, R. B. Daroff, G. M. Fenichel, and J. Jankovic, *Neurology in Clinical Practice*, Butterworth-Heinemann, Elsevier, Philadelphia, Pa, USA, 5th edition, 2008.

[6] F. Assal, M. R. Magistris, and F. J. G. Vingerhoets, "Posttraumatic stimulus suppressible myoclonus of peripheral origin," *Journal of Neurology Neurosurgery and Psychiatry*, vol. 64, no. 5, pp. 673–675, 1998.

[7] O. A. Bamgbade, J. A. Alfa, W. M. Khalaf, and A. P. Zuokumor, "Central neuraxial anaesthesia presenting with spinal myoclonus in the perioperative period: a case series," *Journal of Medical Case Reports*, vol. 3, article 7293, 2009.

[8] B. K. Ray, G. Guha, A. K. Misra, and S. K. Das, "Involuntary jerking of lower half of the body (spinal myoclonus)," *Journal of Association of Physicians of India*, vol. 53, pp. 141–143, 2005.

[9] L. Tyvært, P. Krystkowiak, F. Cassim et al., "Myoclonus of peripheral origin: two case reports," *Movement Disorders*, vol. 24, no. 2, pp. 274–277, 2009.

[10] F. Savrun, D. Uluduz, G. Erkol, and M. E. Kiziltan, "Spinal myoclonus following a peripheral nerve injury: a case report," *Journal of Brachial Plexus and Peripheral Nerve Injury*, vol. 3, article 18, 2008.

[11] H.-W. Shin, B. S. Ye, J. Kim, S. M. Kim, and Y. H. Sohn, "The contribution of a spinal mechanism in developing peripheral myoclonus: a case report," *Movement Disorders*, vol. 22, no. 9, pp. 1350–1352, 2007.

[12] S. M. Russell, *Examination of Peripheral Nerve Injuries: An Anatomical Approach*, Thieme Medical Publishers, New York, NY, USA, 2006.

[13] W. Haymaker and B. Woodhall, *Peripheral Nerve Injuries: Principles of Diagnosis*, W. B. Saunders, Philadelphia, Pa, USA, 2nd edition, 1953.

9

Bladder Explosion during Transurethral Resection of the Prostate with Nitrous Oxide Inhalation

Eiko Hirai,[1] **Joho Tokumine,**[2] **Alan Kawarai Lefor,**[3] **Shinobu Ogura,**[4] **and Miwako Kawamata**[5]

[1]*Department of Anesthesia, Seikei-kai Chiba Medical Center, 1-11-12 Minami-cho, Chuo-ku, Chiba-shi, Chiba 260-0842, Japan*
[2]*Department of Anesthesiology, Kyorin University School of Medicine, 6-20-2 Shinkawa, Mitaka-shi, Tokyo 181-8611, Japan*
[3]*Department of Surgery, Jichi Medical University, 3311-1 Yakushiji, Shimotsuke-shi, Tochigi 329-0498, Japan*
[4]*Department of Anesthesiology, Hakujikai Memorial General Hospital, 5-11-1 Shikahama, Adachi-ku, Tokyo 123-0864, Japan*
[5]*Nippori Clinic, Medical Center East, Tokyo Women's Medical University, Station Port Tower 4th F 2-20-1 Nishinippori, Arakawa-ku, Tokyo 116-0013, Japan*

Correspondence should be addressed to Joho Tokumine; ii36469@wa2.so-net.ne.jp

Academic Editor: Bassem S. Wadie

Bladder explosions are a rare complication of transurethral resection of the prostate. We report a patient who suffered a bladder rupture following transurethral resection of the prostate. Although explosive gases accumulate during the procedure, a high concentration of oxygen is needed to support an explosion. This rare phenomenon can be prevented by preventing the flow of room air into the bladder during the procedure to maintain a low concentration of oxygen inside the bladder.

1. Introduction

An intravesical explosion can occur while using an electrical device such as a resectoscope during transurethral resection of prostate (TURP) [1, 2]. The resectoscope uses electrical energy to remove tissue and cauterize the remaining bladder. Tissue is evaporated by diathermy, which uses high-frequency electrical current and generates a great deal of heat. During TURP, small bubbles on an arc of the resectoscope are usually seen, which include hydrogen, oxygen, and other gases derived from the combustion of tissue and water [3–6]. Some of these gases, especially the hydrogen, are explosive [4, 5]. Occasionally, a "pop" sound can be heard during TURP, which suggests a subclinical intravesical explosion [1]. If the resectoscope causes a sufficient explosion, expansion of the intravesical gas results in increased internal pressure in the bladder which can tear the bladder wall [3–9]. We report a patient who suffered a bladder explosion at the end of a TURP, as well as a review of the literature and summary of the mechanism of explosion, and discuss how to prevent this complication.

2. Case Presentation

A 64-year-old man, ASA physical status class II, was scheduled to undergo TURP for benign prostatic hyperplasia and bladder stones with urinary obstruction.

When the patient entered the operating room, the blood pressure (BP) was 147/95 mmHg, heart rate (HR) was 59 min^{-1}, and hemoglobin saturation (SpO$_2$) was 100%. Spinal anesthesia was administered at the L3-L4 interspinous space, using 3 mL of 0.5% isobaric bupivacaine. The BP gradually decreased to 118/68 mmHg, the pulse was 65 min^{-1}, and SpO$_2$ was 98%. The level of spinal block was assessed with loss of cold sensation and determined to be below the thoracic 11 dermatome level. The patient looked anxious and was somewhat restless. We administrated a sedative using 2 mg of midazolam to induce calm.

The bladder was irrigated with UromaticS (Baxter, Japan) which contains 90 g of D-sorbitol in 3 liters (pH 4.5–6.5, 165 mOsm/L). During the operation, the patient described feeling dull pain. Nitrous oxide 1.5·L·min^{-1} and oxygen 1.5·L·min^{-1} were given by face mask. The pain was alleviated and the operation was performed. The operating time from start to resection of 6 g of the prostate and removal of two bladder stones was 85 mins.

When the resectoscope was removed, a loud "pop" sound was heard at the same time. The BP and the HR were transiently elevated to 147/83 mmHg and 87 min^{-1}, respectively. The surgeon started bladder irrigation which returned bloody fluid. The BP decreased to 96/62 mmHg, and the HR was 65 min^{-1}. The patient then described severe abdominal pain. Exploratory laparotomy was emergently performed. General anesthesia was induced with propofol and rocuronium and maintained with sevoflurane along with mixed air and oxygen. At laparotomy, the bladder was found to be ruptured with a large laceration. Other abdominal organs were not injured. The bladder was primarily repaired, and the operation was completed. During the open procedure, the BP and HR were 138–100/85–64 mmHg and 87–62/min, respectively. The SpO$_2$ was maintained at 98–100% from the beginning of the operation till the procedure was completed.

The postoperative course was uneventful. The patient was discharged without symptoms of urinary dysfunction.

3. Discussion

Bladder explosion is a rare and dreadful complication during TURP. It was first reported in 1926 [10] and there are now 25 patients described in 19 reports [3, 5, 7, 8, 10–24]. Bladder rupture is estimated to occur in approximately 0.02% of transurethral procedures [25]. The degree of bladder injury secondary to an explosion varies from a loud "pop" sound only to a ruptured bladder needing surgical repair [1].

A likely mechanism for the intravesical explosion has been previously described [3, 4, 6, 8, 9]. Gases containing hydrogen are produced by electrolysis of intracellular water. These gases accumulate in the bladder, which contains about 5% oxygen during the procedure. Air from the room can enter the bladder while changing the irrigation bag, or inappropriate handling of the evacuator bulb. Room air is 21% oxygen, which is sufficient to support an explosion. The heated resectoscope in the presence of explosive hydrogen gas with a sufficient amount of oxygen then triggers an explosion.

A variety of conditions in patients suffering intravesical explosions have been reported. In 10 previously reported cases, tumors were present at the bladder dome [4, 7, 12, 15–21]. The occurrence of an explosion may be related to the presence of a gas layer with trapped air at the dome of the bladder. High power electrocautery was used for coagulation in situations with difficult hemostasis (three patients) [7, 10, 24]. In other reported cases, the explosion occurred after evacuating resected tissues (five patients) or changing the irrigation bag (one patient) [3–5, 12, 14]. In each of these cases, room air was noted to have entered the bladder. Bladder rupture was noted at the end of the operation in 11 patients [5, 8, 11, 13, 17, 21, 23]. The explosion may have been related to gas accumulated in the bladder at the end of the procedure.

In previously reported cases, various types of anesthesia have been used. General anesthesia was used in three cases, including two with inhalation agents and one with intravenous anesthesia [5, 11, 12]. Caudal epidural anesthesia was used in two cases [11]. Spinal anesthesia was used in seven cases [18, 19, 22–24]. In the remaining 13 reported cases, the type of anesthesia was not reported. In the present patient, the diagnosis of a major intra-abdominal injury may have been facilitated by the patient's ability to report the sudden onset of severe abdominal pain.

Nitrous oxide was used in one previously reported case [11], in which no explosion occurred. Therefore, the present patient may be the first report of a bladder explosion using nitrous oxide. The instruction manuals of the resectoscope and some investigators have warned not to use nitrous oxide while using the electrocautery [24]. Nitrous oxide may increase the risk of bladder explosion because of its character of combustibility and volume expansion in closed spaces.

The resectoscope is routinely used during TURP. Explosive gases are always present inside the bladder. A prevention strategy should be considered to avoid an increased risk of this serious complication. Furthermore, all members for the surgical team should know their roles to keep the patient safe. Surgeons should limit the power used during coagulation and cutting to the minimum needed for effectiveness, which will lead to accumulation of a smaller volume of explosive gases in the bladder [3–5, 7, 8]. Surgeons should prevent room air from entering the bladder while handling the evacuator bulb [1, 3, 7, 14, 26] and nurses can help to prevent the entry of air into the system while changing the irrigation bag [1, 5]. Background music should be stopped during the operation so that the characteristic "pop" sound could more easily be heard if it occurs [2]. In patients with tumors located at the 12 o'clock position, the anesthesiologist may discuss with the urologist to change the bed angle to avoid accumulation of explosive gases at the bladder dome [2, 15]. The anesthesiologist must be a good communicator in the operating room with all members of the operating room team.

Acknowledgment

The authors thank Dr. Anbe (Department of Anesthesia, Seikei-kai Chiba Medical Center) for helpful advice in preparation of the paper.

References

[1] A. Khan, J. Masood, M. Ghei, Z. Kasmani, A. J. Ball, and R. Miller, "Intravesical explosions during transurethral endoscopic procedures," *International Urology and Nephrology*, vol. 39, no. 1, pp. 179–183, 2007.

[2] G. Oğuz, D. Subaşi, M. Kaya, O. Güven, and S. Ünver, "Intravesical explosion: a rare complication of transurethral resection of prostate," *Journal of Anesthesia*, vol. 27, no. 1, pp. 145–146, 2013.

[3] B. F. Hambleton, R. W. Lackey, and R. E. Van Duzen, "Explosive gases formed during electrotransurethral resections," *The Journal of the American Medical Association*, vol. 105, no. 9, pp. 645–646, 1935.

[4] T. C. Ning Jr., D. M. Atkins, and R. C. Murphy, "Bladder explosions during transurethral surgery," *Journal of Urology*, vol. 114, no. 4, pp. 536–539, 1975.

[5] R. I. Hansen and P. Iversen, "Bladder explosion during uninterrupted transurethral resection of the prostate. A case report and an experimental model," *Scandinavian Journal of Urology and Nephrology*, vol. 13, no. 2, pp. 211–212, 1979.

[6] T. R. C. Davis, "The composition and origin of the gas produced during urological endoscopic resections," *British Journal of Urology*, vol. 55, no. 3, pp. 294–297, 1983.

[7] C. Viville, R. de Petriconi, and L. Bietho, "Intravesical explosion during endoscopic resection. Apropos of a case," *The Journal of Urology (Paris)*, vol. 90, no. 5, pp. 361–363, 1984.

[8] F. Di Tonno, V. Fusaro, R. Bertoldin, and D. Lavelli, "Bladder explosion during transurethral resection of the prostate," *Urologia Internationalis*, vol. 71, no. 1, pp. 108–109, 2003.

[9] A. G. Macdonald, "A brief historical review of non-anaesthetic causes of fires and explosions in the operating room," *British Journal of Anaesthesia*, vol. 73, no. 6, pp. 847–856, 1994.

[10] A. Cassuto, "Explosion dans la vessie au cours d'une électrocoagulation," *The Journal of Urology*, vol. 22, p. 263, 1926.

[11] H. L. Kretschmer, "Intravesical explosions as a complicarion of transurethral electroresection: report of two cases," *The Journal of the American Medical Association*, vol. 103, p. 1144, 1934.

[12] R. M. BOBBITT, "Intravesical rupture of bladder during transurethral prostatic resection.," *The Journal of urology*, vol. 64, no. 2, pp. 338–340, 1950.

[13] N. Dublin, A. H. Razack, and C. S. Loh, "Intravesical explosion during transurethral resection of the prostate," *ANZ Journal of Surgery*, vol. 71, no. 6, pp. 384–385, 2001.

[14] G. Morin, S. Vincendeau, A. Manunta, F. Guillé, B. Lobel, and J.-J. Patard, "Intraperitoneal bladder rupture during transurethral resection of the prostate," *Progres en Urologie*, vol. 13, no. 2, pp. 303–305, 2003.

[15] D. C. Horger and A. Babanoury, "Intravesical explosion during transurethral resection of bladder tumors," *The Journal of Urology*, vol. 172, no. 5, part 1, p. 1813, 2004.

[16] A. Srivastava, A. S. Sandhu, T. Sinha et al., "Intravesical explosion during transurethral resection of prostate—a reminder," *Urologia Internationalis*, vol. 77, no. 1, pp. 92–93, 2006.

[17] M. N. Ribeiro da Silva, A. C. Lopes Neto, J. P. Zambon, and E. R. Wroclawski, "Vesical explosion during transurethral resection of the prostate: report of a case," *Archivos Espanoles de Urologia*, vol. 59, no. 6, pp. 651–652, 2006.

[18] M. M. Rezaee, "Intravesical explosion during endoscopic transurethral resection of prostate," *The Journal of Urology*, vol. 3, pp. 109–110, 2006.

[19] F. Ben Jeddou, S. Ghozzi, M. Ktari, and N. Ben Rais, "Intra vesical explosion during an endoscopic resection of a vesical tumor," *Tunisie Medicale*, vol. 84, no. 6, pp. 377–378, 2006.

[20] K.-P. Dieckmann, R. Gehrckens, and A.-K. Biesewig, "Intravesical explosion with rupture of the bladder wall during transurethral resection," *Der Urologe*, vol. 47, no. 7, pp. 860–862, 2008.

[21] M. Seitz, I. Soljanik, P. Stanislaus, R. Sroka, and C. Stief, "Explosive gas formation during transurethral resection of the prostate (TURP)," *European Journal of Medical Research*, vol. 13, no. 8, pp. 399–400, 2008.

[22] K. T. Adiyat, A. Shetty, and T. Jayakrishnan, "Laparoscopic repair of a rare case of bladder rupture due to intravesical explosion during transurethral resection of the prostate," *Urology Journal*, vol. 11, no. 3, pp. 1692–1694, 2014.

[23] B. Baldvinsdóttir, T. Gíslason, and E. Jónsson, "Explosion of the urinary bladder during transurethral resection of the prostate," *Scandinavian Journal of Urology*, vol. 48, no. 6, pp. 571–572, 2014.

[24] S. Sallami, S. Ben Rhouma, A. Dahmani, K. Cherif, A. Horchani, and Y. Nouira, "Intravesical explosion during endoscopic transurethral resection of a bladder tumor," *Ibnosina Journal of Medicine and Biomedical Sciences*, vol. 3, pp. 215–217, 2011.

[25] A. G. Martov, S. I. Kornienko, B. L. Guschin, D. V. Ergakov, and O. A. Sazonov, "Intraoperative urological complications in transurethral surgical interventions on the prostate for benign hyperplasia," *Urologiia*, no. 4, pp. 3–8, 2005.

[26] H. Takeshita, S. Moriyama, K. Chiba, and A. Noro, "A simple technique for evacuating air bubbles with scum from the bladder dome during transurethral resection of bladder tumor," *Wideochirurgia I Inne Techniki Maloinwazyjne*, vol. 9, no. 4, pp. 619–622, 2014.

10

Tracheal Intubation through the I-gel for Emergency Cesarean Section in a Patient with Multidrug Hypersensitivity: A New Technique

Kartika Balaji Samala,[1,2] **Yuri Uchiyama,**[1] **Yasuyuki Tokinaga,**[1] **Yukitoshi Niiyama,**[1] **Soshi Iwasaki,**[1] **and Michiaki Yamakage**[1]

[1] *Sapporo Medical University School of Medicine, Sapporo, S1W16,Chuo-ku, Sapporo-shi, Hokkaido 060-8543, Japan*
[2] *GSL Medical College and Hospital, Rajahmundry, India*

Correspondence should be addressed to Soshi Iwasaki; soushiiwasaki@gmail.com

Academic Editor: Neerja Bhardwaj

31-year-old female with hypersensitivity to local anesthetics and neuromuscular blocking agents presented for emergency Cesarean section. We successfully performed I-gel-assisted tracheal intubation without using neuromuscular blockers. We believe this method would be helpful in selected situations.

1. Introduction

Allergic reactions to anesthetics, drugs, blood products, and neuromuscular blocking agents (NMBA) have been reported during anesthesia [1]. These are sometimes life threatening and difficult to deal with. Our case report highlights the successful management of a patient who presented for Cesarean section with allergy to both NMBAs and local anesthetics on skin testing. Anesthesia was induced with propofol, fentanyl, and the inhalational agent, sevoflurane. A Parker tracheal tube inserted through an I-gel under fiberoptic bronchoscopy was used to secure the airway. We received permission from the patient and restored in electronic medical record to publish this report.

2. Case Report

A 31-year-old female, 158 cm tall and weighing 73.8 kg who had regular antenatal visits, came for the safe institutional delivery. Her medical history dated back to 5 years, with a history of Steven-Johnson syndrome and allergy to carbamazepine. She reported a past history of allergy to lidocaine, procaine, bupivacaine, chlorpheniramine maleate, diclofenac sodium, serratiopeptidase, latex, raw eggs, crabs, and iodine. She had chronic adrenal insufficiency for which she was treated with steroids, which, however, resulted in osteoporosis. Anesthesiologists, obstetricians, and dermatologists discussed the patient's condition and decided to manage her under general anesthesia if normal vaginal delivery was not possible. As per the guidelines for conduct of general anesthesia [2] in such patients, intradermal skin tests for drug allergies were performed, which were positive for lidocaine, procaine, bupivacaine, suxamethonium, and rocuronium at $1:100$ dilutions as previously reported [3]. The patient was given a trial of normal vaginal delivery in the labor room. However, emergency Cesarean section was required due to nonprogression of labor and fetal distress. Once she arrived in the operating room, oxygen was delivered via a face mask. Anesthesia was induced with 140 mg of propofol, $N_2O:O_2$ in a ratio of $4:2$ l/min, and sevoflurane at an end-tidal concentration of 2%. A supraglottic device, the I-gel size 3, was used to secure the airway, seal pressure being maintained above 20 cm H_2O before the start of surgery. When surgery was commenced, the patient did not show any motor activity, indicating an adequate depth of anesthesia. At the time of the uterine incision, a 6.5 mm Parker tracheal tube (Parker

Flex-tip, Colorado, USA) was inserted through the I-gel under fiberoptic bronchoscopy without any resistance. Six ml of air was used to inflate the cuff and bilateral air entry was confirmed by auscultation of the chest. The baby was successfully delivered and had APGAR scores of 7 and 9 at 1 and 5 min, respectively. The mother was given 200 μg of fentanyl immediately after giving birth of the baby. Suctioning using a 10 Fr catheter (Createmedic, Yokohama, Japan) through the I-gel revealed the presence of 8 mL of gastric juice (Figure 1). Postoperatively, the patient was extubated in the recovery room after emergence from anesthesia. Once she was moved to the ward, she complained of mild itching over the forearm, which was not considered to be significant as she was hemodynamically stable. Postoperatively, both mother and baby did well and were discharged from the hospital after a few days without any complications.

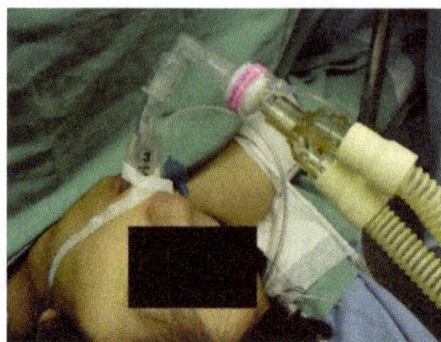

FIGURE 1: Insertion of the Parker tracheal tube and a nasogastric tube through the I-gel.

3. Discussion

Anesthesia-related maternal mortality during Cesarean sections was reported by Hawkins et al. between 1980–90 and 1997–2002. The mortality ratios of general anesthesia to local anesthesia were about 9.8 times [4]. Since local anesthesia very rarely causes severe complications resulting in death, it is preferred over general anesthesia for most surgeries, unless there is an absolute contraindication to its use. General anesthesia is currently adopted when there is no time or when regional anesthesia fails, and it is limited to patients who refuse regional anesthesia or have an abnormal coagulation profile, spinal cord disorders, and allergic reactions to local anesthetics, as in our case.

In our patient, intradermal allergy tests revealed allergy to both ester and amide local anesthetics, limiting their usage. Hence, we selected general anesthesia using drugs that were considered safe in this patient.

Conduct of general anesthesia in parturients can be by (1) rapid sequence induction, (2) awake intubation, or (3) volatile induction. The gold standard for Cesarean section during general anesthesia is rapid sequence induction using thiopentone as the induction agent and suxamethonium as the depolarizing agent to facilitate intubation [5]. Currently, propofol is often used as the induction agent, with rocuronium as the NMBA.

Positive intradermal allergy tests to both depolarizing and nondepolarizing NMBAs in our patient limited their usage, as they are the largest cause of anaphylaxis after induction of anesthesia [2]. We ruled out rapid sequence induction in our patient, as NMBAs could not be used. We also ruled out awake intubation with remifentanil, as the methods would be too slow. Though anaphylaxis cannot be expected in every patient with a positive intradermal test, considering the safety of the patient and her past history of drug allergies, we chose to conduct anesthesia in the manner described here.

Laryngospasm and the risk of aspiration were our main concerns during the conduct of anesthesia in this patient. The sympathetic response to surgery may cause laryngospasm if the depth of anesthesia is inadequate. Use of topical anesthetics to blunt the sympathetic response had to be limited in our patient due to the risk of anaphylaxis. Insertion of the tracheal tube through the I-gel helped overcome this problem, while still maintaining a short time interval between I-gel insertion and intubation. The patient also remained hemodynamically stable during this period. Volatile induction was not considered feasible in our patient since it was an emergency Cesarean section. Our technique enabled avoidance of NMBA usage and showed that, in some difficult airway scenarios during emergency Cesarean section, our technique is easy and saves time.

Opioids are mainly used during general anesthesia to obtund the neuroendocrine stress response and for hemodynamic stability. However, it is not clear how quickly fentanyl crosses the placenta. Hence, keeping in mind the risk of fetal respiratory depression and low APGAR scores, its use was precluded in our patient before delivery of the baby [6]. Halaseh et al. [7] reported that use of the Proseal laryngeal mask airway was effective in protecting against the risk of aspiration in 3000 elective Cesarean section patients with a minimum fasting period of 8 hr. In our patient, we opted to use the I-gel as it has the advantage of more rapid and easier insertion and decreased incidence of gastric insufflation when compared to laryngeal mask airways (LMA), both of which were desirable in our patient. Very few studies or case reports have described use of the I-gel and its advantages over the classic LMA, except for one previous study that supports our work [8]. These reports suggest the utility of supraglottic airway device *per se* in cesarean section. The 2nd generation supraglottic airway device such as proseal LMA(PLMA), intubating LMA(ILMA) could be alternatives in our case. Kleine-Brueggeney reported the success of fibreoptic intubation which was similar between using I-gel and ILMA, and the former was superior to ILMA in terms of time to insertion [9]. Air Q is one supraglottic airway device which could pass tracheal tube as easy as I-gel in the manikin study [10]; however it was necessary to take off the tip which wasted crucial time in scenarios like our patient. So, we choose to use I-gel as a supraglottic device considering our patient's condition. Here, we emphasize that tracheal intubation through the I-gel is a new method in particular for Caesarian section which helps in the progress of anesthesia and surgery at the same time.

Our case report highlights a novel approach of I-gel-assisted tracheal intubation in patients in whom NMBAs cannot be used.

References

[1] K. Chaudhuri, J. Gonzales, C. A. Jesurun, M. T. Ambat, and S. Mandal-Chaudhuri, "Anaphylactic shock in pregnancy: a case study and review of the Literature," *International Journal of Obstetric Anesthesia*, vol. 17, no. 4, pp. 350–357, 2008.

[2] P. M. Mertes, M. C. Laxenaire, A. Lienhart et al., "Reducing the risk of anaphylaxis during anaesthesia: guidelines for clinical practice," *Journal of Investigational Allergology and Clinical Immunology*, vol. 15, no. 2, pp. 91–101, 2005.

[3] E. Macy, M. Schatz, and R. S. Zeiger, "Immediate hypersensitivity to methylparaben causing false-positive results of local anesthetic skin testing or provocative dose testing," *The Permanente Journal*, vol. 6, supplement 1, pp. 17–21, 2002.

[4] J. L. Hawkins, J. Chang, S. K. Palmer, C. P. Gibbs, and W. M. Callaghan, "Anesthesia-related maternal mortality in the United States: 1979–2002," *Obstetrics and Gynecology*, vol. 117, no. 1, pp. 69–74, 2011.

[5] R. S. H. Pumphrey and I. S. D. Roberts, "Postmortem findings after fatal anaphylactic reactions," *Journal of Clinical Pathology*, vol. 53, no. 4, pp. 273–276, 2000.

[6] H. King, S. Ashley, D. Brathwaite, J. Decayette, and D. J. Wooten, "Adequacy of general anesthesia for cesarean section," *Anesthesia & Analgesia*, vol. 77, no. 1, pp. 84–88, 1993.

[7] B. K. Halaseh, Z. F. Sukkar, L. H. Hassan, A. T. H. Sia, W. A. Bushnaq, and H. Adarbeh, "The use of ProSeal laryngeal mask airway in caesarean section: experience in 3000 cases," *Anaesthesia and Intensive Care*, vol. 38, no. 6, pp. 1023–1028, 2010.

[8] A. M. Helmy, H. M. Atef, E. M. El-Taher, and A. M. Heindak, "Comparative study between I-gel, a new supraglottic airway device, and classic laryngeal mask airway in anesthetized spontaneously ventilated patients," *Saudi Journal of Anaesthesia*, vol. 4, pp. 131–136, 2010.

[9] M. Kleine-Brueggeney, L. Theiler, N. Urwyler, A. Vogt, and R. Greif, "Randomized trial comparing the i-gel and Magill tracheal tube with the single-use ILMA and ILMA tracheal tube for fibreoptic-guided intubation in anaesthetized patients with a predicted difficult airway," *British Journal of Anaesthesia*, vol. 107, no. 2, pp. 251–257, 2011.

[10] R. Ueki, N. Komasawa, K. Nishimoto, T. Sugi, M. Hirose, and Y. Kaminoh, "Utility of the Aintree Intubation Catheter in fiberoptic tracheal intubation through the three types of intubating supraglottic airways: a manikin simulation study," *Journal of Anesthesia*, vol. 28, no. 3, pp. 363–367, 2014.

11

Application of Dual Mask for Postoperative Respiratory Support in Obstructive Sleep Apnea Patient

Jahan Porhomayon,[1] Gino Zadeii,[2] Nader D. Nader,[3] George R. Bancroft,[4] and Alireza Yarahamadi[5]

[1] VA Western New York Healthcare System, Division of Critical Care and Pain Medicine, Department of Anesthesiology, State University of New York at Buffalo, School of Medicine and Biomedical Sciences, VA Medical Center, Room 203C, 3495 Bailey Avenue, Buffalo, NY 14215, USA

[2] University of Iowa, Mason City Cardiology, Mason City, IA 50401, USA

[3] VA Western New York Healthcare System, Division of Cardiothoracic Anesthesia and Pain Medicine, Department of Anesthesiology, State University of New York at Buffalo School of Medicine and Biomedical Sciences, Buffalo, NY 14215, USA

[4] Department of Anesthesiology, State University of New York at Buffalo, School of Medicine and Biomedical Sciences, Buffalo, NY 14215, USA

[5] Director of Mercy North-Iowa Neurology and Sleep Laboratory, University of Iowa, Mason City Neurology, Mason City, IA 50401, USA

Correspondence should be addressed to Jahan Porhomayon; jahanpor@buffalo.edu

Academic Editors: U. Buyukkocak, M. Dauri, I.-O. Lee, R. Riley, and E. A. Vandermeersch

In some conditions continuous positive airway pressure (CPAP) or bilevel positive airway pressure (BIPAP) therapy alone fails to provide satisfactory oxygenation. In these situations oxygen (O_2) is often being added to CPAP/BIPAP mask or hose. Central sleep apnea and obstructive sleep apnea (OSA) are often present along with other chronic conditions, such as chronic obstructive pulmonary disease (COPD), congestive heart failure, pulmonary fibrosis, neuromuscular disorders, chronic narcotic use, or central hypoventilation syndrome. Any of these conditions may lead to the need for supplemental O_2 administration during the titration process. Maximization of comfort, by delivering O_2 directly via a nasal cannula through the mask, will provide better oxygenation and ultimately treat the patient with lower CPAP/BIPAP pressure.

1. Introduction

Obstructive sleep apnea (OSA) is a complex medical disorder, characterized by repetitive upper airway collapse during sleep. The disease affects individuals of all ages and predisposes to multiple comorbidities, including increased risk of cardiovascular disease [1].

Perioperative apneas appear to be multifactorial in nature. Sedatives and anesthetics have been shown to decrease pharyngeal muscle tone and therefore predispose to apnea [2]. Meanwhile, the patient's normal arousal responses and reflexes are also compromised by anesthetics [3]. This predisposes to apneic episodes which can be more severe than those associated with natural sleep.

While many patients present for surgery with undiagnosed OSA, it is currently recommended that patients who receive ambulatory CPAP preoperatively should continue to have CPAP administered in the perioperative period. Otherwise, the optimal management of OSA in the perioperative period has yet to be elucidated [4].

2. Case Report

A 51-year-old obese male, with a history of daytime fatigue, presented to the anesthesia holding area for urgent appendectomy. He had previously undergone a sleep study several months before with apnea/hypopnea index (AHI) of 35 and

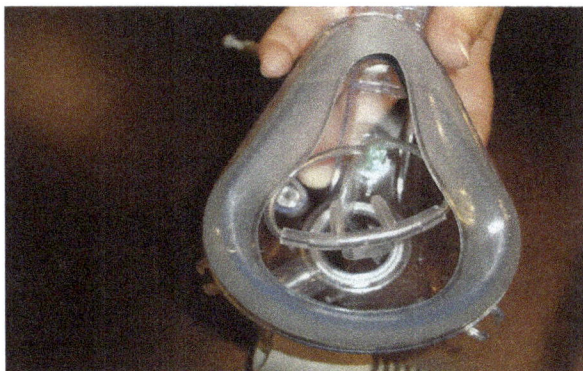

FIGURE 1: Dual mask is easy to apply with inner nasal cannula.

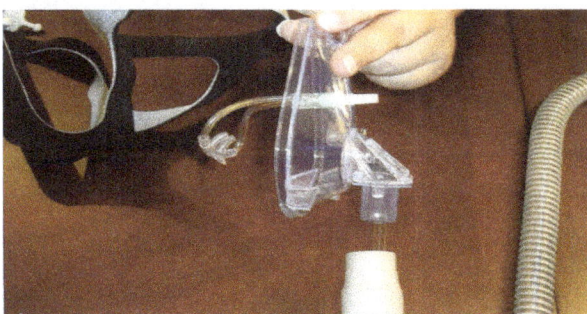

FIGURE 2: Lateral view of dual mask, nasal cannula can be directly applied to the patient nostril and eliminate dilution effect secondary to leak.

a maximum desaturation to the low 60's. Patient vital signs included a blood pressure of 140/85 mm/Hg, heart rate of 95 beats per minute and respiratory rate of 16 per minute with a temperature of 38 centigrade. His pulse oximetry (SaO_2) reading was 91% with 2 liters/minute of nasal oxygen flow. Chest radiography did not show any pathology.

He was brought to operating room, and anesthesia was induced with propofol and succinylcholine in a rapid sequence technique. The trachea was intubated with the aid of a GlideScope. Anesthesia was maintained with mixtures of oxygen/air/desflurane/fentanyl. The patient was extubated without difficulty and was transported to the PACU on supplemental O_2 via mask with SaO_2 of 90%. On arrival to PACU and after the first set of vital signs, his SaO_2 dropped to 88%. As CPAP was applied, he immediately started to have central apneas. Therefore, we started BIPAP therapy with O_2 concentration of 50%. Because the patient was a major mouth breather with full beard, we continued to have difficulty achieving appropriate tidal volumes. The PACU nurses tried multiple full-face masks with or without a chin strap, but low tidal volume alarms continued. At BIPAP pressures of 15/11 cm H_2O and O_2 flow of 4 liters/minutes, we could not

improve the saturation. The nurses were unable to stabilize saturations due to numerous central apneas. We then decided to use the dual mask (Figures 1 and 2) with 2 liters/min of O_2 via nasal cannula. We set the BIPAP machine to pressure of 8/4 cm H_2O and were finally able to adjust the pressure to 12/6 cm H_2O with SaO_2 of 92% and adequate tidal volume.

3. Discussion

The potential for upper airway obstruction remains high postoperatively because of the effects of residual anesthetics, sedatives, and opioids. During the postoperative period, patients with severe obstructive sleep apnea are at increased risk for respiratory and cardiopulmonary complications [5]. If a patient has his or her own CPAP device, it should be available in the recovery room for use immediately upon emergence from anesthesia. Under no circumstances should the patient be left unattended [3, 6]. Close observation is required until stability is established.

The use of higher CPAP/BIPAP pressure can lead to higher leakage, increased nasal drying or congestion, pressure sores on the bridge of the nose, difficulty exhaling, and higher levels of machine noise [7, 8]. Clearly, these are disadvantageous, and lower pressures are preferred.

In current clinical practice O_2 is added to CPAP/BIPAP mask usually from a small hole into the mask or to CPAP/ BIPAP hose. Hence, the added O_2 becomes diluted by CPAP/ BIPAP flow and is also subject to leakage [7]. Patients rarely get the full benefit of supplemental O_2.

Adding O_2 directly to the patient's mask is not practical because it can easily come disconnected when the patient changes position. This is a common source of patient complaints. The pressure can also affect the triggering function of the ventilator [9]. Another disadvantage is having two separate tubes on the bed and two separate machines at the bedside.

Combining the O_2 compressor and CPAP/BIPAP machine as well as combining the CPAP/BIPAP hose and the O_2 hose (dual tube) to occupy less space can provide better convenience. Connecting an adjustable cannula to a full-face or nasal mask and delivering supplemental O_2 directly to the nostrils will provide higher O_2 saturation during inhalation with the help of CPAP/BIPAP pressure [7].

Disclosure

The authors do not have any financial and personal relationships with other people or organizations that could inappropriately influence (bias) their work. Examples of potential conflict of interests include employment, consultancies, stock ownership, honoraria, paid expert testimony, patent applications/registrations, and grants or other funding.

References

[1] D. J. Eckert, A. Malhotra, and A. S. Jordan, "Mechanisms of apnea," *Progress in Cardiovascular Diseases*, vol. 51, no. 4, pp. 313–323, 2009.

[2] G. Dhonneur, X. Combes, B. Leroux, and P. Duvaldestin, "Postoperative obstructive apnea," *Anesthesia and Analgesia*, vol. 89, no. 3, pp. 762–767, 1999.

[3] D. R. Hillman, P. R. Platt, and P. R. Eastwood, "Anesthesia, sleep, and upper airway collapsibility," *Anesthesiology Clinics*, vol. 28, no. 3, pp. 443–455, 2010.

[4] B. Hartmann, A. Junger, and J. Klasen, "Anesthesia and sleep apnea syndrome," *Anaesthesist*, vol. 54, no. 7, pp. 684–693, 2005.

[5] C. Den Herder, J. Schmeck, D. J. K. Appelboom, and N. De Vries, "Risks of general anaesthesia in people with obstructive sleep apnoea," *British Medical Journal*, vol. 329, no. 7472, pp. 955–959, 2004.

[6] J. A. Loadsman and D. R. Hillman, "Anaesthesia and sleep apnoea," *British Journal of Anaesthesia*, vol. 86, no. 2, pp. 254–266, 2001.

[7] D. Samolski, A. Antón, R. Güell, F. Sanz, J. Giner, and P. Casan, "Inspired oxygen fraction achieved with a portable ventilator: determinant factors," *Respiratory Medicine*, vol. 100, no. 9, pp. 1608–1613, 2006.

[8] K. H. Ruhle and G. Nilius, "Mouth breathing in obstructive sleep apnea prior to and during nasal continuous positive airway pressure," *Respiration*, vol. 76, no. 1, pp. 40–45, 2008.

[9] E. Miyoshi, Y. Fujino, A. Uchiyama, T. Mashimo, and M. Nishimura, "Effects of gas leak on triggering function, humidification, and inspiratory oxygen fraction during noninvasive positive airway pressure ventilation," *Chest*, vol. 128, no. 5, pp. 3691–3698, 2005.

12

Emergent Median Sternotomy for Mediastinal Hematoma: A Rare Complication following Internal Jugular Vein Catheterization for Chemoport Insertion

Saptarshi Biswas, Marwa Sidani, and Sunil Abrol

Department of Surgery, Brookdale University Hospital Medical Center, Brooklyn, NY 11212, USA

Correspondence should be addressed to Saptarshi Biswas; saptarshibiswas@comcast.net

Academic Editors: S. Grigoriadis and T. Ho

Mediastinal hematoma is a rare complication following insertion of a central venous catheter with only few cases reported in the English literature. We report a case of a 71-year-old female who was admitted for elective chemoport placement. USG guided right internal jugular access was attempted using the Seldinger technique. Resistance was met while threading the guidewire. USG showed a chronic clot burden in the RIJ. A microvascular access was established under fluoroscopic guidance. Rest of the procedure was completed without any further issues. Following extubation, the patient complained of right-sided chest pain radiating to the back. Chest X-ray revealed a contained white out in the right upper lung field. She became hemodynamically unstable. Repeated X-ray showed progression of the hematoma. Median Sternotomy showed posterior mediastinal hematoma tracking into right pleural cavity. Active bleeding from the puncture site at RIJ-SCL junction was repaired. Patient had an uneventful recovery. Injury to the central venous system is the result of either penetrating trauma or iatrogenic causes as in our case. A possible explanation of our complication may be attributed to the forced manipulation of the dilator or guidewire against resistance. Clavicle and sternum offer bony protection to the underlying vital venous structures and injuries often need sternotomy with or without neck extension. Division of the clavicle and disarticulation of the sternoclavicular joint may be required for optimum exposure. Meticulous surgical technique, knowledge of the possible complications, and close monitoring in the postprocedural period are of utmost importance. Chest X-ray showed to be routinely done to detect any complication early.

1. Introduction

Internal jugular vein catheterization is a fairly common procedure for inserting a chemotherapy port. In fact, more than 5 million central venous catheters are inserted every year in the United States [1]. However, such catheterization may be associated with serious life threatening complications, which have been reported to occur in 6.2–10.7% [2] of patients. Various complications can be encountered including a higher risk of pneumothorax, puncture of the carotid or subclavian artery, cardiac tamponade, or hemothorax. Other less serious risk factors include infection, thrombosis, or factors related to maintenance of the central line.

In this paper we present a case report of a relatively rare complication of mediastinal hematoma following internal jugular vein catheterization for chemoport insertion. We also discuss the relevant literature regarding complications associated with central line placement as well as the various available treatment options.

2. Case Report

A 71-year-old female was admitted under the surgical service for elective chemoport placement. She was known diabetic and hypertensive and well controlled on medications. She was also diagnosed with stage II gastric cancer. She underwent distal gastrectomy and Bilroth II reconstruction several months ago and was scheduled for chemotherapy as part of her management.

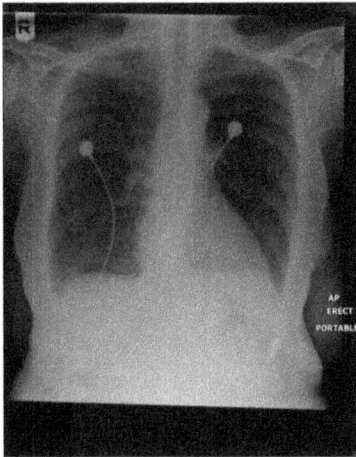

FIGURE 1: Preoperative chest X-ray: essentially normal.

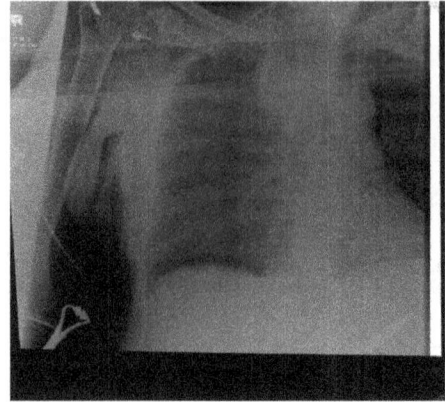

FIGURE 2: Chest X-ray showing right upper lobe whitening.

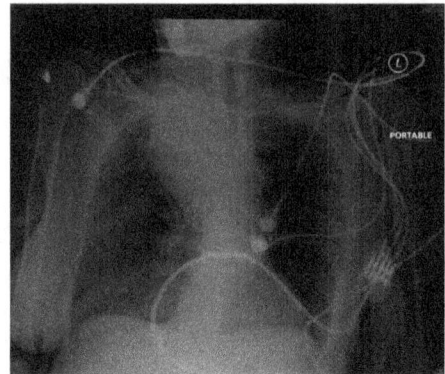

FIGURE 3: Postprocedural chest X-ray showing right mediastinal hematoma. Thoracic and vascular surgery team was consulted immediately and the decision was made to emergently take the patient to the operating room for evacuation of a mediastinal hematoma. Central and arterial access was obtained and transfusion of packed red blood cells (PRBC) was started. The hemodynamic status improved.

Just prior to the procedure the patient developed symptomatic bradycardia manifested as near syncope with her heart rate dropping to 40 beats per minute. Consequently, the procedure was cancelled and the patient was admitted to the medical service for further workup. Cardiology was consulted and she was started on Plavix in addition to the Lovenox she was having for DVT prophylaxis. Workup including transthoracic echocardiography (TTE) was within normal and she was cleared for the procedure. Later Plavix was stopped at the time of the procedure.

The patient was taken to operating room the following day for the placement of a chemoport. Her chest X-ray (Figure 1) was normal and she was asymptomatic. General anesthesia was induced with no complications. The patient was draped and positioned in Trendelenberg. Ultrasound guided insertion of a right internal jugular venous (IJV) access was attempted with a total of 4 trials using Seldinger's technique. Resistance was met while threading the guide wire. Ultrasound examination showed a chronic clot burden in the Right IJV. The vascular surgery team was consulted intra operatively. A right IJV access using a microset access under fluoroscopic guidance was obtained. The procedure was then completed without any further issues. Following extubation, and upon transfer of the patient to the stretcher, she started complaining of right-sided chest pain radiating to the back. She became tachycardic with a heart rate ranging between 105 and 110 beats per minute. CXR was immediately obtained and it revealed a contained white out in the right upper lung field (Figure 2).

Soon after, the patient decompensated with the systolic blood pressure dropping to 60 mm Hg. Volume resuscitation with crystalloids was started and the patient was cross-matched for transfusion of blood products. A third CXR was obtained during this time revealing the progression of a hemothorax in the right side of the chest (Figure 3).

A median sternotomy was performed. Upon exploration of the thorax, a posterior mediastinal hematoma tracking into right pleural cavity was detected. There was active bleeding from the puncture site at IJV-subclavian (SCV) junction. By the end of the surgery, the patient received a total of four

units of (PRBC), two units of fresh frozen plasma (FFP), and one unit of platelets. The patient was transferred to the surgical intensive care unit (SICU) postoperatively intubated and hemodynamically stable. A right pleural chest tube was kept in place for drainage. Postoperative CXR was done showing marked improvement of the right-sided hemothorax (Figure 4). The next morning, the patient was extubated and the mediastinal chest tube was removed. The patient had an unremarkable recovery course and was transferred out of the SICU after removal of the right pleural chest tube.

3. Discussion

Injury to the central venous system in most cases is the result of either penetrating trauma, like gunshot wounds, or iatrogenic causes like central line catheter placement. Penetrating injuries especially secondary to gunshot wounds to the subclavian and innominate veins can often result in rapid exsanguination resulting in significant mortality [3–7] in this patient group.

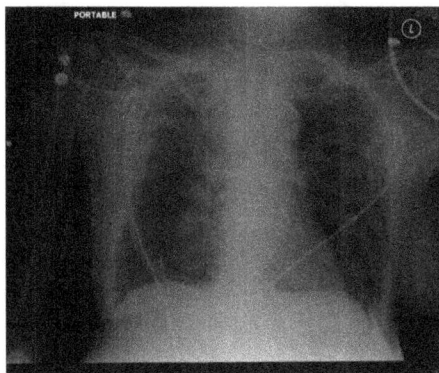

FIGURE 4: Postoperative chest X-ray: significant improvement of the right mediastinal hemothorax.

Right internal jugular vein (RIJV) is often selected as an ideal vein for central venous access for chemoport access because of its straight course, reduced risk of malposition, and thrombosis. However, mechanical complications from central venous catheter insertion are reported to occur in 5 to 19% of patients, infectious complications in 5 to 26%, and thrombotic complications in 2 to 26% [1].

Central venous catheterizations along with erosions are more common causes of injury to the innominate-superior vena cava (SVC) confluence compared to penetrating trauma [3, 8–22]. However, such complications of catheter placement are relatively rare compared to the more common complications like pneumothorax, infection, and intravascular thrombosis [3].

The innominate-SVC junction is in close proximity to the pleural and pericardial spaces. Localized central line perforation within the mediastinal pleura may not cause significant complications if identified early and the catheter removed promptly. However, if the perforation is delayed or missed, hydrothorax communicates to the pleural space. The hydrothorax is usually on the contralateral side of the chest from the central line placement. In some cases, it may be bilateral [22]. Acute perforation of the innominate-SVC junction can result in cardiac tamponade resulting in sudden hemodynamic decompensation [3, 15–17].

Elderly, bed-ridden, debilitated, and malnourished patients with chronic underlying disease processes are predisposed to chronic catheter injury at the innominate-caval junction. Chronic catheter injuries are mostly associated with left sided catheter insertion [22] with the central tip eroding the cephalad portion of SVC. The probable explanation is that the anatomy of the left innominate vein is relatively more horizontal than the right innominate vein and the junction with the SVC is almost at a right angle. Thus, catheter tip inserted through the left side is more likely to impinge on the right caval wall. Abnormal angulation of the catheter relative to the SVC, infusion of hyperosmolar solution and undue flexion, and extension of the patient's neck can result in erosion. Delayed perforation usually results in unilateral right side pleural effusion. However it can be bilateral in 33% of cases [22].

Internal jugular vein central line insertion is widely used as a way for venous access for chemotherapy port. The occurrence of mediastinal hematoma resulting from vascular injury in close proximity to the mediastinum and the need for emergent thoracotomy due to hemodynamic instability is an extremely rare complication. It is documented in the literature in very few case reports [23]. Gupta et al. [23] in a case report published in 2011 mentioned 8 cases of mediastinal hematoma following central line placement.

Arik et al. [24] reported a case of mediastinal hematoma after the insertion of a left subclavian venous catheter in a patient with end stage renal failure for the purpose of hemodialysis. The guide wire most likely penetrated the subclavian vein and caused bleeding that resulted in mediastinal hematoma and eventual death of the patient.

A possible explanation of the mechanism of vascular complication includes forced manipulation of the dilators or guide wires against resistance. In our case, we encountered appreciable resistance while threading the guidewire when it reached the IJ junction. We were able to recognize the difficulty of threading the guidewire into the IJ and to identify a chronic clot burden in the right IJ by using ultrasound examination. We attributed the resistance we met to a thrombus at the IJ junction, although that is considered to be a rare incidence.

Gupta et al. [23] presented a case report of a mediastinal hematoma in a 33-year-old male after placement of a right subclavian central line for intra and postoperative central venous pressure monitoring during a renal transplantation surgery. The mediastinal hematoma was discovered after routine CXR done postoperatively. The right mediastinal hematoma was managed conservatively with repeated chest radiographs. In their discussion, Gupta et al. presented 8 cases of occurrence of mediastinal hematoma after insertion of a central line. Only one case, reported by Doi et al. [25], required a thoracotomy. Three cases presented required coil embolization of the internal mammary artery, two cases were managed with insertion of bilateral intercostal drains for hydrothorax, and two cases were managed conservatively.

Doi et al. [25] described a posterior mediastinal hematoma that developed after right internal jugular cannulation for central venous and PA catheter in a patient undergoing cardiac surgery. The patient experienced hemodynamic instability and stridor on the day following the operation due to tracheal compression by the hematoma. It was speculated to be due to a misplacement of either the internal jugular catheter or the guide wire into the azygous vein. The hematoma was evacuated with a thoracotomy.

Naguib et al. [26] described a case of hydromediastinum and bilateral hydrothorax after a subclavian line insertion in a 28-year old male after multiple fractures due to motor vehicle accident. The left subclavian vein was cannulated intraoperatively. Postoperative CXR was done and was negative for pneumo- or hemothorax. However, three hours later, the patient became hemodynamically unstable, which required further CXR revealing widening of the mediastinum. The patient was managed with bilateral chest tubes for bilateral hydrothorax and the hydromediastinum was managed conservatively.

Also, Chemelli et al. [27] conducted a retrospective analysis of five patients with iatrogenic arterial lesions of the internal mammary artery (IMA). The lesions occurred in three patients from a puncture of the subclavian vein during insertion of a central venous catheter and in two patients from a puncture of the subclavian vein for insertion of a pacemaker lead. Microcoil embolization was performed to control the source of bleeding.

Hohlrieder et al. [28] reported a life-threatening mediastinal hematoma in a 6-month-old girl during surgical correction of scaphocephaly. The left subclavian vein was successfully punctured on the first attempt using the Seldinger technique. The patient showed persistent hemodynamic instability requiring the use of emergent transesophageal echocardiography (TEE) for further investigation. A large mediastinal hematoma compressing the right atrium and the SVC was detected due to dislocation of the left subclavian catheter. The cannula was removed and the patient was managed conservatively.

Innominate-caval injuries are usually related to catheter placement and can result from central line placement at either side. Acute injuries can often cause cardiac tamponade. For innominate-caval confluence exposure, median sternotomy alone is adequate. However, extension of the incision into the neck and resection of the clavicle are necessary for adequate exposure of the subclavian Internal jugular junction. Clamps, ligations or cardiopulmonary bypass can achieve vascular control. Asymptomatic mediastinal hematoma can sometimes be observed and managed conservatively [3].

Moreover, the clavicle as well as the sternum offer bony protection to the vital central venous system. Although some subclavian venous injuries can be managed using only division of the clavicle and disarticulation of the sternoclavicular joint, optimum exposure is achieved when median sternotomy is performed. Thoracotomy does not provide a good exposure of the subclavian-IJ junction. Because of the difficulty of vascular reconstruction at venous confluences some authors recommend simple ligation of the venous injuries at the subclavian-IJ junction. Others like Baumgartner et al. [3], however, prefer primary repair compared to ligation in their series.

4. Conclusion

Meticulous surgical technique, knowledge of the possible complications, and close monitoring of the patient in the perioperative period are required in the management of central line, dialysis catheter, and chemoport placements.

Postprocedural chest radiographs are useful in detecting complications early as in our case and should be done routinely.

Acknowledgment

The authors would like to thank Dr. Richard Fogler MD and Dr. Zeleka Shair MD for their involvement in the clinical management of the patient.

References

[1] I. Raad, "Intravascular-catheter-related infections," *The Lancet*, vol. 351, no. 9106, pp. 893–898, 1998.

[2] D. C. McGee and M. K. Gould, "Preventing complications of central venous catheterization," *The New England Journal of Medicine*, vol. 348, no. 12, pp. 1123–1133, 2003.

[3] F. J. Baumgartner, J. Rayhanabad, F. S. Bongard, J. C. Milliken, C. Donayre, and S. R. Klein, "Central venous injuries of the subclavian-jugular and innominate-caval confluences," *Texas Heart Institute Journal*, vol. 26, no. 3, pp. 177–181, 1999.

[4] P. M. Rao, R. R. Ivatury, P. Sharma, A. T. Vinzons, Z. Nassoura, and W. M. Stahl, "Cervical vascular injuries: a trauma center experience," *Surgery*, vol. 114, no. 3, pp. 527–531, 1993.

[5] E. Degiannis, G. Velmahos, D. Krawczykowski, R. D. Levy, I. Souter, and R. Saadia, "Penetrating injuries of the subclavian vessels," *British Journal of Surgery*, vol. 81, no. 4, pp. 524–526, 1994.

[6] D. Demetriades, B. Rabinowitz, A. Pezikis, J. Franklin, and G. Palexas, "Subclavian vascular injuries," *British Journal of Surgery*, vol. 74, no. 11, pp. 1001–1003, 1987.

[7] J. V. Robbs and E. Reddy, "Management options for penetrating injuries to the great veins of the neck and superior mediastinum," *Surgery Gynecology and Obstetrics*, vol. 165, no. 4, pp. 323–326, 1987.

[8] P. Duntley, J. Siever, M. L. Korwes, K. Harpel, and J. E. Heffner, "Vascular erosion by central venous catheters: clinical features and outcome," *Chest*, vol. 101, no. 6, pp. 1633–1638, 1992.

[9] L. M. Ellis, S. B. Vogel, and E. M. Copeland III, "Central venous catheter vascular erosions. Diagnosis and clinical course," *Annals of Surgery*, vol. 209, no. 4, pp. 475–478, 1989.

[10] T. J. Iberti, L. B. Katz, and M. A. Reiner, "Hydrothorax as a late complication of central venous indwelling catheters," *Surgery*, vol. 94, no. 5, pp. 842–846, 1983.

[11] E. Chute and F. B. Cerra, "Late development of hydrothorax and hydromediastinum in patients with central venous catheters," *Critical Care Medicine*, vol. 10, no. 12, pp. 868–869, 1982.

[12] R. H. Dailey, "Late vascular perforations by CVP catheter tips," *Journal of Emergency Medicine*, vol. 6, no. 2, pp. 137–140, 1988.

[13] C. B. Kapadia, S. O. Heard, and N. S. Yeston, "Delayed recognition of vascular complications caused by central venous catheters," *Journal of Clinical Monitoring*, vol. 4, no. 4, pp. 267–271, 1988.

[14] L. Mukau, M. A. Talamini, and J. V. Sitzmann, "Risk factors for central venous catheter-related vascular erosions," *Journal of Parenteral and Enteral Nutrition*, vol. 15, no. 5, pp. 513–516, 1991.

[15] A. Chabanier, F. Dany, P. Brutus, and H. Vergnoux, "Iatrogenic cardiac tamponade after central venous catheter," *Clinical Cardiology*, vol. 11, no. 2, pp. 91–99, 1988.

[16] B. R. Barton, G. Hermann, and R. Weil III, "Cardiothoracic emergencies associated with subclavian hemodialysis catheters," *Journal of the American Medical Association*, vol. 250, no. 19, pp. 2660–2662, 1983.

[17] G. W. Fischer and R. G. Scherz, "Neck vein catheters and pericardial tamponade," *Pediatrics*, vol. 52, no. 6, pp. 868–871, 1973.

[18] C. W. Armstrong and C. G. Mayhall, "Contralateral hydrothorax following subclavian catheter replacement using a guidewire," *Chest*, vol. 84, no. 2, pp. 231–233, 1983.

[19] P. J. McDonnell, S. J. Qualman, and G. M. Hutchins, "Bilateral hydrothorax as a life-threatening complication of central venous hyperalimentation," *Surgery Gynecology and Obstetrics*, vol. 158, no. 6, pp. 577–579, 1984.

[20] M. K. Agarwal, A. S. Banner, and W. W. Addington, "Bilateral hydrothorax from unilateral subclavian vein catheterization," *Journal of the American Medical Association*, vol. 239, no. 3, pp. 190–191, 1978.

[21] M. E. Flatley and R. M. Schapira, "Hydropneumomediastinum and bilateral hydropneumothorax as delayed complications of central venous catheterization," *Chest*, vol. 103, no. 6, pp. 1914–1916, 1993.

[22] P. K. Li, C. W. Taylor III, and R. S. Chung, "Delayed hydrothorax: a complication of central venous catheterization," *Surgical Rounds*, vol. 20, pp. 462–468, 1997.

[23] P. Gupta, S. Guleria, and S. Sharma, "Mediastinal haematoma: a rare complication following insertion of central venous catheter," *The Indian Journal of Chest Diseases & Allied Sciences*, vol. 53, no. 4, pp. 225–228, 2011.

[24] N. Arik, T. Akpolat, F. Demirkan et al., "Mediastinal hematoma: a rare complication of subclavian catheterization for hemodialysis," *Nephron*, vol. 63, no. 3, p. 354, 1993.

[25] A. Doi, H. Iida, Y. Saitoh, T. Sunazawa, and Y. Tajika, "A posterior mediastinal hematoma causing tracheal obstruction after internal jugular cannulation for cardiac surgery," *Journal of Cardiothoracic and Vascular Anesthesia*, vol. 23, no. 5, pp. 682–683, 2009.

[26] M. Naguib, H. Farag, and R. N. Joshi, "Bilateral hydrothorax and hydromediastinum after a subclavian line insertion," *Canadian Anaesthetists Society Journal*, vol. 32, no. 4, pp. 412–414, 1985.

[27] A. P. Chemelli, I. E. Chemelli-Steingruber, N. Bonaros et al., "Coil embolization of internal mammary artery injured during central vein catheter and cardiac pacemaker lead insertion," *European Journal of Radiology*, vol. 71, no. 2, pp. 269–274, 2009.

[28] M. Hohlrieder, R. Oberhammer, I. H. Lorenz, J. Margreiter, G. Kühbacher, and C. Keller, "Life-threatening mediastinal hematoma caused by extravascular infusion through a triple-lumen central venous catheter," *Anesthesia and Analgesia*, vol. 99, no. 1, pp. 31–35, 2004.

13

A Multidisciplinary Approach to Anesthetic Management of a Parturient with Severe Aortic Stenosis

Kalpana Tyagaraj,[1] David A. Gutman,[1] Lynn Belliveau,[1] Adnan Sadiq,[2] Alok Bhutada,[3] and Dennis E. Feierman[1]

[1]*Department of Anesthesiology, Maimonides Medical Center, 4802 10th Avenue, Brooklyn, NY 11219, USA*
[2]*Department of Cardiology, Maimonides Medical Center, 4802 10th Avenue, Brooklyn, NY 11219, USA*
[3]*Department of Neonatology, Maimonides Medical Center, 4802 10th Avenue, Brooklyn, NY 11219, USA*

Correspondence should be addressed to Kalpana Tyagaraj; kalpana_tyagaraj@msn.com

Academic Editor: Maria Jose C. Carmona

In order to optimize anesthetic management and avoid adverse maternal and fetal outcomes, a clear understanding of the changes in cardiovascular physiology that occur during pregnancy is paramount. The effects of normal gestation on the cardiovascular system are particularly significant in a parturient with cardiac valvular pathology. We present a case of a 27-year-old G2P0 at 37 weeks with a past medical history of diabetes, macrosomia, congenital bicuspid aortic valve with severe stenosis (valve area 0.7 cm^2) who was scheduled for elective C-section. A multidisciplinary discussion involving cardiologists, cardiac surgeons, obstetric surgeons, neonatal intensivists, perfusion staff, anesthesiologists, and nursing staff was held to formulate a plan for the perioperative management of this parturient. Also, contingency plans were formulated and discussed with the care providers, in the event of acute decompensation of the mother and baby and possible need for emergency aortic valvuloplasty and/or aortic valve replacement.

1. Introduction

Anesthetic management of parturients with significant cardiac valvular pathology can be challenging. Marked hemodynamic changes during normal pregnancy account for signs and symptoms that can mimic those of heart disease (Table 2). The cardiovascular changes of normal pregnancy, including increased hear rate, stroke volume, cardiac output, increased circulating blood volume, and decreased systemic vascular resistance, place the myocardium under stress. This is well tolerated in a healthy young parturient but often compromised myocardium can fail, placing the patient and her fetus at risk. The myocardium can fail any time during the antepartum, intrapartum, and postpartum periods. Parturients with cardiac valvular disease have greater mortality and morbidity compared to their healthy counterparts without cardiac disease. The incidence of cardiac disease in pregnancy has remained stable (0.1–4%) [1]. Though rare, nonobstetrical maternal death as a result of cardiac disease accounts for approximately 15% of all maternal obstetrical mortality.

Peripartum maternal morbidity for parturients with aortic stenosis and New York Heart Association (NYHA) functional classes III and IV symptoms is 10% [2] as compared to 0.4% for those in NYHA functional classes I and II.

2. Case Presentation

A 27-year-old G2P0 with a past medical history of insulin dependent diabetes (since the age of 9) and congenital bicuspid aortic valve presents at 37 weeks' gestation to the Labor and Delivery Suite. On physical exam it was noted that she had a grade 4 mummer at the right sternal boarder and +2 bilateral edema. She denied shortness of breath, dyspnea on exertion, or chest pain. Fourteen months before presentation, her valve area was 0.9 cm^2. She presented at this time for poorly controlled diabetes and fetal macrosomia for induction of labor. Secondary to her history of bicuspid aortic valve with an area that was 0.9 cm^2, she was sent to the cardiothoracic intense care unit for monitoring. A transthoracic echo revealed an even more stenotic valve with

TABLE 1: Hemodynamic changes associated with pregnancy.

Cardiovascular changes	% change	Implication for severe AS
Blood volume	↑30–40%	Potential volume overload
Plasma volume	↑40%	
Red cell mass	↑30%	
Hematocrit	↓29–34%	↓ oxygen delivery
Blood pressure	↓20%	↓ coronary perfusion
Systolic	↓5%	
Diastolic	↓15%	
SVR	↓15%	↓ coronary perfusion
CVP pressures	↓30%	
PA pressures	↓30%	
Heart rate	↑15–20%	↓ coronary perfusion time
Stroke volume	↑15–20%	Fixed in AS → ↓↓ in BP

EKG: electrocardiogram; SR: sinus rhythm; FHR: fetal heart rate.

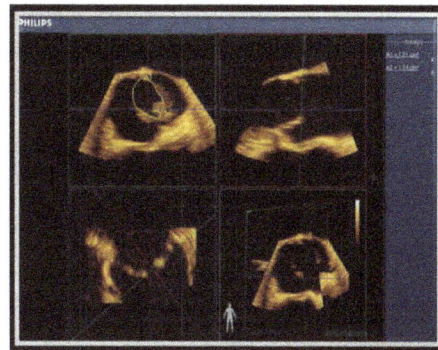

FIGURE 1: TEE 3D image (Philips Qlab) of the aortic valve using the planimetry method to measure the aortic valve area. TEE = Transesophageal echocardiography.

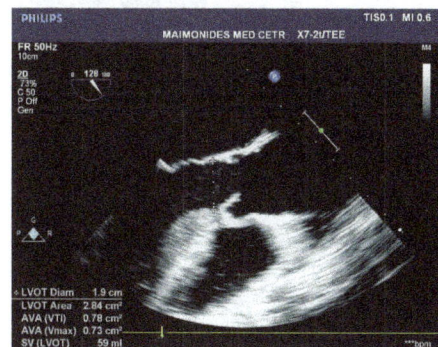

FIGURE 2: TEE image of the midesophageal aortic valve long axis (ME AV LAX) view measuring the LVOT diameter (one of three measurements used to calculate the aortic valve area using the continuity equation). LVOT = left ventricular outflow tract.

an area of $0.7 \, cm^2$, with an estimated peak gradient of 64 and mean gradient of 38. A multidisciplinary discussion was held with interventional cardiologists, cardiac surgeons, obstetric surgeons, neonatal intensivists, perfusion staff, anesthesiologists, and nursing staff. A C-section was planned.

The patient received 30 mL of nonparticulate antacid orally and metoclopramide 10 mg intravenously 30 minutes prior to the planned procedure. The patient was brought to the hybrid operating room. Standard ASA monitors were applied. Two large bore antecubital IVs (18 g in the right upper extremity and 16 in the left upper extremity) and left radial arterial line were placed. Induction was initiated with two 1 mg boluses of Midazolam, followed by a remifentanil infusion started at 0.3 mcg/kg/min. Esmolol 20 mg boluses were used to titrate the heart rate to a target heart rate of 70–80. A rapid sequence induction was performed with a combination of 14 mg of etomidate, 80 mg of propofol, and 120 mg succinylcholine and the airway was secured. Maintenance of anesthesia consisted of remifentanil infusion and sevoflurane 2%. Midazolam 2 mgs and fentanyl 100 mcgs were administered after the delivery of the baby. The baby was delivered within 3 minutes of intubation. A transesophageal echo probe was inserted. Intraoperative TEE findings were aortic stenosis with $0.8 \, cm^2$ valve area (Figures 1 and 2), mild AI, mild MR, peak transaortic valvular gradient of 38 and mean transaortic valvular gradient of 20 (Figure 3), and mild pulmonary valve regurgitation. The rest of the intraoperative course was unremarkable. The mother was successfully extubated at end of the procedure with careful titration of a beta-blocker for heart rate and blood pressure control (Table 2). The patient was transferred to cardiothoracic intensive care unit (CTICU) for close monitoring. Postoperative pain management consisted of IV PCA hydromorphone, intravenous ketorolac, and intravenous acetaminophen. The postoperative course was uneventful and the patient was discharged on post-op day 3. The patient returned 11 months later and underwent successful minimally invasive aortic valve replacement.

The NICU staff was present for the delivery and the baby was taken to the NICU for close monitoring. The initial APGAR score was 2 and the baby was floppy and apneic. After initial positive pressure ventilation, the baby was intubated. APGAR scores quickly improved to 5 and then 8 at which point the baby was extubated. The baby was observed in the NICU for a few days with an initial diagnosis of respiratory distress. The baby was treated with C-PAP for one day and the diagnosis of apnea and transient tachypnea of the newborn baby of a diabetic mother was made. Chest X-ray was unremarkable and, after one day on IV glucose solutions, the baby was able to maintain normal glucose levels. The apnea improved and the baby was discharged to the nursery on day 4.

3. Discussion

Aortic stenosis is typically seen in the elderly population; when encountered in the younger population, it is usually attributed to congenital bicuspid aortic valve. Maternal and perinatal mortality of 17% and 32% respectively have been reported in parturients with severe aortic stenosis. During pregnancy, a parturient undergoes many physiologic changes to best prepare for the needs of the growing fetus and the

TABLE 2: Intrapartum and postpartum hemodynamic measurements.

	Before induction 8:45	Induction 9:40	Intubation 9:44	Delivery 9:46	Postpartum		
					After 15 min 9:51	Extubation 11:06	CTICU 11:38
Blood pressure (mmHg)	149/90	136/92	103/75	120/79	111/74	148/104	153/87
Heart rate (beats/min)	94	83	80	75	69	93	84
SpO$_2$ (%)	100	100	100	100	100	100	100
EKG	SR	SR	SR	SR	SR	SR	SR
FHR (beats/min)	130	130					
FHR tracing category	I	I					

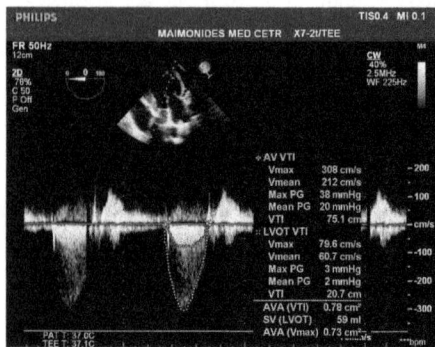

FIGURE 3: TEE image of the deep transgastric long axis (Deep TG LAX) view measuring the gradient through the aortic valve and LVOT (two of three measurements used to calculate the aortic valve area using the continuity equation).

placenta. One of the biggest changes during pregnancy is the increase in cardiac output secondary to an increase in heart rate and stroke volume, up to a 75% increase above prelabor values (Table 1). These normal physiological changes of pregnancy can precipitate heart failure in patient with severe AS. The increase in cardiac output and blood volume attributable to uterine contractions during labor, in face of the fixed stroke volume of aortic stenosis, may precipitate tachycardia. Tachycardia is worsened further by the pain-induced sympathetic stimulation and acute decompensation can set in.

4. Obstetric Management of a Parturient with Aortic Stenosis

Patients who are symptomatic or who have a peak out-flow gradient of more than 50 mm Hg are advised to delay conception until after surgical correction. Termination of pregnancy should be strongly considered if the patient is symptomatic before the end of the 1st trimester. Aortic valve replacement and palliative aortic balloon valvuloplasty have been performed during pregnancy with associated maternal and fetal risk. Vaginal delivery is preferred, facilitated by instrumental delivery to avoid hemodynamic changes associated with the Valsalva maneuver. The option of Cesarean Section is reserved for maternal and fetal indications.

5. Anesthetic Management of a Parturient with Aortic Stenosis

It is controversial whether general or neuraxial anesthesia is more appropriate for parturients with aortic stenosis. The choice should not be made depending on the severity of stenosis or the transvalvular gradient, rather the preanesthetic assessment of the symptoms and signs, right and left heart function, function of the other cardiac valves, and presence or absence of pulmonary hypertension. Hemodynamic monitoring with A-line and CVP/PAC may be indicated.

Epidural analgesia is ideal for labor pain management since it provides adequate pain control and also minimizes blood volume and cardiac output increases after delivery. It is prudent to avoid epinephrine "test dose" and careful titration of dosing the epidural catheter to avoid sudden decreases in SVR is essential. Dilute local anesthetics with opioids are preferred to minimize sympathectomy and the decrease in SVR.

If Cesarean Section is indicated in a patient with severe aortic stenosis, general anesthesia has traditionally been advocated and remains the gold standard. There are published case reports which have described administration of neuraxial techniques successfully; publication bias cannot be ruled out. Goals of anesthetic management are as follows:

(1) Maintenance of a normal heart rate and sinus rhythm: since patients with severe AS do not tolerate bradycardia and can decompensate with tachycardia, the overall anesthetic consideration with respect to heart rate is to maintain a normal to slightly elevated heart rate. Patients with severe AS can decompensate with tachycardia, since the noncompliant, hypertrophic ventricle needs time to fill and the increased heart's demand for oxygen associated with tachycardia in the face of limited supply secondary to decreased diastolic time (and coronary perfusion time) can result in myocardial ischemia which can increase LVEDP and even further decrease myocardial perfusion. Development of atrial fibrillation with rapid ventricular response decreases the diastolic filling time and eliminates the atrial component of left ventricular filling. Prompt restoration of sinus rhythm is vital to avoid hypotension or ventricular failure.

(2) Maintenance of intravascular volume and preload: the stroke volume, hence cardiac output, is maintained if the end diastolic volume is maintained via adequate venous return.

(3) Maintenance of systemic vascular resistance: decreases in systemic vascular resistance, typically found in pregnancy, can lead to decreased myocardial perfusion that, coupled with ventricular hypertrophy, can result in myocardial ischemia leading to left ventricular failure. Careful, close monitoring of blood pressure with an arterial line and heart rate is paramount.

(4) Avoidance of myocardial depression: agents like propofol and thiopental are to be avoided to minimize myocardial depression.

(5) Avoid aortocaval compression.

Opioid based induction and maintenance are preferred to achieve and maintain the hemodynamic goals. Potential fetal depression warrants the immediate presence of neonatal resuscitation team.

Careful planning using a multidisciplinary approach is essential for optimal maternal and neonatal outcomes. The key to manage this patient was to control the heart rate, thus decreasing the heart's demand for oxygen in the face of limited supply secondary to the ramifications to the aortic valve stenotic pathology.

References

[1] W. N. van Mook and L. Peeters, "Severe cardiac disease in pregnancy, part I: hemodynamic changes and complaints during pregnancy, and general management of cardiac disease in pregnancy," *Current Opinion in Critical Care*, vol. 11, pp. 430–434, 2005.

[2] http://www.clevelandclinicmeded.com/medicalpubs/disease-management/cardiology/pregnancy-and-heart-disease/#assessment.

14

Anesthesia and Intensive Care Management in a Pregnant Woman with PRES

Ismail Demirel,[1] Ayse Belin Ozer,[1] Mustafa K. Bayar,[1] and Salih Burcin Kavak[2]

[1] Department of Anaesthesiology and Reanimation, Faculty of Medicine, Firat University, 23119 Elazig, Turkey
[2] Department of Obstetrics and Gynecology, Faculty of Medicine, Firat University, 2311 Elazig, Turkey

Correspondence should be addressed to Ismail Demirel, ismaildemirel23@gmail.com

Academic Editors: D. A. Story and E. A. Vandermeersch

Posterior reversible encephalopathy syndrome (PRES) is a temporary condition that is diagnosed clinically, neurologically, and radiologically. Its symptoms vary, and nonspecific headaches, confusion, impairment of consciousness, nausea, vomiting, and visual impairment may occur. Acute hypertension often accompanies these symptoms. Patients can also suffer from convulsions, cortical visual impairment, and coma. Diagnosis can be difficult due to focal neurologic signs. Nevertheless, knowing the clinical risk factors can lead to the right diagnosis. It has been reported that this condition may also occur during organ transplantation, immunosuppressive treatment, and autoimmune diseases and chemotherapy, and also patients with eclampsia. In this paper, a 21-year-old, 31-week pregnant woman, who had been diagnosed with PRES and thanks to early diagnosis and treatment had fully recovered and discharged from the intensive care unit, is presented, and the relevant literature is discussed.

1. Introduction

Originally described in 1996 as a disease of the posterior cerebrum PRES is the clinical syndrome of vasogenic edema in the central nervous system. It is a cerebral vascular autoregulation deficiency resulting from sudden changes in blood pressure. It is characterized by headaches, generalized seizures, vision impairment, lethargy, confusion, stupor, changes in mental status, and focal neurologic signs. Diagnosis is made by piecing together clinical and radiological findings [1]. The etiologic factors of this condition are hypertensive encephalopathy, eclampsia/preeclampsia, drug use, renal disease (acute and chronic), thrombotic thrombocytopenic purpura, systemic lupus erythematosus, hemolytic uremic syndrome, and diseases that cause immune system deficiency (leukemia, lymphoma) [2, 3]. With early diagnosis and treatment, patients can recover clinically in a few weeks. If not treated in time, the condition can get worse, resulting in cerebral ischemia, infarcts, and even death. As there are no clinically specific signs for the syndrome, it can often be confused with other clinical conditions, leading to unnecessary and/or wrong treatments [4].

Preeclampsia is a syndrome characterized by hypertension, edema, proteinuria, and the activation of coagulation mechanisms after the 20th week of pregnancy. Many hypotheses have been suggested regarding the mechanism of the disease process, and it is stated that the condition occurs due to issues regarding placental location and trophoblastic invasion. Severe systemic vasospasm, which is the most significant physiological change in the patients, causes reduced perfusion of all organs. Other reasons for the hypoperfusion are hemoconcentration and third-space loss. Moreover, inappropriate endothelial activation and increased inflammatory response can be observed [5]. If preeclampsia is not treated or does not respond to treatment, it can lead to a more serious condition, that is, eclampsia condition that covers all the symptoms of pre-eclampsia with the addition of seizures. PRES can occur during pregnancy and in the postpartum state. Radiological findings of PRES resulting from pregnancy are identical to the radiological findings in other etiologic causes of PRES. The most important differential diagnosis that one must keep in mind about these patients is dural sinus thrombosis.

Magnetic resonance imaging (MRI) typically shows hyperintensity in the bilateral parieto-occipital areas in sequences T2A and FLAIR, consistent with vasogenic edema. In atypic involvements of PRES, frontal lobe, basal ganglia,

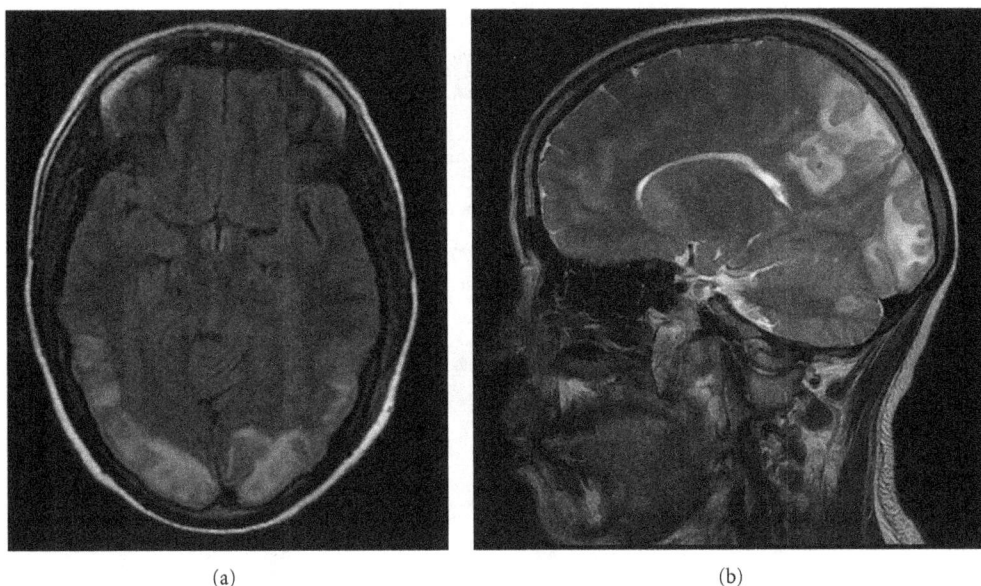

(a)   (b)

FIGURE 1: The patient MRI findings in postoperative first day.

brain stem, and deep white matter are affected [6, 7]. Recurrent attacks of PRES are mainly related with eclampsia, and their incidence is proportional to recurrent eclampsia [8]. With this paper, we wanted to draw attention to the fact that an eclamptic patient 31 weeks pregnant, who developed PRES, was treated in the intensive care unit after an early diagnosis and was discharged fully recovered, and that there are more than one disease entity that may result in PRES.

2. Case Report

A 21-year-old, 31-week pregnant, gravida 1, para 0 case was confused with a moderately poor general condition and was admitted to the obstetric clinic. When the patient came to the hospital, her arterial blood pressure was 210/130 mmHg, and anamnesis from her relatives revealed that she had a generalized seizure 1 hour prior to admission. On bedside ultrasound, normal amniotic fluid volume and one viable fetus with a body size consistent with 29 weeks were found. The patient had 4+ proteinuria and was diagnosed as eclamptic and given a loading dose of magnesium sulphate (4 grams). Three minutes after magnesium sulphate was administered, the patient had another generalized convulsion and was given diazepam (10 mg i.v.). The patient had respiratory distress and was intubated orotracheally and taken to the operating room for an emergency Cesarean section. Thiopental sodium (250 mg, Pental) and cisatracurium (4 mg, Nimbex) was administered for induction of anesthesia followed by 50% O_2 + 50% N_2O and 0.75% MAC isoflurane. One viable female baby in breech presentation was delivered by Cesarean section. The baby's birth weight was 1100 gr and height was 36 cm with a 1-minute APGAR score of 7. After the operation, the patient, still entubated, was taken to the intensive care unit, and mechanical ventilation was initiated (SIMV, f: 12/min, FiO$_2$: 60, TV: 500 mL, I : E = 1 : 2). In the intensive care unit, her blood pressure tended to

increase (180/110 mmHg) so nitroglycerin (10 μg/kg/h) and magnesium sulfate (2 gr/h) infusion was continued. The patient was administered dexamethasone (32 mg/day) and an oral antihypertensive amlodipine (Norvasc 10 mg/day). As she regained consciousness and spontaneous breathing, the patient was extubated. But 15 min after extubation, the patient had another convulsion and was reintubated. Biochemical values of the case were as follow: Hb: 13.5 gr/dL, Htc: %37, WBC: 16590/mm^3, PLT: 50.000/mm^3, AST: 375 U/L, and ALT: 183 U/L, LDH: 1213 U/L, and her coagulation parameters were Prothrombin time (PT): 52,1 secs, activated prothrombin time (APTT): 25,2 secs, INR: 1,44. With these findings, the patient was diagnosed as having HELLP syndrome and eclampsia, and neurologic examination showed no lateralization. The patient was administered Thiopental sodium (100 mg bolus followed by a continuous infusion of 250 mg/h i.v.), and her convulsions were reduced considerably. Therefore, first day after surgery thiopental sodium was stopped, and after approximately 6 hours, the patient was extubated. Magnesium sulfate infusion was continued. The patients, postoperative first-day MRI showed increased intensity lesions on sequences T2, FLAIR, DAG, and ADC in bilateral basal ganglia, at the level of centrum semiovale on the frontal areas, bilateral parietotemporal, occipital regions, and left cerebellum (Figure 1). The patient was diagnosed as having PRES. The patient was treated with magnesium sulfate for 48 hours, and her platelet counts were 44,000/mm^3 on the first day after the operation. Her liver enzyme and LDH levels were elevated. As her general condition improved, the patient was taken to the obstetric clinic on the second postoperative day. Her liver enzyme and LDH levels started to decrease starting from the second postoperative day. Her platelet counts were 97,000/mm^3 on the second day after surgery. Her drains were removed on the third day after the surgery and sutures were removed on the 7th postpartum day. The patient was discharged with

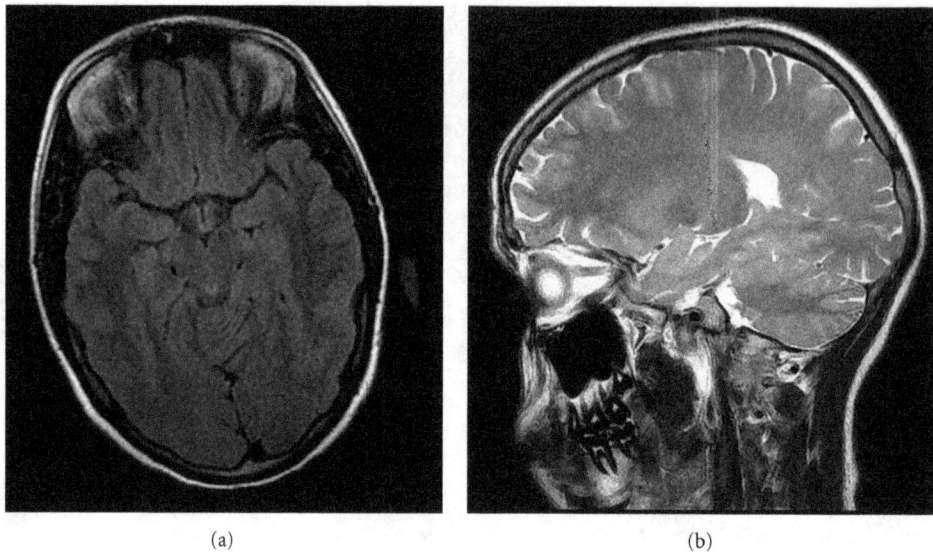

(a)

(b)

FIGURE 2: The patient MRI findings in one month later.

suggestions after that. Her MRI was taken after a month and was totally normal (Figure 2).

3. Discussion

PRES is a clinical condition that causes neurological symptoms such as variable consciousness, seizures, and vision impairment, and its symptoms and imaging findings are generally reversible. Many diseases such as hypertension, eclampsia/preeclampsia, immunosuppresive drugs (cyclosporine), various antineoplastic agents, hypercalcemia, thrombocytopenic syndromes, Henoch-Schönlein purpura, hemolytic uremic syndrome, systemic lupus erythematosus, amyloid angiopathy, and renal failure can cause PRES. The pathophysiology of PRES is unclear. The generally accepted theory is edema formation in subcortical white matter as a result of the extravasation due to sudden changes in blood pressure and/or toxins that damage the endothelium and disrupt the blood brain barrier. Another opinion is that vasospasm is the underlying cause with resulting cytotoxic edema in affected areas [9].

The typical MRI findings of PRES are symmetric increases of the signals in the bilateral parieto-occipital areas, subcortical white matter of bilateral frontal and temporal lobe, posterior segments, and sometimes the cortex in sequences FLAIR and T2. In diffusion MRI images, increased diffusion consistent with vasogenic edema is detected. Lesions due to vasogenic edema are reversible. However, in some cases, lesions with reduced diffusion due to cytotoxic edema can be determined, and these lesions generally heal leaving a sequel. In atypic presentations, high-contrast lesions and hemorrhage can be seen in the thalamus, basal ganglia, brain stem, and cerebellum [9]. Our patient had increased intensity of the lesions on sequence T2 in the bilateral basal ganglia, at the level of centrum semiovale in the frontal areas, bilateral parietotemporal, occipital regions and left cerebellum.

PRES is a condition that rapidly responds to aggressive treatment. Clinical and radiological findings are reversible. Its clinical symptoms are similar to many neurological diseases. The following disorders must be considered in differential diagnosis: demyelinating diseases, basilar artery embolism, and venous sinus thrombosis. The first step in treatment must be correcting the underlying etiological factors. Preventing hypertension and other triggers (cytotoxic conditions, immunosuppressive drugs, sepsis, and the like) is the key. For our patient, the etiology was thought to be eclampsia as a result of her pregnancy and encephalopathy because of disturbed blood pressure autoregulation. Her condition rapidly changed for the better once the convulsions stopped, and her blood pressure was normalised. This is why the condition is called posterior "reversible" encephalopathy syndrome [10]. Oral and i.v. antihypertensive agents, sedative hypnotics, and diuretics can be used to treat the hypertension [11–14]. Our patient had a generalized seizure on her 31st week of pregnancy, was admitted to the hospital, was started on magnesium sulfate infusion, and after her second generalized seizure was given additionally diazepam and was taken for a Cesarean section after being orotracheally intubated. When the patient had another generalized seizure in the intensive care unit after the operation, the patient was reintubated orotracheally and was administered thiopental sodium in addition to magnesium and i.v. antihypertensive agents. The patient was diagnosed with PRES that responded to early treatment. Magnesium sulphate is widely used for preeclamptic patients to prevent eclamptic seizures. Generally, 4–6 gr i.v. is administered in the first 20 minutes continued with 1-2 gr/h. During the treatment, the patient's deep tendon reflexes, respiratory rate, heart rate, blood pressure, and urine output must be monitored closely. Magnesium shows its central anticonvulsant effect by antagonizing glutamate's attachment to n-methyl-d-aspartate (NMDA) receptors. It reduces postsynaptic membrane sensitivity and muscle membrane stimulation by decreasing the calcium transport in the presynaptic space and the release of acetylcholine. During general anesthesia, even in patients taking standard doses of magnesium sulphate, the effect of neuromuscular blocking agents can be potentialized, and their duration can be prolonged [15, 16]. Drugs with low biotransformation rates (like isoflurane), low renal clearance, short half-life, and low active metabolites (like atracurium) must be chosen for general anesthesia. Nitroglycerin and magnesium sulphate are suggested to prevent hypertensive attacks that can occur during the induction of anesthesia [17, 18]. We used isoflurane for anesthesia maintenance and cisatracurium as a neuromuscular blocking agent.

Striano et al. retrospectively analyzed 3000 cases, who were reviewed in order to identify subjects with a clinical history of PRES, in their study, and came across 8 cases with PRES. Five of these cases had eclampsia, and 2 of them had postpartum eclampsia [19]. Although magnesium sulphate is routinely used in eclampsia, it is reported that prophylactic use of magnesium sulphate has limited effect in preventing postpartum eclampsia [20]. After PRES did occur, magnesium sulphate can be inadequate for the treatment of postpartum eclampsia. Magnesium sulphate suppresses the seizures by regulating the Ca^{++}-Mg^{++} metabolism and relaxing the muscles. It decreases cerebral edema formation after brain injury an has neuroprotective and anticonvulsant property. In addition to this, there are cerebral ischemic and edematous areas in PRES that cause the seizures. Antiedematous, antiepileptic, and sedative hypnotic must be added to treatment for cases like this. In patients with PRES as a result of Burkitt's lymphoma, there can be seizures that do not respond to dexamethasone, phenytoin, and valproic acid. Thiopental sodium is successfully used to treat this kind of generalized seizure [21]. In our patient, generalized tonic-clonic seizures occurred while she was under the treatment of magnesium sulphate, and with the addition of thiopental sodium infusion, her condition rapidly regressed. Furosemide and dexamethasone were additionally given.

In conclusion, PRES is a condition that is caused by multifactorial etiological factors, and its clinical presentation may vary. The diagnosis can be confirmed by radiological imaging studies. With early diagnosis, the syndrome may reverse without sequels. If mental status disorders and generalized seizures in the prepartum period, during the delivery, and in the postpartum period are present in the presence or absence of preeclampsia/eclampsia, must suspect the possibility of PRES and investigated. Our patient with PRES secondarily to eclampsia on the 31st week of pregnancy was diagnosed early and treated in the intensive care unit with good result. This paper is intended to remind critical care specialists of the etiology and differential diagnosis of PRES, which is a relatively rare condition.

References

[1] T. Kinoshita, T. Moritani, D. A. Shrier et al., "Diffusion-weighted MR imaging of posterior reversible leukoencephalopathy syndrome: a pictorial essay," *Clinical Imaging*, vol. 27, no. 5, pp. 307–315, 2003.

[2] L. M. Brubaker, J. K. Smith, Y. Z. Lee, W. Lin, and M. Castillo, "Hemodynamic and permeability changes in posterior reversible encephalopathy syndrome measured by dynamic susceptibility perfusion-weighted MR imaging," *American Journal of Neuroradiology*, vol. 26, no. 4, pp. 825–830, 2005.

[3] P. Mukherjee and R. C. McKinstry, "Reversible posterior leukoencephalopathy syndrome: evaluation with diffusion-tensor MR imaging," *Radiology*, vol. 219, no. 3, pp. 756–765, 2001.

[4] W. S. Bartynski, "Posterior reversible encephalopathy syndrome, Part 2: controversies surrounding pathophysiology of vasogenic edema," *American Journal of Neuroradiology*, vol. 29, no. 6, pp. 1043–1049, 2008.

[5] G. A. Dekker and B. M. Sibai, "Etiology and pathogenesis of preeclampsia: current concepts," *American Journal of Obstetrics and Gynecology*, vol. 179, no. 5, pp. 1359–1375, 1998.

[6] K. J. Ahn, W. J. You, S. L. Jeong et al., "Atypical manifestations of reversible posterior leukoencephalopathy syndrome: findings on diffusion imaging and ADC mapping," *Neuroradiology*, vol. 46, no. 12, pp. 978–983, 2004.

[7] H. Kitaguchi, H. Tomimoto, Y. Miki et al., "A brainstem variant of reversible posterior leukoencephalopathy syndrome," *Neuroradiology*, vol. 47, no. 9, pp. 652–656, 2005.

[8] J. M. Sweany, W. S. Bartynski, and J. F. Boardman, "'Recurrent' posterior reversible encephalopathy syndrome: report of 3 cases–PRES can strike twice!," *Journal of Computer Assisted Tomography*, vol. 31, no. 1, pp. 148–156, 2007.

[9] A. M. McKinney, J. Short, C. L. Truwit et al., "Posterior reversible encephalopathy syndrome: incidence of atypical regions of involvement and imaging findings," *American Journal of Roentgenology*, vol. 189, no. 4, pp. 904–912, 2007.

[10] T. Uwatoko, K. Toyoda, Y. Hirai et al., "Reversible posterior leukoencephalopathy syndrome in a postpartum woman without eclampsia," *Internal Medicine*, vol. 42, no. 11, pp. 1139–1143, 2003.

[11] W. S. Bartynski, J. F. Boardman, Z. R. Zeigler, R. K. Shadduck, and J. Lister, "Posterior reversible encephalopathy syndrome in infection, sepsis, and shock," *American Journal of Neuroradiology*, vol. 27, no. 10, pp. 2179–2190, 2006.

[12] S. C. Won, S. Y. Kwon, J. W. Han, S. Y. Choi, and C. J. Lyu, "Posterior reversible encephalopathy syndrome in childhood with hematologic/oncologic diseases," *Journal of Pediatric Hematology/Oncology*, vol. 31, no. 7, pp. 505–508, 2009.

[13] W. S. Bartynski, "Posterior reversible encephalopathy syndrome, Part 1: fundamental imaging and clinical features," *American Journal of Neuroradiology*, vol. 29, no. 6, pp. 1036–1042, 2008.

[14] H. M. Hefzy, W. S. Bartynski, J. F. Boardman, and D. Lacomis, "Hemorrhage in posterior reversible encephalopathy syndrome: imaging and clinical features," *American Journal of Neuroradiology*, vol. 30, no. 7, pp. 1371–1379, 2009.

[15] S. L. Sipes, C. P. Weiner, T. M. Gellhaus, and J. D. Goodspeed, "The plasma renin-angiotensin system in preeclampsia: effects of magnesium sulfate," *Obstetrics and Gynecology*, vol. 73, no. 6, pp. 934–937, 1989.

[16] J. R. Kambam, S. Mouton, S. Entman, B. V. R. Sastry, and B. E. Smith, "Effect of pre-eclampsia on plasma cholinesterase activity," *Canadian Journal of Anaesthesia*, vol. 34, no. 5, pp. 509–511, 1987.

[17] M. D. Lindheimer and A. I. Katz, "Hypertension in pregnancy," *New England Journal of Medicine*, vol. 313, no. 11, pp. 675–680, 1985.

[18] S. P Gatt, "Gestational proteinuric hypertension," *Current Opinion in Anaesthesiology*, vol. 5, pp. 354–359, 1992.

[19] P. Striano, S. Striano, F. Tortora et al., "Clinical spectrum and critical care management of Posterior Reversible Encephalopathy Syndrome (PRES)," *Medical Science Monitor*, vol. 11, no. 11, pp. CR549–CR553, 2005.

[20] B. M. Sibai, "Diagnosis, prevention, and management of eclampsia," *Obstetrics and Gynecology*, vol. 105, no. 2, pp. 402–410, 2005.

[21] B. Malbora, Z. Avci, F. Dönmez et al., "Posterior reversible leukoencephalopathy syndrome in children with hematologic disorders," *Turkish Journal of Hematology*, vol. 27, no. 3, pp. 168–176, 2010.

15

Paravertebral Block Combined with Sedation for a Myasthenic Patient Undergoing Breast Augmentation

Betul Kozanhan, Betul Basaran, Leyla Kutlucan, and Sadık Ozmen

Department of Anesthesiology and Reanimation, Konya Training and Research Hospital,
Meram Yeniyol Street No. 97, Meram, 42090 Konya, Turkey

Correspondence should be addressed to Betul Kozanhan; betulkozanhan@gmail.com

Academic Editor: Richard Riley

Paravertebral block is a unilateral analgesic technique that can provide adequate surgical anesthesia and great advantages in many types of surgery with a low side-effect profile. In this case we present combination of bilateral thoracic paravertebral block under ultrasound guidance with sedation which provides complete anesthesia and postoperative analgesia in a myasthenic patient undergoing cosmetic breast surgery. In myasthenic patients paravertebral blocks may be a better option for breast surgery with avoiding the need for muscle relaxants and opioids and risk of respiratory failure in postoperative period.

1. Introduction

Thoracic paravertebral block (TPVB) is a regional anesthesia technique that involves injection of a local anesthetic alongside the thoracic vertebral body close to where the spinal nerves emerge from the intervertebral foramen [1]. This produces unilateral, segmental, somatic, and sympathetic nerve blockade in multiple adjacent thoracic dermatomes [1]. Combined with sedation, TPVB provides effective surgical anesthesia for patients undergoing oncological breast procedures and breast augmentation [2]. We report here the use of ultrasound-guided bilateral TPVB with sedation as a primary anesthetic technique, in a patient with myasthenia gravis (MG) undergoing bilateral cosmetic breast augmentation.

2. Case Presentation

A 28-year-old female (60 kg; 165 cm; ASA II) presented for bilateral cosmetic breast augmentation. Ten years prior to this presentation she had been diagnosed with MG with respiratory dysfunction and mild generalized weakness and classified as Osserman stage III. At the time of diagnosis she underwent thymectomy. After the operation tracheal intubation was performed and remained for 7 postoperative days due to myasthenic crisis. During preoperative evaluation her neurological examination was normal and there were no symptoms of MG. She was not receiving medication. Preoperative pulmonary function tests revealed her forced vital capacity (FVC) 3.51 L, with 1 s forced expiratory volume (FEV1) of 2.95 L. The patient's baseline vital signs were a heart rate of 76 bpm and blood pressure of 130/70 mmHg. After discussions with the patient about options for anesthesia a decision was made to proceed with TPVB.

In order to provide better consistency in the spread of the local anesthetic and produce a more reliable sensory block, we planned to perform multiple level injections TPVB [3]. On the day of surgery, standard ASA monitors were applied, intravenous access was established, and crystalloid infusion was started. While the patient was in the sitting position, Th2–Th5 spinous processes were identified and marked by palpating and counting down from vertebra prominens (C7). Under aseptic conditions, local anesthesia with 2% lidocaine was performed to skin and subcutaneous tissues. Linear array probe (Esaote MyLab 5, Genova, Italy) was placed longitudinally in sagittal plane at a point 2-3 cm lateral to the midline. Both transverse processes were visualized as two hyperechoic lines and the parietal pleura was visualized as a bright structure running deep to the adjacent transverse processes. If the pleura was not clearly delineated probe was slightly tilted laterally. The distance from the skin to the paravertebral space was measured (38, 41, and 43 mm at Th3, Th4, and Th5, resp.) and a 22-gauge, echogenic peripheric block needle (Pajunk, Germany) was inserted using in-plane technique in caudad to cephalad direction. The tip of needle was advanced until the superior costotransverse ligament punctured. The proper placement of the needle in the paravertebral space was confirmed with hydrolocation after negative aspiration of blood or air local anesthetic was slowly injected. Spread of local anesthetic was visualized with displacement of the pleura anteriorly. The same procedure was repeated at both bilateral Th2–Th5 levels and total 30 mL of 0.5% levobupivacaine was divided equally in paravertebral spaces. During the block procedure verbal contact was maintained with the patient and there were no signs of local anesthetic toxicity. Also no difficulty of breath or desaturation occurred. Loss of sensation to cold and pinprick of chest wall from Th2 to Th6 dermatomes was verified 20 min following block placement. Intraoperative sedation (Ramsay score of 2-3) was provided with continuous infusion of propofol 30–50 mcg/kg/min (total given was 266 mg). The patient remained hemodynamically stable throughout the 115 min of surgery. At the end of the procedure she was comfortable and pain management consisted of oral acetaminophen 500 mg every 6 h as the postoperative routine. She remained pain-free overnight and did not require any opioids for analgesia. She received tenoxicam 20 mg intravenous for a pain score of 4 (visual analog scale (0 = no pain and 10 = the worst pain)) at the postoperative 15 h. Her lung function capacity was assessed after 24 h and FVC was 3.12 L. She was discharged home on the second postoperative day without any complications.

3. Discussion

Myasthenia gravis (MG) is an autoimmune neuromuscular disease characterized by a decrease in acetylcholine receptors secondary to their destruction or inactivation by circulating IgG antibodies causing weakness and fatigue in ocular, bulbar, limb, and respiratory muscles due to repetitive use [4]. Anesthesia in patients with MG requires special attention, because of an abnormal response to muscle relaxants, increased sensitivity to sedatives, and a restricted respiratory capacity [5, 6]. These patients are more sensitive to the effects of nondepolarizing neuromuscular blockers and resistant to the effects of succinylcholine [4, 5]; therefore some clinicians avoid muscle relaxants and prefer deep inhalational anesthesia for facilitating tracheal intubation. However, inhalational anesthetics would be a factor for depression of neuromuscular function in myasthenic patients [5]. Asymptomatic myasthenic patients should be assumed to be sensitive to the effect of neuromuscular blocking agents and volatile anesthetics [6]. In addition, effectively blocking pain pathways is important to reduce the acute surgical stress response which can worsen disease symptoms and may trigger myasthenic crisis [4, 5]. Postoperative respiratory compromise may be associated with pain. In this way opioid usage could be a factor for central respiratory depression. So relatively opioid free anesthetic modalities are accepted and convenient for this type of patients [4, 5].

TPVB can be used with excellent effect for analgesia but it is also suitable as a sole anesthetic technique. Studies have shown that paravertebral block has been associated with an improved postoperative pain scores with reduced requirements for opioid analgesics, decreased incidence of nausea and vomiting, quicker discharge times, and greater patient satisfaction when compared to general anesthesia [2, 7]. Bilateral TPVB may cause blockade of intercostal muscles. This leads to concern about respiratory depression in myasthenic patients. However, when compared to thoracic epidural analgesia, TPVB provides comparable analgesia with epidural blockade and is associated with a significantly better postoperative pulmonary function, earlier mobilization, less urinary retention, and hypotension [8, 9].

Paravertebral block is generally associated with low and acceptable side effects and complications. Hypotension, theoretic high blood concentrations of local anesthetic, and epidural or spinal spread of local anesthetic and pneumothorax are the possible controversial issues related to the bilateral PVB [10]. Ultrasound has been used to improve efficacy and reduce complications via real-time visualization of the intended anatomic space, surrounding structures, and the approaching needle. Though bilateral PVB caused an eightfold increase in the rate of the pneumothorax [11], the study using in-plane ultrasound technique did not indicate any pleural puncture from paravertebral block [12]. We performed TPVB under ultrasound guidance and measured the distance from the skin to paravertebral space to potentially minimize the risk of pneumothorax. We used multiple injections slowly with low doses of local anesthetic at each level to prevent the spread of anesthetic from paravertebral to epidural space. Beside these we also used low dose amide local anesthetic levobupivacaine because its metabolism is independent of pseudocholinesterase function with long-term continuing analgesia into the postoperative period. Our patient's postoperative respiratory function has limited deterioration possibly due to used opioid sparing anesthetic technique.

We demonstrate that administering bilateral TPVB is a safe and useful procedure for performing cosmetic breast augmentation for patients when general anesthesia is not desirable. The procedure is advantageous in that the use of muscle relaxants, volatile anesthetic agents can be avoided. The risk of perioperative respiratory depression caused by high dose opioid usage can be minimized. Performing the block with ultrasound guidance by an anesthesiologist who is experienced in this technique, the chance of pneumothorax will be extremely low.

References

[1] M. K. Karmakar, "Thoracic paravertebral block," *Anesthesiology*, vol. 95, no. 3, pp. 771–780, 2001.

[2] Y. Tahiri, D. Q. H. Tran, J. Bouteaud et al., "General anaesthesia versus thoracic paravertebral block for breast surgery: a meta-analysis," *Journal of Plastic, Reconstructive & Aesthetic Surgery*, vol. 64, no. 10, pp. 1261–1269, 2011.

[3] Z. M. Naja, M. El-Rajab, M. A. Al-Tannir et al., "Thoracic paravertebral block: influence of the number of injections," *Regional Anesthesia and Pain Medicine*, vol. 31, no. 3, pp. 196–201, 2006.

[4] B. M. Conti-Fine, M. Milani, and H. J. Kaminski, "Myasthenia gravis: past, present, and future," *The Journal of Clinical Investigation*, vol. 116, no. 11, pp. 2843–2854, 2006.

[5] L. Blichfeldt-Lauridsen and B. D. Hansen, "Anesthesia and myasthenia gravis," *Acta Anaesthesiologica Scandinavica*, vol. 56, no. 1, pp. 17–22, 2012.

[6] V. Erden and Delatioglu H, "Anesthesia of a patient with cured myasthenia gravis," *Anesthesia & Analgesia*, vol. 96, pp. 1842–1843, 2003.

[7] A. Schnabel, S. U. Reichl, P. Kranke, E. M. Pogatzki-Zahn, and P. K. Zahn, "Efficacy and safety of paravertebral blocks in breast surgery: a meta-analysis of randomized controlled trials," *British Journal of Anaesthesia*, vol. 105, no. 6, Article ID aeq265, pp. 842–852, 2010.

[8] R. G. Davies, P. S. Myles, and J. M. Graham, "A comparison of the analgesic efficacy and side-effects of paravertebral vs epidural blockade for thoracotomy—a systematic review and meta-analysis of randomized trials," *British Journal of Anaesthesia*, vol. 96, no. 4, pp. 418–426, 2006.

[9] X. Ding, S. Jin, X. Niu, H. Ren, S. Fu, and Q. Li, "A comparison of the analgesia efficacy and side effects of paravertebral compared with epidural blockade for thoracotomy: an updated meta-analysis," *PLoS ONE*, vol. 9, no. 5, Article ID e96233, 2014.

[10] J. Richardson, P. A. Lönnqvist, and Z. Naja, "Bilateral thoracic paravertebral block: potential and practice," *British Journal of Anaesthesia*, vol. 106, no. 2, pp. 164–171, 2011.

[11] Z. Naja and P.-A. Lönnqvist, "Somatic paravertebral nerve blockade: incidence of failed block and complications," *Anaesthesia*, vol. 56, no. 12, pp. 1184–1188, 2001.

[12] W. Zhang, C. Fang, J. Li et al., "Single-dose, bilateral paravertebral block plus intravenous sufentanil analgesia in patients with esophageal cancer undergoing combined thoracoscopic-laparoscopic esophagectomy: a safe and effective alternative," *Journal of Cardiothoracic and Vascular Anesthesia*, vol. 28, no. 4, pp. 978–984, 2014.

16

Nosocomial Methemoglobinemia Resulting from Self-Administration of Benzocaine Spray

Christopher Hoffman, Hawa Abubakar, Pramood Kalikiri, and Michael Green

Drexel University College of Medicine, Hahnemann University Hospital, Philadelphia, PA 19102, USA

Correspondence should be addressed to Michael Green; michael.green@drexelmed.edu

Academic Editor: Renato Santiago Gomez

Methemoglobinemia is life-threatening and bears pathognomonic signs difficult to diagnose in real time. Local anesthetics are widely used and are known for eliciting this condition. We report a case of methemoglobinemia secondary to self-administered use of benzocaine spray. A 27-year-old woman was found to be in respiratory distress during postoperative recovery. After desaturation persisted, arterial blood gas yielded a methemoglobin level of 47%. The patient was successfully treated with intravenous methylene blue. Review of the events revealed self-administered doses of benzocaine spray to alleviate discomfort from a nasogastric tube. We review this case in detail in addition to discussing methemoglobinemia and its relevant biochemistry, pathophysiology, clinical presentation, and medical management. Given the recognized risk of methemoglobinemia associated with benzocaine use, we recommend its removal from the market in favor of safer alternatives.

1. Introduction

Methemoglobin arises when the ferrous ($Fe2+$) iron moiety of the heme group within hemoglobin is converted to the ferric ($Fe3+$) state. This occurs in the setting of oxidative stress and converts the heme group into a non-oxygen binding state. If allowed to persist in high concentration, significant hindrance of oxygen delivery to tissue occurs leading to hypoxia, lactic acidosis, and death [1, 2]. The red blood cell, as the primary oxygen carrier, is constantly exposed to oxidative stress with the concomitant risk of methemoglobinemia development.

Local anesthetics enhance methemoglobin formation as much as 1000-fold mainly through the oxidizing activity of their metabolites [3, 4]. Severity and frequency vary among anesthetics; a 2009 retrospective search of 242 reported episodes of methemoglobinemia yielded 159 cases with benzocaine, 68 cases with prilocaine, and 12 cases with lidocaine, among others [5]. The methemoglobinemia that arises leads to functional anemia and inadequate tissue oxygen delivery can result in symptoms observable even in the setting of modest increases in percent methemoglobin. Breakdown of symptom presentation to corresponding percentage methemoglobin values can be found in Table 1 [6].

Given the nonspecific nature of the presenting symptoms, diagnosis can be particularly challenging. If methemoglobinemia is allowed to continue unrecognized by cooximetry or arterial blood gas and untreated by methylene blue, significant morbidity and mortality can result from tissue hypoxia. This requires a heightened index of suspicion when relevant exogenous substances like local anesthetics are incorporated into therapy. We report an episode of methemoglobinemia in which clinical diagnosis was challenging given lack of cues pointing towards a diagnosis.

2. Case Presentation

A 27-year-old 100 kg woman presented for low anterior resection for endometriosis. The patient's history included anemia and obesity for which she previously underwent a gastric banding procedure. The surgical procedure was completed under general anesthesia with no relevant complications and the patient was transferred to the surgical intensive care unit. Recovery was complicated by an episode of ileus on postoperative day 6, necessitating nasogastric tube placement.

On day 7, the patient's oxygen saturation decreased to 82% and she reported headaches, drowsiness, and abdominal

TABLE 1: Expected signs and symptoms for a given percentage methemoglobin level assuming normal starting hemoglobin [6, 7].

Percentage methemoglobin	Expected symptoms
<10%	None
10–20%	Peripheral and central cyanosis
20–30%	Anxiety, tachycardia, lightheadedness, and headache
30–50%	Confusion, dizziness, fatigue, tachypnea, and worsening tachycardia
50–70%	Acidosis, arrhythmia, seizures, and coma
>70%	Death

pain. The patient denied increased work of breathing but was noted to be tachypneic with a respiratory rate at 22–25 breaths per minute. Unchanged on 100% oxygen via nonrebreather mask, an arterial blood gas sample yielded chocolate brown colored blood. The blood gas result was as follows: pH 7.49, PCO_2 37, PO_2 138, HCO_3 28, BE +4, O_2 saturation 98%, and methemoglobin level 47%. Upon further investigation, it was ascertained that a bottle of benzocaine spray had been left at the bedside to assist in the patient's tolerance of the nasogastric tube. The patient admitted using the spray 4 times over a 5-hour period and estimated each spray to be 2 seconds in length. The patient received 120 mg (1.2 mg/kg) IV methylene blue. Three hours later, arterial blood sampling on 27% oxygen yielded similar blood gas except for a methemoglobin level of 1.3% with resolution of prior symptoms.

3. Discussion

Methemoglobinemia presents with a variety of clinical features. Our patient's methemoglobin level was 47% where confusion, dyspnea, tachypnea, and tachycardia would be expected. A 30% circulating methemoglobin level is routinely cited as the critical value for initiation of methylene blue therapy (1-2 mg/kg of 1% solution) for methemoglobinemia; however, there are patients that do become symptomatic at circulating methemoglobin as low as 8% [5].

Several endogenous pathways have developed to correct for methemoglobinemia by reducing the oxidized heme group. These processes rely on the presence of reduced NADH and NADPH and maintain methemoglobin concentrations below 1% of total hemoglobin [8]. The major mechanism is reduction via cytochrome b5 reductase, accounting for 95–99% activity. Minor pathways that utilize NADPH methemoglobin reductase, reduced flavin, tetrahydropterin, cysteamine, and reduced cysteine on protein molecules are also in existence. Of note is the NADPH methemoglobin reductase pathway which has a particular affinity for dyes. It is this affinity that is exploited with the use of methylene blue in the treatment of methemoglobinemia [3, 4]. As would be expected, methemoglobin levels increase when these pathways are exhausted, when enzymes are deficient, or when methemoglobin production abnormally increases. The latter occurs when exogenous substances or their metabolites

are potent oxidizers that induce excessive methemoglobin formation.

Given that methemoglobin is formed as part of a redox reaction, intuitively one can conclude that high oxidative states would predispose to the development of methemoglobinemia. This reasoning appears to hold true as septic patients have an increased risk of developing methemoglobinemia with concomitant use of benzocaine [9–11]. Other predisposing factors include baseline anemia, cancer, gastric acid suppression, and gastric mucosa inflammation [7, 9, 12].

The link between benzocaine use and methemoglobinemia has long been recognized with the FDA issuing a public advisory warning in 2006 which was later updated in 2011 advising both the public and clinicians to be judicious in their use of benzocaine following reports of 319 cases of benzocaine induced methemoglobinemia with three reported deaths [13]. Benzocaine comes in a variety of preparations including Hurricane, Cetacaine, Exactacain, and Topex. The above patient self-administered Hurricane spray (20% benzocaine spray (200 mg/mL)). The manufacturer's package insert states that a 3-4-second spray is equivalent to 1 mL of aerosolized 20% benzocaine. In terms of dosing, they recommend a 0.5-second spray, which may be repeated up to a maximum of four times a day. When used correctly, this technique should deliver a 30 mg dose. The manufacturer strongly advises against sprays in excess of two seconds [14]. Our patient admitted administering 4 sprays each 2 seconds in duration. This would result in a total dose of 120 mg per spray with a five-hour total dose of 480 mg. Keeping in mind that benzocaine toxicity is reported at doses as low as 100 mg, this patient received 4.8 times more in a relatively short time span.

Overuse of benzocaine is thought to be the most likely risk factor for development of benzocaine induced methemoglobinemia; however, current evidence suggests that this may not necessarily be the case. Methemoglobinemia has been noted to develop with as little as a one-second spray [15, 16]. Likely contributing to this is the fact that orientation of the canister appears to have an effect on the total administered dose. According to Khorasani et al. [17], the dose of benzocaine administered when specifically using the Hurricane canister is highly dependent on orientation with upright positioning resulting in larger doses compared to horizontal or upside down positioning with the resultant dose per second spray varying from less than 76 mg to 212 mg [17].

Quick recognition and evaluation of the patient's complaints allow for this case to be an effective teaching tool instead of something more catastrophic. A raised index of suspicion should be met with attempts to improve oxygenation, even with assisting ventilation if necessary. Diagnosis can be made with cooximetry or methemoglobin levels and the treatment of choice is methylene blue. Adjustments to therapy are required in the event of G6PD deficiency as methylene blue is simply ineffective due to low levels of NADPH. In G6PD deficiency, the use of ascorbic acid is advocated with the caveat that it would take longer for clinical resolution to occur.

Expanding outside the realm of clinical management, cases like this demand attention towards more practical means of preventing adverse events. With the advent of electronic medical records and electronic prescribing, perhaps this case highlights the important role of medication tracking. Given that methemoglobinemia presents in a nonspecific way, tracking of benzocaine administration via barcode scanning into the electronic medication administration record would have allowed for identification of methemoglobinemia as a potential diagnosis even prior to blood gas analysis.

The FDA as discussed earlier has long recognized safety concerns with regard to the use of benzocaine. This case highlights the ease with which adverse outcomes can result from simple mistakes. Fortunately, this patient was in a monitored environment where prompt identification and treatment were possible. It is not difficult to imagine a similar clinical scenario unfolding in a patient's home resulting in significant morbidity or even mortality. This risk warrants the development of a more practical means of external control. Potential solutions would include reconfiguring benzocaine spray canisters to allow for a maximum of 100 mg only per canister. Alternatively, the bottles could be redesigned to include metered dosing for more predictable total dose actuation. However, the question still remains whether benzocaine should be available at all on the market. As discussed earlier, lidocaine, an alternative to benzocaine, is comparatively much safer. It is available as a topical aerosolized spray with an attachable atomizer for use in hard-to-reach places such as the back of the throat. These bottles also feature metered dosing for predictable dose actuation per spray. Patient safety must take precedence above all else and perhaps it is time that the use of benzocaine is reconsidered in favor of safer alternatives.

References

[1] R. C. Darling and J. W. Roughton, "The effect of methemoglobin on the equilibrium between oxygen and hemoglobin," *The American Journal of Physiology—Legacy Content*, vol. 137, no. 1, pp. 56–68, 1942.

[2] S. Kurapati, A. C. Mehta, and P. Jain, "Benzocaine-induced methemoglobinemia," *Journal of Bronchology*, vol. 14, no. 1, pp. 41–44, 2007.

[3] E. R. Jaffé, "Methemoglobin pathophysiology," *Progress in Clinical and Biological Research*, vol. 51, pp. 133–151, 1981.

[4] S. McLean, B. P. Murphy, G. A. Starmer, and J. Thomas, "Methaemoglobin formation induced by aromatic amines and amides," *Journal of Pharmacy and Pharmacology*, vol. 19, no. 3, pp. 146–154, 1967.

[5] J. Guay, "Methemoglobinemia related to local anesthetics: a summary of 242 episodes," *Anesthesia & Analgesia*, vol. 108, no. 3, pp. 837–845, 2009.

[6] R. O. Wright, W. J. Lewander, and A. D. Woolf, "Methemoglobinemia: etiology, pharmacology, and clinical management," *Annals of Emergency Medicine*, vol. 34, no. 5, pp. 646–656, 1999.

[7] C. M. Anderson, K. J. Woodside, T. A. Spencer, and G. C. Hunter, "Methemoglobinemia: an unusual cause of postoperative cyanosis," *Journal of Vascular Surgery*, vol. 39, no. 3, pp. 686–690, 2004.

[8] J. C. Bloom and J. T. Brandt, "Toxic responses of the blood," in *Casarett and Doull's Toxicology: The Basic Science of Poisons Online*, C. D. Klaassen, Ed., chapter 11, McGraw-Hill, 6th edition, 2001.

[9] G. C. Kane, S. M. Hoehn, T. R. Behrenbeck, and S. L. Mulvagh, "Benzocaine-induced methemoglobinemia based on the Mayo Clinic experience from 28 478 transesophageal echocardiograms: incidence, outcomes, and predisposing factors," *Archives of Internal Medicine*, vol. 167, no. 18, pp. 1977–1982, 2007.

[10] B. Krafte-Jacobs, R. Brilli, C. Szabó, A. Denenberg, L. Moore, and A. L. Salzman, "Circulating methemoglobin and nitrite/nitrate concentrations as indicators of nitric oxide overproduction in critically ill children with septic shock," *Critical Care Medicine*, vol. 25, no. 9, pp. 1588–1593, 1997.

[11] K. Ohashi, H. Yukioka, M. Hayashi, and A. Asada, "Elevated methemoglobin in patients with sepsis," *Acta Anaesthesiologica Scandinavica*, vol. 42, no. 6, pp. 713–716, 1998.

[12] G. M. Novaro, H. D. Aronow, M. A. Militello, M. J. Garcia, and E. M. Sabik, "Benzocaine-induced methemoglobinemia: experience from a high-volume transesophageal echocardiography laboratory," *Journal of the American Society of Echocardiography*, vol. 16, no. 2, pp. 170–175, 2003.

[13] FDA Drug Safety Communication: FDA Continues to Receive Reports of a Rare, but Serious and Potentially Fatal Adverse Effect with the Use of Benzocaine Sprays for Medical Procedures, April 2011.

[14] Package Insert, "Hurricaine topical anesthetic—benzocaine spray," Physician's Desk Reference PDR Search. HurriCaine Topical Anesthetic Spray, Beutlich Pharmaceuticals, July 2015, http://www.pdr.net/drug-summary/hurricaine-topical-anesthetic-spray?druglabelid=2182.

[15] S. E. Guerriero, "Methemoglobinemia caused by topical benzocaine," *Pharmacotherapy*, vol. 17, no. 5, pp. 1038–1040, 1997.

[16] W. J. O'Donohue Jr., L. M. Moss, and V. A. Angelillo, "Acute methemoglobinemia induced by topical benzocaine and lidocaine," *Archives of Internal Medicine*, vol. 140, no. 11, pp. 1508–1509, 1980.

[17] A. Khorasani, K. D. Candido, A. H. Ghaleb, S. Saatee, and S. K. Appavu, "Canister tip orientation and residual volume have significant impact on the dose of benzocaine delivered by hurricaine spray," *Anesthesia & Analgesia*, vol. 92, no. 2, pp. 379–383, 2001.

17

BIS-Guided Total Intravenous Anesthesia for Orchiopexy and Circumcision in a Child with Severe Autism

Selçuk Okur, Müge Arıkan, Gülşen Temel, and Volkan Temel

Department of Anesthesiology, Karabük State Hospital, Karabük, Turkey

Correspondence should be addressed to Müge Arıkan, mugearikan@hotmail.com.tr

Academic Editors: A. Apan, A. Kaki, and J.-j. Yang

Autistic children are very difficult to manage in the hospital setting because they react badly to any change in routine. We describe a case of 10-year-old male patient with severe autism undergoing orchidopexy and circumcision. Following premedication, anesthesia was induced with remifentanil, propofol, atracurium, and maintained with total intravenous anesthesia (propofol and remifentanil). The Bispectral Index System was monitored for determination of the depth of anesthesia. After surgery, all infusions were discontinued. The patient was then transferred to the postanesthetic care unit. There were no adverse events observed during the anesthetic management. The patient was discharged from the hospital on the second postoperative day. Bispectral Index System-guided Total Intravenous Anesthesia can provide some advantages for patient with autism, such as hemodynamic stability, early and easy recovery, to facilitate faster discharge, to optimize the delivery of anesthetic agents, to minimize its adverse effects, and to maximize its safety.

1. Introduction

Autism is an heterogeneous developmental disorder mainly characterized by three domains of impairments: communication-language, social interaction, and behavioral oddities [1]. There is a great variation in the severity of autism and hospital needs of these children. Patients with impaired ability to understand and communicate can be difficult to manage perioperatively [2, 3]. Various agents and methods have been tried in these patients. Autistic patients scheduled to surgical procedures demand special care, such as detailed preanesthetic evaluation with history and specific physical evaluation and careful choice of anesthetic technique [2]. There appears to be little literature in paediatric anaesthetic practice relevant to children suffering with autism. Recent findings suggest a need for rigorous study of the potential problems that autistic children may have when undergoing an anaesthetic [4].

Patients with autism present many potential problems in terms of management of anesthesia. This case aimed at reporting a case of Bispectral Index System-guided TIVA in autistic patient.

2. Case Report

After his family written consent, a 10-year-old male child (32 kg), classified as American Society of Anesthesiologists physical status III (with severe autism, mild mental retardasyon, language disability-stage 5, musculo-skeletal and nervous system weakness, and hearing loss in the left ear). Preoperative laboratory tests were abnormal. Patient was scheduled for orchidopexy and circumcision under general anesthesia.

Upon arrival in the operating room, standard monitoring, including EKG, pulse oximetry, end-tidal capnography, Bispectral Index (BIS vista, Aspect Medical Systems, The Netherlands), and Train-of-four monitor (TOF watch, Organon, Ireland) were applied. Preoperative vital signs included blood pressure of 86/52 mmHg, a heart rate of 130 beats/min, oxygen saturation rate of 98%, and sinus rhythm on the electrocardiogram.

After establishing an intravenous access, he was given midazolam 1 mg (iv). The patient's fluid level was maintained with crystalloid solution. Anaesthesia was induced with remifentanil (1 μg/kg), propofol (2 mg/kg). Atracurium

(0.5 mg/kg) was used to intubate the patient. After to reach Train-of-four ratio (T4/T1) at 0, he was intubated with an internal diameter 5.5 mm endotracheal tube under direct laryngoscopy. No problems were encountered during tracheal intubation and the breathing sound was clear at both lung fields. The patient was mechanically ventilated in the pressure control mode, and the end-tidal carbon dioxide levels were monitored and maintained at the range of 30–32 mmHg. Anesthesia was maintained with oxygen (1 L/min), medical air (1.5 L/min), and continuous infusion of 100–150 µg/kg/min of propofol and 0.2–0.4 µg/kg/min of remifentanil using an infusion pump (AS50 Auto Syringe Infusion Pump, Baxter International Inc. Deerfield, IL, USA). The infusions of propofol and and remifentanil were adjusted in order to keep BIS as 50 ± 10. To maintain T1 in the TOF ratio (T4/T1) at 25%, atracurium (0.2 mg/kg) was intravenously injected with the top-up dose.

Oxygen saturation, heart rate, noninvasive hemodynamometer, and BIS values were recorded at 5 min intervals intraoperatively. Vital signs were stable throughout the procedure. Total procedure time was 45 min. After skin closure, all infusion drugs were stopped and antagonism of residual neuromuscular block was carried out by 35 µg/kg neostigmine together with 20 µg/kg atropine when T4/T1 ratio reached 75% or higher followed by tracheal extubation (3.51 min). The time from stoppage of propofol and remifentanil infusions until BIS level raised to 80 was considered as the recovery time (6 min). The patient was then transferred to the postanesthetic care unit. The patient was discharged from the hospital on the second postoperative day.

3. Discussion

Mental disability is a term which is used when an individual's intellectual development is significantly lower than average, limiting his or her ability to adapt to the environment [5]. Autism is a neurobehavioral and cognitive disorder characterized by impaired development of interpersonal and communication skills, limited interests, and repetitive behaviors. The incidence of autism is about 0.2% [6]. There are enormous variations in the behavioral patterns and the severity of illness among individuals with autism. Mental retardation is evident in approximately 70% of individuals with autism. The behavioral symptoms in children include temper tantrums, hyperactivity, short attention span, impulsivity, agitation, anger, and a tendency for aggressive and self-injurious behaviors [7]. Disorders of language and social communication, poor response to external stimulation, tendency to isolate themselves, and poor eye-to-eye contact are well-recognized symptoms.

Patients with impaired ability to understand and communicate can be difficult to manage perioperatively. They frequently require lateral thinking on the part of the anesthesiologists to make the induction process as smooth as possible. The main targets of these patients are rapid recovery, smooth postoperative pain, early discharge and low stress during the peroperative period [8].

Solak et al. reported that TIVA can be valuable alternative to inhalation anesthesia for children [9]. The bispectral index is a pharmacodynamic measure of the effect of anesthesia on the central nervous system. Messieha et al. announced that monitoring anesthesia with BIS promotes earlier extubation and discharge for pediatric dental patients who receive general anesthesia [10]. Park et al. aimed that their study was to investigate the relationship between BIS index and predicted plasma concentration of propofol delivered by target-controlled infusion during emergency in children. As a result they concluded that when respiration returned, mean BIS was 77.2 ± 5.3 and propofol plasma concentration 1.6 ± 0.3 µg/kg and when a verbal command was obeyed, BIS was 82.4 ± 5.6 and propofol plasma concentration 1.5 ± 0.3 µg/kg and BIS moderately correlated with the predicted plasma concentration of propofol [11]. Zhang et al. reported that BIS effectively monitors the depth of intravenous anesthesia with remifentanil and propofol [12].

Asahi et al. suggested that autistic patients have greater propofol requirements for anaesthesia during ordinary dental treatment compared with intellectually impaired patients [13].

In our patient, anesthesia was induced with propofol and remifentanil and maintained with propofol and remifentanil infusions. The dosages of propofol and remifentanil were adjusted in order to keep BIS as 50 ± 10. Vital signs were stable throughout his procedure.

Bispectral Index System-guided TIVA can provide some advantages for patient with autism, such as hemodynamic stability, early and easy recovery, to facilitate faster discharge, to optimize the delivery of TIVA, to minimize its adverse effects, and to maximize its safety.

References

[1] American Psychiatric Association, *Psychiatric Association the Diagnostic and Statistical Manual of Psychiatric Disorders*, American Psychiatric Association, Washington, DC, USA, 4th edition, 1994.

[2] J. H. Walt and C. Moran, "An audit of perioperative management of autistic children," *Paediatric Anaesthesia*, vol. 11, no. 4, pp. 401–408, 2001.

[3] M. Bagshaw, "Anaesthesia and the autistic child," *Journal of Perioperative Practice*, vol. 21, no. 9, pp. 313–317, 2011.

[4] L. Rainey and J. H. van der Walt, "The anaesthetic management of autistic children," *Anaesthesia and Intensive Care*, vol. 26, no. 6, pp. 682–686, 1998.

[5] J. A. Weddell, B. J. Sanders, and J. E. Jones, "Dental problems of children with disabilities," in *Dentistry for the Child and Adolescent*, R. E. McDonald, D. R. Avery, and J. A. Dean, Eds., p. 540, Mosby, St. Louis, Mo, USA, 8th edition, 2004.

[6] J. Veenstra-Vanderweele, E. H. Cook Jr., and P. J. Lombroso, "Genetics of childhood disorders: XLVI. Autism, part 5: genetics of autism," *Journal of the American Academy of Child and Adolescent Psychiatry*, vol. 42, no. 1, pp. 116–118, 2003.

[7] A. H. Friedlander, J. A. Yagiela, V. I. Paterno, and M. E. Mahler, "The pathophysiology, medical management, and dental implications of autism," *Journal of the California Dental Association*, vol. 31, no. 9, pp. 681–686, 2003.

[8] S. Shah, S. Shah, J. Apuya, S. Gopalakrishnan, and T. Martin, "Combination of oral ketamine and midazolam as a premedication for a severely autistic and combative patient," *Journal of Anesthesia*, vol. 23, no. 1, pp. 126–128, 2009.

[9] A. Solak, A. Tavlan, S. Tuncer, A. Yosunkaya, R. Reisli, and S. Okesli, "Comprasion of total intravenous anesthesia using remifentanil and propofol with sevoflurane and nitrous oxide anesthesia in children," *Turkiye Klinikleri Journal of Anesthesiology Reanimation*, vol. 2, no. 3, pp. 130–136, 2004.

[10] Z. S. Messieha, R. C. Ananda, W. E. Hoffman, I. C. Punwani, and H. M. Koenig, "Bispectral index system (BIS) monitoring reduces time to extubation and discharge in children requiring oral presedation and general anesthesia for outpatient dental rehabilitation," *Pediatric Dentistry*, vol. 27, no. 6, pp. 500–504, 2005.

[11] H. J. Park, Y. L. Kim, C. S. Kim, S. D. Kim, and H. S. Kim, "Changes of bispectral index during recovery from general anesthesia with 2% propofol and remifentanil in children," *Paediatric Anaesthesia*, vol. 17, no. 4, pp. 353–357, 2007.

[12] J. M. Zhang, F. Wang, Z. Xin, and H. Lü, "Effectiveness of bispectral index in intravenous anesthesia with remifentanil and propofol in children," *Zhonghua yi xue za zhi*, vol. 88, no. 41, pp. 2904–2906, 2008.

[13] Y. Asahi, K. Kubota, and S. Omichi, "Dose requirements for propofol anaesthesia for dental treatment for autistic patients compared with intellectually impaired patients," *Anaesthesia and Intensive Care*, vol. 37, no. 1, pp. 70–73, 2009.

18

Iatrogenic Left Main Bronchus Injury following Atraumatic Double Lumen Endotracheal Tube Placement

William R. Hartman, Michael Brown, and James Hannon

Department of Anesthesiology, Mayo Clinic, Rochester, MN, USA

Correspondence should be addressed to William R. Hartman; hartman.william@mayo.edu

Academic Editors: N. Bhardwaj and C.-H. Hsing

Tracheobronchial disruption is an uncommon but severe complication of double lumen endotracheal tube placement. The physical properties of a double lumen tube (large external diameter and length) make tracheobronchial injury more common than that associated with smaller single lumen endotracheal tubes. Here we present the case of an iatrogenic left main bronchus injury caused by placement of a double lumen tube in an otherwise unremarkable airway.

1. Introduction

Thoracic surgery procedures requiring lung isolation are often performed with the assistance of a double lumen endotracheal tube (DLT). While placement of DLTs is routine and safe in experienced hands, it is not without risk. A rare complication is airway rupture, perhaps due to DLTs having a larger external diameter compared to a single lumen tube and a stiff stylette used for ease of proper endotracheal tube placement [1, 2]. Early recognition of airway rupture, evaluation of the defect, and repair of the airway are critical to optimal patient outcome [3].

Here we present the case of a 52-year-old woman who presented to the operating room for removal of a right upper lobe mass via right thoracotomy. Despite a seemingly atraumatic intubation with a 35-French left double lumen endotracheal tube, a significant tear in her left main bronchus was identified intraoperatively.

2. Case Report

A 158 cm, 93 kg (BMI 37.4), 52-year-old woman presented to a tertiary care center for evaluation of a Merkel cell tumor in her right forearm. Wide resection of this forearm tumor and an axillary lymph node dissection were successfully performed. During the course of her evaluation, however, a suspicious mass in her right upper lobe was identified on chest X-ray, and a $2.7 \times 2.2 \times 2.9$ cm hypermetabolic solid nodule in the right apex was confirmed with CT imaging. The patient was asymptomatic. Preoperative pulmonary function tests were normal. Patient was deemed to be optimized for a thoracic surgical procedure and was brought to the operating room.

After routine intravenous sedation with Midazolam and Fentanyl, an epidural was placed at the T6-7 vertebral interspace. Patient was returned to the supine position where general anesthesia was induced intravenously with fentanyl, lidocaine, propofol, and succinylcholine. Her airway was secured via direct laryngoscopy (grade one view) and placement of a styleted 35-French left double lumen endotracheal tube without difficulty. Once the tracheal cuff had passed through the cords, the stylette was removed and bilateral breath sounds were confirmed. Proper placement of the bronchial lumen of the tube in the left main bronchus was confirmed with fiberoptic bronchoscopy. The patient was placed in lateral position for her surgical procedure, and proper placement of the DLT was once again confirmed with the fiberoptic bronchoscope. No blood or signs of bronchial or tracheal trauma were observed.

Following initiation of single lung ventilation, a surgical decision was made to proceed with a right upper lobectomy which was performed in the usual fashion. Individual branches of the pulmonary artery to the right upper lobe were identified and doubly ligated with 2-0 silk suture. Right

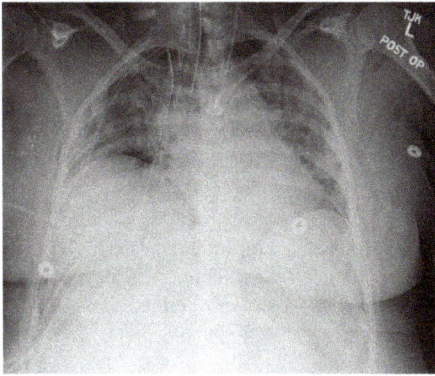

FIGURE 1: Postoperative chest X-ray. Seen are a single lumen ETT (DLT was replaced with SLT for bronchoscopy), three right chest tubes, and tiny right apical and basilar pneumothoraces. Infiltrate is observed throughout both lungs.

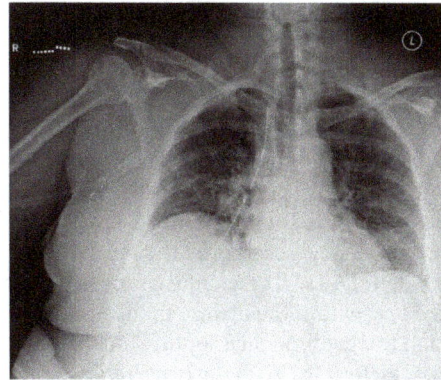

FIGURE 3: Postoperative day 7 chest X-ray. No evidence of left sided air leak or residual left main bronchus rupture.

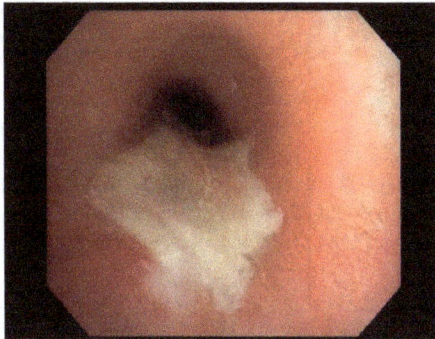

FIGURE 2: Endobronchial view of left main bronchus repair.

superior pulmonary vein was mobilized. Branches going to the right upper lobe were identified and divided with silk stick ties and free ties. The fissures between the middle lobe and upper lobe were completed with multiple firings of a GIA stapler. All interlobar lymph nodes were resected. The right upper lobe bronchus was sharply dissected free. The right lung was reinflated and the bronchial stump was competent to 40 cm pressure; however, with positive pressure ventilation and the right hemithorax filled with saline, a small air leak was identified. Further evaluation revealed the air leak to be arising from a long linear tear located along the left mainstem bronchus and extending from the carina as far down the left mainstem bronchus as could be visualized. The double-lumen endotracheal tube was identified in the region of injury. This left main bronchus injury was not evident during the course of the case because the bronchial balloon had successfully isolated the left lung. The injury and resultant air leak only became apparent with deflation of the bronchial balloon and the resumption of right lung ventilation.

Due to the location of the injury and concern that the current exposure would not provide adequate visualization for surgical repair, a right thoracotomy was performed. The bronchial lumen of the DLT was inserted distal to the defect with the use of a flexible bronchoscope and surgeon observation. With the ability to ventilate the lung distal to the

airway rupture, the defect was repaired with a combination of a pericardial patch and pleural flap. No air leak was identified upon completion of the repair, and the chest was closed in the usual fashion.

The patient was returned to the supine position, and the anesthesiologist removed the double lumen endotracheal tube under direct vision with a video laryngoscope and placed a single lumen endotracheal tube (Figures 1 and 3). At this time, a bronchoscopist conducted a thorough examination of the airway, revealing findings consistent with a right upper lobectomy with intact surgical stump. The remainder of the visible tracheobronchial tree on the right side was normal and fully patent. Examination of the left tracheobronchial tree, findings consistent with a left mainstem bronchial injury beginning approximately 0.5 cm below the main carina and along its medial wall and continuing down to approximately 1 cm above the intermediate carina separating the take-offs to the left upper and lower lobes. The injury itself included a portion of bronchial mucosa emanating into the airway although the airway was fully patent. There was no evidence of residual injury, or leak and distal airways were fully patent (Figure 2). A single blood clot was evacuated from the airway.

The patient was allowed to emerge from anesthesia in the postanesthesia care unit and was making excellent respiratory effort with adequate tidal volumes. She was successfully extubated and observed for any signs of respiratory difficulty in the PACU for approximately 2 hours. She was discharged to the ICU for observation and recovered without any further complication.

3. Discussion

In 1949, the Carlens double lumen endotracheal tube [4] was developed and successfully used to separate lungs and facilitate single lung ventilation. Since that time, DLTs have been widely used for isolated lung ventilation in thoracic and cardiac surgeries as well as in cases of single lung trauma or infection. Placement of these endotracheal tubes is relatively simple in experienced hands and rarely is associated with complications. However, because of the large external tube diameter and the stiff stylette, placement of a DLT is not completely without risk.

Tracheobronchial rupture during DLT placement is a potentially life-threatening complication but occurs very rarely, likely less than 0.2% of DLT intubations [5]. In fact, between 1998 and 2010, only six reported cases of tracheobronchial injury were published [6–8]. Most commonly, injuries were associated with the distal trachea and/or left main bronchus, likely because of the strong preference to place left sided DLTs. These injuries usually occur as a longitudinal tear within the membranous portion of the trachea. Though tracheobronchial rupture incidence is very low, possible risk factors for such an occurrence might include placement by an inexperienced airway manager, multiple intubation attempts, placement of the stylette through the DLT in such a way that the tip emerges from the luminal tip, overinflation of the cuff, too large of a tube size, incompletely anesthetized patient, weakened membranous trachea secondary to chemotherapy, steroid use or radiation therapy, and previous tracheomalacia.

When a tracheobronchial tear does occur, it can result in life-threatening complications. Symptoms of bronchial rupture recognized during a surgical procedure can include tension pneumothorax or subcutaneous emphysema. If unrecognized during surgery, this type of tear can result in thoracic cavity infection or sepsis. Early recognition of tracheobronchial tear and prompt repair are essential for optimal patient outcome. Anesthesia provider recognition might include abrupt changes in vital signs, difficulty with ventilation, and the onset of a significant and unexplainable ventilatory leak.

In the case presented here, the tear was not initially recognized presumably because of ongoing successful ventilation of the injured lung due to correct placement of the inflated bronchial balloon below the distal portion of the tear. In the absence of ventilation difficulty or vital sign changes, we did not suspect any problem to have occurred. A large air leak following deflation of the bronchial cuff manifested by persistent air bubbles in the surgical field alerted the surgeon of a potential airway disruption. Concurrently, we detected a large leak in our ventilatory circuit. Prompt identification of the bronchial tear and proper patching of the defect prevented further sequela from the injury. In addition, inspection of the bronchus by an experienced bronchoscopist was necessary to exclude the possibility of a distal tear that was not observed in the initial surgical repair. As in most cases of recognized tracheobronchial tears caused by DLT placement, our patient experienced a favorable outcome.

In conclusion, a tracheal rupture after intubation with a double lumen endotracheal tube during an operation is very rare. Prompt recognition and repair are important to optimal patient outcome and prevention of further endobronchial as well as systemic complications. Immediate inspection of the airway by an experienced bronchoscopist is necessary to ensure that proper repair has occurred and no further airway injury is present. Finally, prompt extubation of the patient is preferred to avoid further injury by either positive pressure ventilation or movement of the endotracheal tube causing disruption of the repair.

Acknowledgments

The authors acknowledge the support by the Foundation for Anesthesia Education and Research (FAER) (WRH) and Department of Anesthesiology, Mayo Clinic, Rochester.

References

[1] H. Liu, J. S. Jahr, E. Sullivan, and P. F. Waters, "Tracheobronchial rupture after double-Lumen endotracheal intubation," *Journal of Cardiothoracic and Vascular Anesthesia*, vol. 18, no. 2, pp. 228–233, 2004.

[2] G. Massard, C. Rougé, A. Dabbagh et al., "Tracheobronchial lacerations after intubation and tracheostomy," *Annals of Thoracic Surgery*, vol. 61, no. 5, pp. 1483–1487, 1996.

[3] A. Mussi, M. C. Ambrogi, G. Menconi, A. Ribechini, and C. A. Angeletti, "Surgical approaches to membranous tracheal wall lacerations," *Journal of Thoracic and Cardiovascular Surgery*, vol. 120, no. 1, pp. 115–118, 2000.

[4] E. Carlens, "A new flexible double-lumen catheter for bronchospirometry," *The Journal of Thoracic Surgery*, vol. 18, no. 5, pp. 742–746, 1949.

[5] K. Ceylan, S. Kaya, O. Samancilar et al., "Intraoperative management of tracheobronchial rupture after double-lumen tube intubation," *Surgery Today*, vol. 43, no. 7, pp. 757–762, 2013.

[6] T. B. Gilbert, C. W. Goodsell, and M. J. Krasna, "Bronchial rupture by a double-lumen endobronchial tube during staging thoracoscopy," *Anesthesia and Analgesia*, vol. 88, no. 6, pp. 1252–1253, 1999.

[7] R. R. Jha, S. Mishra, and S. Bhatnagar, "Rupture of left main bronchus associated with radiotherapy-induced bronchial injury and use of a double-lumen tube in oesophageal cancer surgery," *Anaesthesia and Intensive Care*, vol. 32, no. 1, pp. 104–107, 2004.

[8] R. C. Bessa Júnior, J. C. Jorge, A. F. Eisenberg et al., "Ruptura brônquica após intubação com tubo de duplo lúmen: relato de caso," *Revista Brasileira de Anestesiologia*, vol. 55, pp. 660–664, 2005.

19

A Common Anesthesiology Procedure for a Patient with an Uncommon Combination of Diseases

Aliki Tympa,[1] Dimitrios Hassiakos,[2] Nikolaos Salakos,[2] and Aikaterini Melemeni[1]

[1] *1st Department of Anesthesiology, Aretaieion University Hospital, 76 Vas. Sofias Avenue, 11528 Athens, Greece*
[2] *1st Department of Obstetrics and Gynecology, Aretaieion University Hospital, 76 Vas. Sofias Avenue, 11528 Athens, Greece*

Correspondence should be addressed to Aliki Tympa, tympaaliki@yahoo.gr

Academic Editors: S. Faenza, R. S. Gomez, and S. Grigoriadis

Administering neuraxial anesthesia to a patient with an underlying neurological disease and a combination of four other pathological disorders can be challenging. We report in this paper the case of a 45-year-old woman with neurological deficit due to ischemic brain infarct, multiple sclerosis, antiphospholipid syndrome, and β-heterozygous thalassemia that was subjected to abdominal hysterectomy and bilateral salpingoophorectomy under epidural anesthesia for ovarian cancer.

1. Introduction

The choice of anesthetic technique in patients with preexisting neurological disease may be a specific concern for anesthetists [1]. Neurological deficits appearing after spinal or epidural anesthesia have cast additional doubt on the benefit of neuraxial anesthesia in these patients [2, 3]. If administering neuraxial anesthesia to a patient with an underlying neurological disease is puzzling, then the conduct of anesthesia in a patient with preexisting neurological deficit and a combination of four other pathological disorders is undoubtedly challenging. Safely caring for the health, comfort, and quality of life of a patient with neurological disease and several other comorbidities is a difficult task that extends beyond the operating and recovery room.

2. Case Presentation

A 45-year-old, ASA physical status IV woman (78 kg, 172 cm) with ovarian cancer was scheduled for abdominal hysterectomy and bilateral salpingoophorectomy with epidural anesthesia, after her refusal for general anesthesia. The patient had been successfully subjected to cesarean section under epidural anesthesia four years ago.

Her clinical history revealed an ischemic infarct of the left frontal lobe since the age of 19, multiple sclerosis since the age of 20, antiphospholipid syndrome (heterozygote for the methylenetetrahydrofolate reductase (MHTFR) gene), and heterozygous β-thalassemia. On her admission, normotensive sinus tachycardia (115 bpm), fever and intense lower abdominal pain along with ascites and nausea were noted. The patient presented with 26.5% hematocrit, a platelet count of 465.000/L, and normal bleeding tests. Neurological examination revealed right hemiparesis, dropping of the left corner of the mouth, impaired oropharyngeal function with dysphagia to both solids and liquids, and altered walking gait. The patient had been receiving cinnarizine 10 mg daily, bromazepam 3 mg three times per day, and paracetamol occasionally.

In the operating room, with the patient positioned in the left lateral decubitus position, a 18-gauge Tuohy needle was inserted at L_1-L_2 intervertebral space; the epidural space was found using the loss-of-resistance technique. A polyamide catheter was easily introduced and placed at the 12 cm catheter mark. A test dose of 3 mL of 2% lidocaine was injected. After catheter placement the patient turned supine and was given 15 mL of ropivacaine 0.75% and 100 μg fentanyl. A sensory block to T_3 was established 15 minutes later. During the 2-hour surgery, another 5 mL of ropivacaine 0.75% and 10 mL of lidocaine 2% were given as the patient complained of discomfort during peritoneal traction. Entonox inhalation was used to alleviate patients' discomfort during peritoneal traction and abdominal wall closure. At the recovery room, 1/2 an hour after the last epidural dose, the patient experienced severe pain and was administered 8 mL of ropivacaine 0.2% and 2 mg of preservative free morphine followed by 6 mL of ropivacaine 0.375% fifteen minutes later. A sensory block to T_{12} was present $1^{1/2}$ hours later with no motor block at recovery.

Postoperative analgesia with 8 mL ropivacaine 0.2% four times daily, 2 mg morphine twice a day, and rescue dose of 6 mL ropivacaine 0.375% failed and the regimen was replaced by a continuous epidural pump, set to infuse 2 mL of ropivacaine 0.2% and 8 μg fentanyl hourly. The patient also received 3 g of paracetamol daily and triple antiemetic drug combination (metoclopramide 30 mg, 5HT$_3$ antagonist 12 mg, and dexamethasone 8 mg). On the second postoperative day, pain was effectively managed with the continuous pump infusion but nausea persisted. Neurological examination revealed no signs of deterioration of the preexisting disease. The epidural catheter was removed on the fifth postoperative day. Nausea was not alleviated despite rigorous treatment. The patient developed paralytic ileus on the sixth postoperative day that resolved spontaneously two days later.

3. Discussion

Neurological deficit, chronic neuropathic cancer pain, antiphospholipid syndrome, and hematological disorders along with the patients' refusal for general anesthesia form a noteworthy clinical profile, challenging for every anesthetist.

In the present case, we report the anesthetic management and the medical questions raised during the clinical course of a patient with the combination of the abovementioned uncommon diseases.

Worsening of neurological symptoms in patients with preexisting neural compromise has always been a fear for the neuraxial anesthesia and analgesia performing anesthetist [1–3]. Disorders of the central nervous system such as multiple sclerosis have historically been a relative contraindication to spinal and epidural anesthesia. Dripps and Vandam [4] were the first to report exacerbation of preexisting neurological disease after spinal anesthesia. Several years later, Brinkmeier et al. [5] provided evidence that an endogenous pentapeptide in patients with multiple sclerosis has a higher blocking efficacy than that of 50 μM of lidocaine and may well contribute to the fast changes of symptoms.

Epidural anesthesia is commonly thought to be less harmful than spinal anesthesia; however secondary parameters such as local anesthetic neurotoxicity and needle or catheter induced trauma may cause relapse of the dormant underlying neurologic pathology. Furthermore, many perioperative factors such as fever, infection, stress, fatigue, and the operation itself may result in deterioration of the preexisting neural compromise. To this direction, Hebl et al. [1]

in their retrospective review of 136 patients with preexisting central nervous system disorders suggest that the risks commonly associated with epidural or spinal anesthesia and analgesia may not be as frequent as once thought.

The patient has also been diagnosed with antiphospholipid syndrome; an autoimmune disorder characterized by vascular thrombosis. The need for anticoagulant therapy for the patient with antiphospholipid syndrome may prove higher postoperatively and this unanticipated anticoagulation regimen explains the reluctancy in performing neuraxial blockade [6].

Given the intense postoperative pain experienced by the patient in the recovery room and the ward along with the patients' characteristics, the roles of opioid-induced hyperalgesia and preemptive analgesia come into question. The cancer patient with neurological deficit gathers several potential preoperative risk determinants of postsurgical pain; anxiety, depression, and catastrophising personality along with impaired pain modulation have been postulated as primary causal factors leading to postsurgical pain [7]. The intensity of perioperative pain—which in this case was not negligible—has also been suggested as a key risk factor to postoperative pain [7–9]. Acute opioid-induced hyperalgesia (resulting from the desensitization of antinociceptive pathways) in the perioperative period may be an explanation for the postsurgical pain; opioid-induced hyperalgesia can occur in various, low-dose, high-dose, or maintenance-dose regimens of opioids [7]. Hyperalgesia induced to patients with preexisting neurological deficits and chronic pain is a matter that remains to be elucidated in the future.

Preemptive analgesia could probably play a role in the clinical setting of this patient [8–11]; however NSAIDs carry the risk of precipitating thromboembolic events to patients with antiphospholipid syndrome [6] while gabapentin may eventually deteriorate the underlying neurological pathology. Alternative methods of preemptive analgesia including a$_2$ agonists or ketamine [10] could have been used to improve analgesia while reducing opioid-related side effects. Of course, the role of preemptive analgesia in patients with preexisting neurological deficit or antiphospholipid syndrome has not been studied, but identification of the problem is the first step to improving outcomes after surgery.

Another skepticism that emerges from this case report is whether spinal anesthesia with profound sensory and motor block intraoperatively could have resulted in reduced postoperative pain. Recent studies on spinal anesthesia in patients with preexisting central nervous system disorders report complication-free procedures with patient satisfaction [1].

Although epidural anesthesia to this patient may have been a common final procedure, balancing the risks and benefits of the anesthetic technique and critically questioning the problems raised by her clinical course was a copious work in the hope that definitive conclusions will be made after new prospective studies.

References

[1] J. R. Hebl, T. T. Horlocker, and D. R. Schroeder, "Neuraxial anesthesia and analgesia in patients with preexisting central nervous system disorders," *Anesthesia and Analgesia*, vol. 103, no. 1, pp. 223–228, 2006.

[2] P. Lirk, B. Birmingham, and Q. Hogan, "Regional anesthesia in patients with preexisting neuropathy," *International Anesthesiology Clinics*, vol. 49, pp. 144–165, 2011.

[3] J. A. Aldrete, M. Reza-Medina, O. Daud et al., "Exacerbation of preexisting neurological deficits by neuraxial anesthesia: report of 7 cases," *Journal of Clinical Anesthesia*, vol. 17, no. 4, pp. 304–313, 2005.

[4] R. D. Dripps and L. D. Vandam, "Exacerbation of pre-existing neurologic disease after spinal anesthesia," *The New England Journal of Medicine*, vol. 255, no. 18, pp. 843–849, 1956.

[5] H. Brinkmeier, P. Aulkemeyer, K. H. Wollinsky, and R. Rüdel, "An endogenous pentapeptide acting as a sodium channel blocker in inflammatory autoimmune disorders of the central nervous system," *Nature Medicine*, vol. 6, no. 7, pp. 808–811, 2000.

[6] K. W. Park, "The antiphospholipid syndrome," *International Anesthesiology Clinics*, vol. 42, pp. 45–57, 2004.

[7] C. L. Wu and S. N. Raja, "Treatment of acute postoperative pain," *The Lancet*, vol. 377, no. 9784, pp. 2215–2225, 2011.

[8] D. J. Kelly, M. Ahmad, and S. J. Brull, "Preemptive analgesia II: recent advances and current trends," *Canadian Journal of Anesthesia*, vol. 48, no. 11, pp. 1091–1101, 2001.

[9] E. G. VanDenKerkhof, W. M. Hopman, D. H. Goldstein et al., "Impact of perioperative pain intensity, pain qualities, and opioid use on chronic pain after surgery: a prospective cohort study," *Regional Anesthesia and Pain Medicine*, vol. 37, pp. 19–27, 2012.

[10] G. Blaudszun, C. Lysakowski, N. Elia, and M. R. Tramèr, "Effect of perioperative systemic $\alpha 2$ agonists on postoperative morphine consumption and pain intensity: systematic review and meta-analysis of randomized controlled trials," *Anesthesiology*, vol. 116, pp. 1312–1322, 2012.

[11] M. Karanikolas, D. Aretha, I. Tsolakis et al., "Optimized perioperative analgesia reduces chronic phantom limb pain intensity, prevalence, and frequency: a prospective, randomized, clinical trial," *Anesthesiology*, vol. 114, no. 5, pp. 1144–1154, 2011.

20

Postanesthetic Severe Oral Angioedema in Patient's Taking Angiotensin-Converting Enzyme Inhibitor

Acílio Marques, Carla Retroz-Marques, Sara Mota, Raquel Cabral, and Matos Campos

Anaesthesiology Department, Coimbra University Hospital Center, Praceta Mota Pinto, 3001-301 Coimbra, Portugal

Correspondence should be addressed to Acílio Marques; a917557752@gmail.com

Academic Editor: Eugene A. Vandermeersch

Angiotensin-converting enzyme (ACE) inhibitors are the leading cause of a drug-induced angioedema. This occurrence is frequently underdiagnosed, but its relapse can be life-threatening. The authors' intention in reporting this clinical case is to sound a warning about reviewing attitudes and surveillance to try to improve patient perioperative safety.

1. Introduction

Angiotensin-converting enzyme (ACE) inhibitors are widely prescribed and are the leading cause of a drug-induced angioedema [1]. However, contrary to what may happen with other drugs, this adverse reaction is frequently missed because it can start years after beginning the treatment and recurs erratically but with increased morbidity severity or even mortality [2].

The management of these severe adverse reactions has been discussed but still missing consensus about perioperative surveillance guidelines in patients taking ACE inhibitors [3–6]. However, it is obviously unquestionable that the quality of perioperative care is crucial to the patient's safety, and all medical surveillance decisions must be carefully planned and implemented.

The severity of this case legitimizes it being reported to raise the awareness of health care professionals and propose preventive attitudes for discussion that could improve the perioperative safety of patients.

The patient reviewed the case report and gave permission for the authors to publish.

2. Case Description

We report the case of a male Caucasian, 81-year-old, weighing 90 kg, and 175 cm tall. He was hospitalized in the Burn Intensive Care Unit (BICU) with a third-degree burn of the foot and he was proposed for surgical cleaning with skin grafting. The patient was conscious and oriented but with amnesia regarding his medical history. The anesthetic risk by the American Society of Anesthesiologists classification was grade III due to hypertension, and he had NYHA class II heart failure. The usual pharmacological therapy was perindopril, furosemide, finasteride, and pantoprazole.

We performed a combined anesthesia: femoral/sciatic nerve blocks with ropivacaine associated to general anesthesia with propofol, fentanyl, and sevoflurane. For airway patency, we used a nontraumatic supraglottic device (Igel), and the patient was in spontaneous ventilation all the time. There were no abnormal or unexpected incidents during the operation. The overall perioperative period was spent in the BICU with constant medical surveillance.

Five hours later, the patient developed dysphagia and mild respiratory distress. He was aware and oriented but anxious with polypnea and tachycardia. The main clinical sign was oropharyngeal edema involving the tongue (Figure 1).

The upper airways were nebulized with epinephrine. Intravenous drugs were given: 250 mg methylprednisolone and 2 mg clemastine. We opted to keep the patient under strict medical surveillance without additional specific drug therapy but keeping a possible emergency tracheostomy in mind. The daily therapy was reviewed, and the ACE inhibitor, perindopril, was suspended. Laboratory blood levels of IgE and tryptase were normal.

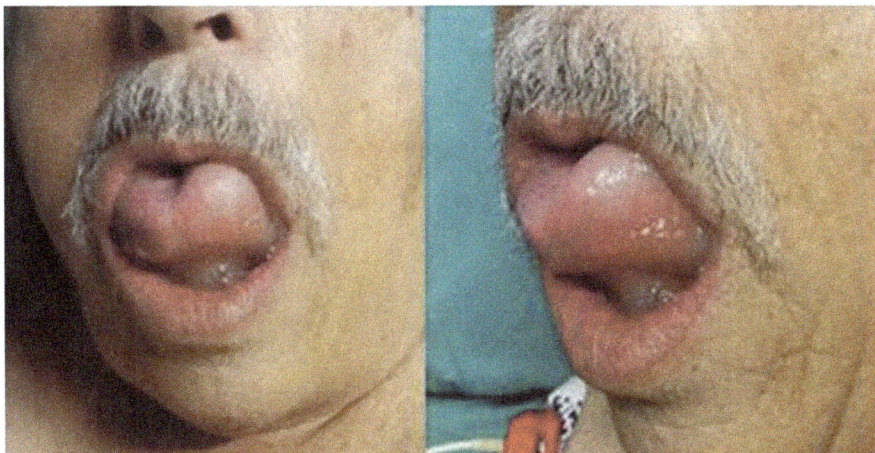

FIGURE 1: Oropharyngeal edema involving the tongue.

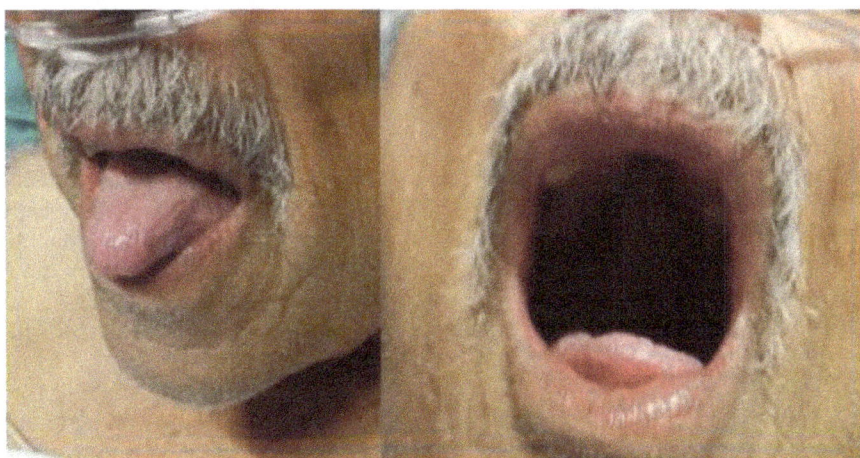

FIGURE 2: After 24 hours of ACE inhibitor suspension.

After 24 hours of ACE inhibitor suspension there was a clinical improvement (Figure 2). There were no new episodes in the six-month follow-up period.

3. Discussion

ACE inhibitors are the most common cause of nonhereditary angioedema (25–39%). The probability that a patient taking an ACE inhibitor will go on to develop angioedema is 0.1–0.7% [7–9]. However and unlike other cases of drug-related angioedema, this adverse reaction is frequently missed because it can start years after beginning the treatment and recurs erratically while treatment continues. Another clinical concern is that the severity of adverse reactions increases with each recurrence and can be life-threatening [10–13].

The bradykinin receptor and its active metabolites have been demonstrated experimentally as humoral mechanisms of angioedema due to increased levels of nitric oxide, prostacyclin PG12, and neuropeptide substance P and a consequent increase in vascular permeability. The inactivation of kinins is mainly caused by angiotensin-converting enzyme (ACE),

but other important enzymes are aminopeptidase (APP), dipeptidyl peptidase IV (DPP-IV), and neutral endopeptidase (NEP) [3].

Patients taking other drugs that are also bradykinin-degrading enzyme inhibitors are at increased risk. Diabetic patients have new drug therapies that are DPP-IV inhibitors (sitagliptin, saxagliptin, and vildagliptin). Transplant recipients with immunosuppressant medications should receive inhibition of DPP-IV enzyme activity to improve graft survival success [3].

In addition to the amount of bradykinin, individual sensitivity is an important factor to trigger angioedema. In the presence of clinical angioedema, we should exclude hereditary autosomal dominant disease typified by a deficiency or dysfunction of the C1-esterase inhibitor [14].

Perioperative patients taking ACE inhibitors have mainly been studied in relation to anesthetic hemodynamic stability [15, 16]. The possibility of severe angioedema must be discussed enough for the best practices improvement [17].

In perioperative medicine, preventive attitudes begin with preoperative evaluation, anesthetic-surgery planning, and appropriate postoperative recovery care [18]. These surveillance attitudes do not necessarily mean more medical care but are essential for a better health care.

In the case reported here, the first main concern was the hypothesis of an anaphylactic reaction to surgical/anesthetic procedures and the inherent therapy. However, the painless, nonpruritic mucosal edema was restricted to the oral cavity localized, with only slight response to the antianaphylactic drugs, and the blood tests were normal. The only drug discontinued was the ACE inhibitor, while the other drugs were administered daily, and there was a late but sustained clinical improvement without further episodes in the following months. We conclude that the patient had a severe life-threatening angioedema with high probability that the etiology was directly related to the previous treatment with an ACE inhibitor [7].

There are risk factors for oral angioedema that should be evaluated in patients taking ACE inhibitors: older age, femal sex, Hispanic race, or African-American ancestry. Also, patients should be screened for positive smoking history, coexistent cardiopulmonary disease, class III or above of Anesthesiologist's American Society, previous allergic reactions, and cough or taking other drugs that are also bradykinin-degrading enzyme inhibitors [19, 20].

This patient had several risk factors for severe angioedema: the therapy with ACE inhibitor which was not stopped, older age, Hispanic race, class III of Anesthesiologist's American Society, and coexistent cardiopulmonary disease.

The patient's therapy with ACE inhibitor, perindopril, was not stopped before surgery because the patient had no previous adverse reactions, and postoperatively he will stay in Burn Intensive Care Unit under safety vigilance. The ACE inhibitors intake suspension or replacement remains a dilemma. Researchers of Toronto General Hospital reviewed data from more than 61,000 perioperative patients and concluded that therapy with ACE inhibitors does not have additional morbidity or mortality. Although this evidence is encouraging, randomized prospective confirmatory trials must confirm that conclusion [21]. The American College of Physicians issued recommendations on the perioperative management of patients stating that clinicians should consider holding or reducing the usual dose of ACE inhibitors for better perioperative patient's hemodynamic stability [22, 23].

In the absence of adverse reactions, drug discontinuations have to be carefully planned and weighted [24, 25]. If patients have been recommended to discontinue ACE inhibitor and replace it, upon advice of a physician, such exchange should take place as early as possible. However, some studies revealed that patients are still at risk of developing angioedema during several months after therapeutic stop [26]. The patients with adverse reactions to ACE inhibitors can have safer alternatives with angiotensin II receptor blockers (ARBs) or calcium channel blockers [27, 28]. Although, there are reports that 10% of patients with previous ACE inhibitors angioedema also develop this adverse reaction after changing the medication to ARBs [29, 30].

The anesthetic airway manipulations are an additional risk factor for oropharyngeal edema. Although trauma may trigger angioedema, the intensity and time to onset are

not clear [31]. This patient had a nontraumatic supraglottic device (Igel); however we cannot exclude this etiology for angioedema trigger. Whenever possible, avoiding airway manipulating should be one of the angioedema preventive anesthetic attitudes for patients taking ACE inhibitor.

The postoperative vigilance is the main key for the anesthetic plan and safety of these patients. The oral edema severity of this case occurred five hours after the operation. Fortunately, the patient was under medical supervision in a specialized intensive care unit. Therefore, patients with recent ACE inhibitor intake should have postoperative surveillance suited to their conscientious autonomy and accessibility to emergency care units.

Our report raises the awareness of health care professionals for preventive attitudes. Probably in the near future the pharmacogenomics and personalized medicine applications can improve patient safety and prevent morbidity [32, 33].

4. Conclusions

Perioperative ACE inhibitor angioedema is a rare occurrence but can be life-threatening. Unfortunately, there is no specific test that can predict that adverse reaction. ACE inhibitor intake withdrawn is the main treatment and the only prophylactic measure to avoid the drug-induced angioedema.

Preoperative risk stratification aims to determine probabilities, optimize medical therapy, and modify risk factors. Before the surgery, patients with increased risk factors for severe cases of angioedema should withdraw ACE inhibitor as early as possible.

After the ACE inhibitors withdraw, the probability of angioedema lowers with the passing time. However the occurrence of angioedema should always be adequately surveyed.

References

[1] Audit INP, *Top Therapeutic Classes by Prescriptions*, MS National Prescription Audit PLUS, 2011, http://www.imshealth.com/deployedfiles/ims/Global/Content/Corporate/PressRoom/Top-LineMarketData&Trends/2011Top-lineMarketData/Top_Therapy_Classes_by_RX.pdf.

[2] T. Hoover, M. Lippmann, E. Grouzmann, F. Marceau, and P. Herscu, "Angiotensin converting enzyme inhibitor induced angio-oedema: a review of the pathophysiology and risk factors," *Clinical & Experimental Allergy*, vol. 40, no. 1, pp. 50–61, 2010.

[3] L. Stojiljkovic, "Renin-angiotensin system inhibitors and angioedema: anesthetic implications," *Current Opinion in Anaesthesiology*, vol. 25, no. 3, pp. 356–362, 2012.

[4] P. Sarkar, G. Nicholson, and G. Hall, "Brief review: Angiotensin converting enzyme inhibitors and angioedema: anesthetic implications," *Canadian Journal of Anesthesia*, vol. 53, no. 10, pp. 994–1003, 2006.

[5] D. A. Sica and H. R. Black, "Current concepts of pharmacotherapy in hypertension: ACE inhibitor-related angioedema: can angiotensin-receptor blockers be safely used?" *The Journal of Clinical Hypertension*, vol. 4, no. 5, pp. 375–380, 2002.

[6] S. Al-Khudari, M. J. Loochtan, E. Peterson, and K. L. Yaremchuk, "Management of angiotensin-converting enzyme inhibitor-induced angioedema," *Laryngoscope*, vol. 121, no. 11, pp. 2327–2334, 2011.

[7] A. P. Kaplan and M. W. Greaves, "Angioedema," *Journal of the American Academy of Dermatology*, vol. 53, no. 3, pp. 373–388, 2005.

[8] H. Makani, F. H. Messerli, J. Romero et al., "Meta-analysis of randomized trials of angioedema as an adverse event of renin-angiotensin system inhibitors," *The American Journal of Cardiology*, vol. 110, no. 3, pp. 383–391, 2012.

[9] D. R. Miller, S. A. Oliveria, D. R. Berlowitz, B. G. Fincke, P. Stang, and D. E. Lillienfeld, "Angioedema incidence in US veterans initiating angiotensin-converting enzyme inhibitors," *Hypertension*, vol. 51, no. 6, pp. 1624–1630, 2008.

[10] G. M. Gabb, P. Ryan, L. M. Wing, and K. A. Hutchinson, "Epidemiological study of angioedema and ACE inhibitors," *Australian & New Zealand Journal of Medicine*, vol. 26, no. 6, pp. 777–782, 1996.

[11] N. J. Brown, M. Snowden, and M. R. Griffin, "Recurrent angiotensin-converting enzyme inhibitor-associated angioedema," *The Journal of the American Medical Association*, vol. 278, no. 3, pp. 232–233, 1997.

[12] H. Wernze, "ACE inhibitor-induced angioedema: remarkable new perspectives for intensive care/emergency medicine," *Anasthesiol Intensivmed Notfallmed Schmerzther*, vol. 33, no. 10, pp. 637–641, 1998.

[13] G. Peltekis, D. Palaskas, M. Samanidou et al., "Severe migratory Angioedema due to ACE inhibitors use," *Hippokratia*, vol. 13, no. 2, pp. 122–124, 2009.

[14] O. Roche, A. Blanch, T. Caballero, N. Sastre, D. Callejo, and M. López-Trascasa, "Hereditary angioedema due to C1 inhibitor deficiency: Patient registry and approach to the prevalence in Spain," *Annals of Allergy, Asthma and Immunology*, vol. 94, no. 4, pp. 498–503, 2005.

[15] P. Coriat, C. Richer, T. Douraki et al., "Influence of chronic angiotensin-converting enzyme inhibition on anesthetic induction," *Anesthesiology*, vol. 81, no. 2, pp. 299–307, 1994.

[16] D. W. Pigott, C. Nagle, K. Allman, S. Westaby, and R. D. Evans, "Effect of omitting regular ACE inhibitor medication before cardiac surgery on haemodynamic variables and vasoactive drug requirements," *British Journal of Anaesthesia*, vol. 83, no. 5, pp. 715–720, 1999.

[17] Reducing and Preventing Adverse Drug Events to Decrease Hospital Costs, Agency for Healthcare Reasearch and Quality, U.S. Department of Health & Human Services, http://archive.ahrq.gov/research/findings/factsheets/errors-safety/aderia/ade.html.

[18] A. K. Jaffer and F. A. Michota, "Why perioperative medicine matters more than ever," *Cleveland Clinic Journal of Medicine*, vol. 73, supplement 1, p. S1, 2006.

[19] P. A. Loftus, M. Tan, G. Patel et al., "Risk factors associated with severe and recurrent angioedema: an epidemic linked to ACE-inhibitors," *The Laryngoscope*, 2014.

[20] T. Hoover, M. Lippmann, E. Grouzmann, F. Marceau, and P. Herscu, "Angiotensin converting enzyme inhibitor induced angio-oedema: a review of the pathophysiology and risk factors," *Clinical and Experimental Allergy*, vol. 40, no. 1, pp. 50–61, 2010.

[21] A. McCook, "ACE inhibitors before surgery may do no harm patients on blood pressure drugs experienced lower 30-day mortality," *Clinical Anesthesiology*, vol. 37, article 6, 2011.

[22] J. K. Ghali, "How to Keep Your Surgeon Out of Trouble. Perioperative Medicine: Risk Stratification," American College of Physicians, http://www.acponline.org/about_acp/chapters/ga/13-ghali.pdf.

[23] A. Prochazka, *Preoperative Evaluation Update*, American College of Physicians, 2014, http://www.acponline.org/about_acp/chapters/co/prochazka08.pdf.

[24] A. Ahmed, "Chronic heart failure in older adults," *Medical Clinics of North America*, vol. 95, no. 3, pp. 439–461, 2011.

[25] S. Beggs, A. Thompson, R. Nash, A. Tompson, and G. Peterson, "Cardiac failure in children," in *Proceedings of the 17th Expert Committee on the Selection and Use of Essential Medicines*, World Health Organization, Geneva, Switzerland, March 2009, http://www.who.int/selection_medicines/committees/expert/17/application/paediatric/Paed_Cardiac_Failure_Review.pdf.

[26] L. Beltrami, A. Zanichelli, L. Zingale, R. Vacchini, S. Carugo, and M. Cicardi, "Long-term follow-up of 111 patients with angiotensin-converting enzyme inhibitor-related angioedema," *Journal of Hypertension*, vol. 29, no. 11, pp. 2273–2277, 2011.

[27] J. Wang, S. Surbhi, and J. W. Kuhle, "Receipt of angiotensin-converting enzyme inhibitors or angiotensin II receptor blockers among Medicare beneficiaries with diabetes and hypertension," *Journal of Pharmaceutical Health Services Research*, vol. 5, no. 1, pp. 67–74, 2014.

[28] J. Alfie, L. S. Aparicio, and G. D. Waisman, "Current strategies to achieve further cardiac and renal protection through enhanced renin-angiotensin-aldosterone system inhibition," *Reviews on Recent Clinical Trials*, vol. 6, no. 2, pp. 134–146, 2011.

[29] P. Campo, T. D. Fernandez, G. Canto, and C. Mayorga, "Angioedema induced by angiotensin-converting enzyme inhibitors," *Current Opinion in Allergy and Clinical Immunology*, vol. 13, no. 4, pp. 337–344, 2013.

[30] M. Cicardi, L. C. Zingale, L. Bergamaschini, and A. Agostoni, "Angioedema associated with angiotensin-converting enzyme inhibitor use: outcome after switching to a different treatment," *Archives of Internal Medicine*, vol. 164, no. 8, pp. 910–913, 2004.

[31] D. Sondhi, M. Lippmann, and G. Murali, "Airway compromise due to angiotensin-converting enzyme inhibitor-induced angioedema: clinical experience at a large community teaching hospital," *Chest*, vol. 126, no. 2, pp. 400–404, 2004.

[32] M. Bochud, M. Burnier, and I. Guessous, "Top three pharmacogenomics and personalized medicine applications at the nexus of renal pathophysiology and cardiovascular medicine," *Current Pharmacogenomics and Personalized Medicine*, vol. 9, no. 4, pp. 299–322, 2011.

[33] P. J. S. Jacques and M. N. Minear, "Improving Perioperative Patient Safety Through the Use of Information Technology," http://www.ahrq.gov/professionals/quality-patient-safety/patient-safety-resources/resources/advances-in-patient-safety-2/vol4/Advances-StJacques_105.pdf.

21

Ambulatory Anesthesia in an Adult Patient with Corrected Hypoplastic Left Heart Syndrome

Jennifer Knautz, Yogen Asher, Mark C. Kendall, and Robert Doty Jr.

*Department of Anesthesiology, McGaw Medical Center, Feinberg School of Medicine,
Northwestern University, Chicago, IL 60611, USA*

Correspondence should be addressed to Jennifer Knautz, j-knautz@fsm.northwestern.edu

Academic Editors: M. Dauri, C.-H. Hsing, D. Lee, and I.-O. Lee

With recent advancements in clinical science, an increasing number of patients with congenital heart defects are surviving into adulthood and presenting for noncardiac surgeries. We describe one such example of a 26-year-old patient with corrected hypoplastic left heart syndrome presenting for knee arthroscopy and performed under general anesthesia with preoperative ultrasound guided saphenous nerve block. In this case, we review the anesthetic implications of corrected single ventricle physiology, anesthetic implications, as well as discuss the technique and role of saphenous nerve block in patients undergoing knee arthroscopy.

1. Introduction

Congenital heart defects occur in approximately 4–9/1000 live births. Advances in clinical science have resulted in an expected survival rate into adulthood of approximately 85% [1]. This allows adult patients with surgically corrected congenital heart defects to present for noncardiac surgery. A thorough understanding of their complex physiology is essential for safe anesthetic management. We present a case of a young adult patient with Fontan physiology who presented for ambulatory knee arthroscopy.

2. Case Report

A 26-year-old female with hypoplastic left heart syndrome (HLHS) presented to our ambulatory surgery center for knee arthroscopy for worsening knee pain. Her cardiac surgical history included undergoing a Norwood procedure at birth, Glen procedure at age 4 months, and Fontan procedure at age 5 years. Other medical history included hypertension, pacemaker insertion for sick sinus syndrome, lung arteriovenous malformations, and cirrhosis. Her exercise tolerance was greater than 4 metabolic equivalents, and her baseline oxygen saturation was 92–94% on room air. A summary of her preoperative evaluation can be seen in Table 1.

Preoperative consultation with the surgical team indicated the desire to maintain motor function of the leg post op. The anesthetic plan was thus a general anesthetic with laryngeal mask airway (LMA) and a preoperative mid-thigh saphenous nerve block for postoperative analgesia. After peripheral intravenous (IV) access and standard monitors were placed, she received 250 mL of 5% albumin, 1 mg midazolam, and 2 liters oxygen via nasal cannula. After chlorhexidine prep, a mid-thigh, ultrasound-guided saphenous nerve block was performed with a 22 gauge 90 millimeter (mm) Pajunk block needle. Bupivacaine 0.5% 10 mL with epinephrine 1:300 k added was injected without complication (see Figure 1 for sonoanatomy of saphenous nerve). The patient was pre-oxygenated, and general anesthesia was induced with 50 mcg of fentanyl and propofol in IV increments of 50 mg (total 200 mg). An LMA was placed with immediate return of spontaneous ventilation; anesthesia was maintained with 1 MAC of sevoflurane, oxygen, and air. The patient remained hemodynamically stable during the case (blood pressure and heart rate were maintained within 20% of preoperative baseline values). An additional 250 mL of 5% albumin was infused during the case. At the end of the case the LMA was removed without complication. The patient was transferred to the PACU, and following anesthesia recovery, was discharged home after approximately

TABLE 1: Preoperative evaluation.

PMH	Hypoplastic left heart
	Sick sinus with pacemaker
	Hypertension
	Cirrhosis
	Lung arteriovenous malformations
PSH	Norwood (at birth)
	Glen (at 4 m)
	Fontan (at 5 y)
	Cholecystectomy
	Tonsillectomy
	Wrist surgery
	Esophagogastroduodenoscopy
	Cardiac cath
Meds	Spironolactone
	Digoxin
	Atenolol
	Aspirin
	Hydrochlorothiazide
	Losartan
	Pantoprazole
	Potassium chloride
Labs	Hemoglobin 17.5, platelets of 100 [nadir 50]
	AST 49, ALT 70
	INR of 1.3
	Na 123, K 3.7, Cr 0.73, HCO_3 23
	Albumin 4.8, total protein 7.2
EKG	Heart rate 79 bpm, atrial-paced with 1° AV block, right access deviation,
	incomplete right bundle branch block, right ventricular hypertrophy,
	ST depression in precordial leads with T wave inversion (nonacute)
Echo	Grossly adequate myocardial function, no Fontan obstruction, unobstructed atrial septal defect, mild aortic regurgitation
Cardiac Cath	Patent superior vena cava to right pulmonary artery conduit with a saturation of 88%, mean pressure of 14 mmHg,
	inferior vena cava to left pulmonary artery conduit with a saturation of 85%, mean pressure of 14 mmHg

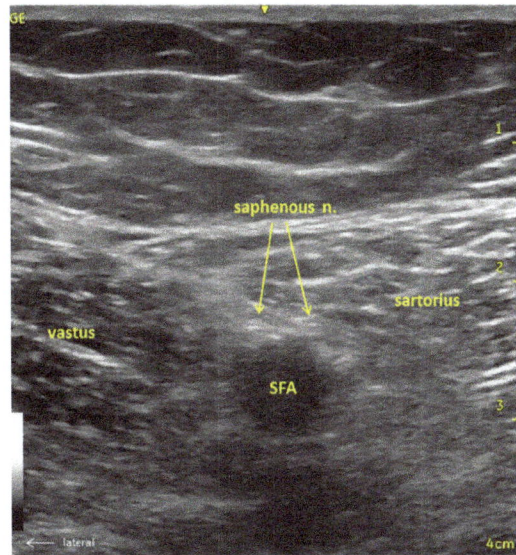

FIGURE 1: Sonoanatomy of saphenous nerve at mid-thigh.

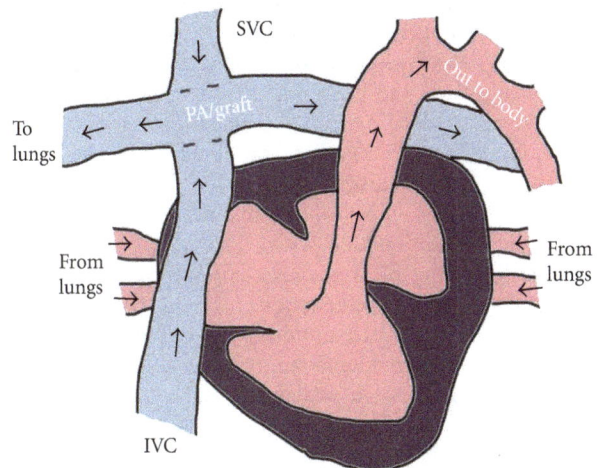

FIGURE 2: Simplified schematic depicting extracardiac Fontan physiology in HLHS. Deoxygenated blood is directly shunted to the lungs via graft to pulmonary arteries, then returned to heart via pulmonary veins where oxygenated blood can be pumped to the rest of the body.

90 minutes without the need for additional opioids. The patient denied any nausea, had no episodes of emesis, and her pain was well controlled. Her hemodynamics remained stable postoperatively. Her pacemaker, interrogated before and after the procedure, remained functioning during the entire perioperative period.

3. Discussion

Hypoplastic left heart syndrome is frequently repaired in 3 stages, with the final stage called a Fontan procedure where venous return is passively routed to the pulmonary arteries (see Figure 2). The cardiac output and pulmonary blood flow are determined by the transpulmonary gradient (the pressure difference between the systemic venous return and the pulmonary pressure). For this physiology to be effective, the goal systemic venous pressure should be approximately 10–15 mmHg with a pulmonary pressure of 5–10 mmHg, creating a driving pressure of 5–8 mmHg [2]. Because filling is passive, there must be adequate preload without obstruction to blood flow (patent grafts). Additionally, maintenance of sinus rhythm and a competent aortic valve are essential for adequate cardiac function.

Goals for our anesthetic management include maintenance of adequate preload, adequate oxygenation/ventilation to prevent pulmonary hypertension, adequate pain control, and avoiding nausea/vomiting, which could lead to dehydration and decreased preload postoperatively. While positive pressure has been used successfully in the past, its use may contribute to decreased venous return and increase pulmonary resistance, thus spontaneous ventilation should be used whenever possible. Approximately 4% of Fontan patients have a protein losing enteropathy that occurs via the GI tract. Thus, albumin was chosen for volume replacement in this case in order to maintain intravascular volume and to prevent third spacing of fluid given the diminished oncotic pressure from protein losing enteropathy. Hepatic dysfunction is common resulting from sluggish conduits and passive filling, and may necessitate evaluation prior to regional anesthesia.

The saphenous nerve is a distal branch of the posterior division of the femoral nerve, and branches into the infrapatellar branch (innervation to knee) and distal branches (antero-medial innervation of the lower leg/ankle). Midthigh, it lies between the vastus medialis and sartorius muscles adjacent to the superficial femoral artery (SFA). Saphenous nerve blocks have been used successfully to decrease pain scores and opioid consumption in patients undergoing knee arthroscopy [3] without interfering with quadricep function. In this case, the block was paramount in achieving intra- and postoperative pain control to avoid both the respiratory depressant and proemetic effects of opioids. In addition, given the possibility of liver dysfunction and increased risk of bleeding in this patient, this block is peripherally located. If bleeding was to occur from the block, compression could be used to control bleeding.

The combined effect of maintaining optimal cardiac function of this adult patient with HLHS under general anesthesia with diligent fluid management combined with preoperative placement of a saphenous nerve block to minimize the need for postoperative opioid use in the immediate peroperative period, provided a smooth uneventful course for an otherwise common outpatient surgical procedure.

References

[1] P. D. Bailey Jr. and D. R. Jobes, "The fontan patient," *Anesthesiology Clinics*, vol. 27, no. 2, pp. 285–300, 2009.

[2] P. Khairy, N. Poirier, and L. A. Mercier, "Univentricular heart," *Circulation*, vol. 115, no. 6, pp. 800–812, 2007.

[3] T. Akkaya, O. Ersan, D. Ozkan et al., "Saphenous nerve block is an effective regional technique for post-menisectomy pain," *Knee Surgery, Sports Traumatology, Arthroscopy*, vol. 16, no. 9, pp. 855–858, 2008.

22

Anesthetic Approach for a Patient with Jeune Syndrome

Mehmet I. Buget,[1] Emine Ozkan,[1] Ipek S. Edipoglu,[2] and Suleyman Kucukay[1]

[1]*Department of Anesthesiology, Istanbul Medical Faculty, Istanbul University, Fatih, 34093 Istanbul, Turkey*
[2]*Department of Anesthesiology, Suleymaniye Obstetrics & Pediatrics Training and Research Hospital, Zeytinburnu, 34116 Istanbul, Turkey*

Correspondence should be addressed to Mehmet I. Buget; mbuget@yahoo.com

Academic Editor: Mark Coburn

Jeune syndrome (JS) is an autosomal recessive disease also known as asphyxiating thoracic dystrophy. A narrow bell-shaped thoracic wall and short extremities are the most typical features of the syndrome. Prognosis in JS depends on the severity of the pulmonary hypoplasia caused by the chest wall deformity. Most patient deaths are due to respiratory problems at early ages. Herein, we report a case of JS patient, who was scheduled for femoral extension under general anesthesia. The severity of respiratory problems in JS patients is thought to diminish with age. Our case supported this theory, and we managed the anesthetic process uneventfully.

1. Introduction

Jeune syndrome (JS) was defined by Jeune et al. [1] in 1955 and is a rare form of skeletal dysplasia with an incidence of 1 in every 100,00–130,000 live births [2]. Jeune syndrome patients typically present with a narrow bell-shaped rib cage, a distended abdomen, and short arms and legs. Radiological examination often shows narrow chest cage, short and horizontal ribs, bicycle handlebar-shaped clavicle, pronounced costochondral junctions, short extremities, hypoplastic pelvic iliac wings, and acetabular bone protrusions (trident acetabulum) [3–5]. While the main characteristics of this syndrome are chest wall deformities and short extremities, renal, hepatic, pancreatic, and ocular involvements are also common [3, 6]. The structure of the thorax results in serious respiratory problems for JS patients [3]. During early childhood, they often die owing to respiratory distress. The severity of the thoracic deformity is the main prognostic factor [4, 7]. Infants with mild JS often present with recurrent respiratory infections. Renal and hepatic involvements are common among patients who survive the early childhood manifestations of JS, and these involvements often determine the prognosis [7, 8].

In this report, we present a case of JS in a 5-year-old boy who was scheduled for femur-lengthening surgery.

2. Case Description

We obtained written and oral informed consent from the patient's parents for the publication of the report. The patient was a 5-year-old boy born at term (weight: 3140 g; height: 47 cm). After birth, he was mechanically ventilated for 15 days and placed in the intensive care unit (ICU) for 23 days. He had tuberculosis at the age of 2 years and was prescribed antituberculosis drugs for 6 months. Until the age of 3 years, he had recurrent respiratory infections and underwent frequent hospitalizations. One year prior to this presentation, he underwent surgery for polydactyly and was in the ICU for a day.

His present medical examination showed height and weight of 85 cm and 16 kg, respectively, and a normal mental status. He had a long, narrow chest wall and bilateral short extremities (Figure 1). His respiratory examination showed normal results. Renal, hepatic, and ocular functions also were normal. Radiologic presentation showed a long and narrow thorax, short and horizontal costae, and bicycle handlebar-shaped clavicles (Figure 2).

Pulse oximetry and electrocardiogram (ECG) were performed, and arterial blood pressure was monitored. We preferred to use an inhalational agent for anesthetic induction, did not detect any respiratory problem or desaturation events. He was transferred to the ward after his modified Aldrete Score was 10.

3. Discussion

Jeune syndrome is one of the ciliopathies, and diagnosis is mostly based on clinical and radiological findings [4, 7]. Cilia are microtubule structures that support cell proliferation and differentiation, neural development, and tissue integrity. In ciliary disorders, multiple tissues and organs are often involved [9]. In our case, genetic analysis of the TCTEX1D2 gene, which is associated with JS and ciliopathies, revealed a homozygotic change [10, 11]. In the antenatal period, skeletal changes characteristic of JS can be identified by ultrasonography (USG) and subsequently diagnosed with genetic amniocentesis [12, 13]. Our patient was similarly diagnosed during the pregnancy.

Most JS patients die because of respiratory problems caused by chest deformities in early childhood. As the severity of the chest wall deformity is important for patient prognosis and because JS patients are often treated for recurrent respiratory infections preoperative anesthetic examination should be thorough and clinicians should be vigilant during respiratory examination. A chest radiograph, laboratory tests, and physical examinations should be performed. If a respiratory impairment is detected, blood gas analysis and spirometry are also advisable. In the preoperative settings, JS patients' lung volumes are reduced due to pulmonary hypoplasia, and, with positive-pressure ventilation, barotrauma and pneumothorax may occur [14, 15]. Additionally, increased thoracic pressure can decrease venous return and diminish cardiac output [2]. For these reasons, JS patients' ventilation settings and regular follow-ups are very important. The lowest possible peak pressure ventilation should be provided. Hence, Saletti et al. suggested pressure-controlled ventilation and Şahin et al. suggested low tidal volume (7 mL/kg and 16/min frequency) strategies in their reports [2, 14]. Both strategies were applicable to our case. We used pressure-controlled ventilation and the lowest possible peak pressure, and we managed to avoid any barotrauma risks.

Different surgical techniques are available to facilitate chest wall volume increases in the management of JS, although the success of the treatment depends on the level of the pulmonary hypoplasia [3, 16].

De Vries et al., in their case series involving 13 patients, proposed that JS patients who survive early childhood present with relatively diminished respiratory problems later in life [3]. They reported that 11 of their 13 patients had milder respiratory problems at older ages than they did in early childhood, possibly because the mechanical properties of the thorax get sufficiently altered with growth [3]. Our case supports this hypothesis. In our case, artificial respiration was needed for postpartum respiratory failure resulting from pulmonary hypoplasia. After 1 month of respiratory support, intensive care was no longer needed. Until 3 years of age, he was hospitalized for intermittent respiratory infections, for which he received treatments. At the age of 5, he underwent the surgical procedure described herein, without any serious

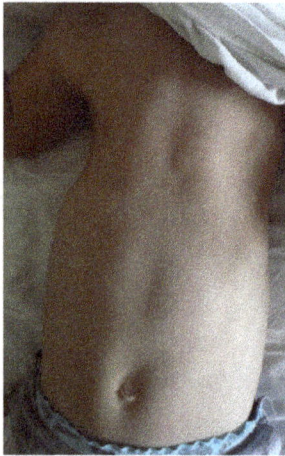

Figure 1: Narrow, long rib cage.

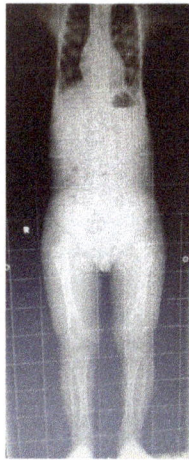

Figure 2: Radiography of patient. A long and narrow thorax, short and horizontal costae, and short extremities.

because his Mallampati score was 1. We induced general anesthesia with 8% sevoflurane and mask ventilation. Once the mask ventilation was successful, we placed an intravenous catheter for fentanyl (2 μg/kg) and rocuronium (0,6 mg/kg) administration. We intubated the trachea with a 5.0 cuffed endotracheal tube. We did not detect any problems during the intubation. We preferred pressure-controlled mechanical ventilation for our patient. The anesthesia was maintained with 2% sevoflurane, 40% oxygen, and 60% nitrogen. The operation was uneventful. The perioperative ventilation parameters were as follows: 20 mmHg peak pressure and 110 mL tidal volume with a frequency of 18/min. His arterial blood gas analyses showed the following: pH, 7,38; pO_2, 164 mmHg; pCO_2, 42 mmHg; and oxygen saturation, 99%. Length of the operation was 135 minutes. We did not use muscle relaxation monitor for our patient because to our knowledge we could not detect any association between JS and delayed recovery from muscle relaxants in the literature. The patient's trachea was successfully extubated after we ensured sufficient respiratory efforts. He was under observation for an hour in the postanesthesia care unit (PACU). We adverse events. We acknowledge that an absolute conclusion about the diminishing of JS-related respiratory problems with age is not possible, noting that Leroy et al. presented a case of JS in a 13-year-old patient with respiratory problems [17].

Thirty percent of JS patients are thought to have renal insufficiency [3]. Kidney involvement, which can be detected by clinical and objective findings, typically would be seen after 2 years of age [3]. In our case, recent kidney function tests and radiological studies were unremarkable. In JS, complications characterized by increases in transaminase levels, hepatomegaly, liver involvement, and pancreatic insufficiency, sometimes resulting in portal hypertension, can occur [3, 6]. In our patient, there were no clinical and radiological findings of any liver and pancreatic insufficiency. Jeune syndrome patients can show various kinds of ocular involvement such as retinitis pigmentosa. We did not detect any eye problems in our patient.

We suggest a thorough anesthetic profiling for patients with JS, because the disorder can involve different organs. Respiratory evaluation is of utmost importance for these patients, as it can have fatal consequences, especially in younger patients. We believe that patients with JS would be better suited for comprehensive surgeries at older ages than at early childhood given that respiratory complications can diminish with age in most cases.

References

[1] M. Jeune, C. Béraud, and R. Carron, "Dystrophie thoracique asphyxiante de caractère familial," *Archives Françaises de Pédiatrie*, vol. 12, pp. 886–891, 1955.

[2] D. Saletti, T. R. Grigio, D. Tonelli, O. D. Ribeiro Júnior, and F. Marini, "Case report: anesthesia in patients with asphyxiating thoracic dystrophy: Jeune syndrome," *Revista Brasileira de Anestesiologia*, vol. 62, no. 3, pp. 424–431, 2012.

[3] J. De Vries, J. L. Yntema, C. E. Van Die, N. Crama, E. A. M. Cornelissen, and B. C. J. Hamel, "Jeune syndrome: description of 13 cases and a proposal for follow-up protocol," *European Journal of Pediatrics*, vol. 169, no. 1, pp. 77–88, 2010.

[4] F. Oberklaid, D. M. Danks, V. Mayne, and P. Campbell, "Asphyxiating thoracic dysplasia. Clinical, radiological, and pathological information on 10 patients," *Archives of Disease in Childhood*, vol. 52, no. 10, pp. 758–765, 1977.

[5] C. Poggiani, M. C. Gasparoni, G. Mangili, and A. Colombo, "Asphyxiating thoracic dysplasia in a lethal form: radiological and sonographic findings," *Minerva Pediatrica*, vol. 52, no. 1-2, pp. 63–66, 2000.

[6] S. N. Reddy, B. A. Seth, and P. Colaco, "Jeune syndrome with neonatal cholestasis," *Indian Journal of Pediatrics*, vol. 78, no. 9, pp. 1151–1153, 2011.

[7] A. Verma and H. S. Gurudatta, "Jeune syndrome," *Indian Pediatrics*, vol. 41, no. 9, pp. 954–955, 2004.

[8] P. Labrune, M. Fabre, P. Trioche et al., "Jeune syndrome and liver disease: report of three cases treated with ursodeoxycholic acid,"

American Journal of Medical Genetics, vol. 87, no. 4, pp. 324–328, 1999.

[9] C. Huber and V. Cormier-Daire, "Ciliary disorder of the skeleton," *American Journal of Medical Genetics Part C: Seminars in Medical Genetics*, vol. 160, no. 3, pp. 165–174, 2012.

[10] M. Schmidts, H. H. Arts, E. M. H. F. Bongers et al., "Exome sequencing identifies DYNC2H1 mutations as a common cause of asphyxiating thoracic dystrophy (Jeune syndrome) without major polydactyly, renal or retinal involvement," *Journal of Medical Genetics*, vol. 50, no. 5, pp. 309–323, 2013.

[11] Y. Çelik, B. Akbas, M. Keçeli, and A. E. Arslanköylü, "A rare cause of respiratory failure in a newborn: Jeune Syndrome," *Türk Toraks Dergisi*, vol. 14, pp. 161–163, 2013.

[12] C.-P. Chen, S.-P. Lin, F.-F. Liu, S.-W. Jan, S.-Y. Lin, and C.-C. Lan, "Prenatal diagnosis of asphyxiating thoracic dysplasia (Jeune syndrome)," *American Journal of Perinatology*, vol. 13, no. 8, pp. 495–498, 1996.

[13] N. S. Den Hollander, S. G. F. Robben, A. J. M. Hoogeboom, M. F. Niermeijer, and J. W. Wladimiroff, "Early prenatal sonographic diagnosis and follow-up of Jeune syndrome," *Ultrasound in Obstetrics and Gynecology*, vol. 18, no. 4, pp. 378–383, 2001.

[14] N. Şahin, H. Kara, F. Ertuğrul, T. Aydogdu Titiz, and E. İçel, "Jeune syndrome and anesthesia: case report," *Turkiye Klinikleri Journal of Anesthesiology Reanimation*, vol. 5, pp. 150–153, 2007.

[15] L. M. Borland, "Anesthesia for children with Jeune's syndrome (asphyxiating thoracic dystrophy)," *Anesthesiology*, vol. 66, no. 1, pp. 86–88, 1987.

[16] F. Özçay, M. Derbent, B. Demirhan, K. Tokel, and Ü. Saatçi, "A family with Jeune syndrome," *Pediatric Nephrology*, vol. 16, no. 8, pp. 623–626, 2001.

[17] P. Leroy, M. Martens, N. Schott, and N. Cobben, "Late respiratory failure in Jeune syndrome," *European Journal of Pediatrics*, vol. 169, no. 3, pp. 375–376, 2010.

23

Uncommon Cause of Trigeminal Neuralgia: Tentorial Ossification over Trigeminal Notch

Sun Woo Bang,[1] **Kyung Ream Han,**[2] **Seung Ho Kim,**[2] **Won Ho Jeong,**[2]
Eun Jin Kim,[2] **Jin Wook Choi,**[3] **and Chan Kim**[2]

[1]*Department of Radiology, Kim Chan Hospital, 228 Hyowon-ro, Gwonseon-gu, Suwon 441-822, Republic of Korea*
[2]*Department of Pain Medicine, Kim Chan Hospital, 228 Hyowon-ro, Gwonseon-gu, Suwon 441-822, Republic of Korea*
[3]*Department of Cardiovascular Surgery, Kim Chan Hospital, 228 Hyowon-ro, Gwonseon-gu, Suwon 441-822, Republic of Korea*

Correspondence should be addressed to Sun Woo Bang; mdrbsw@gmail.com

Academic Editor: Alparslan Apan

Ossification of the tentorium cerebelli over the trigeminal notch is rare, but it may cause compression of the trigeminal nerve, leading to trigeminal neuralgia (TN). We were unable to find any previously reported cases with radiological evaluation, although we did find one case with surgically proven ossification of the tentorium cerebelli. Here, we present a case of TN caused by tentorial ossification over the trigeminal notch depicted on magnetic resonance imaging (MRI) and computed tomography (CT).

1. Introduction

Calcifications or ossifications in the free edges of the tentorium cerebelli, in the so- called tentorial notch, are frequent and age-related physiologic and neurodegenerative changes [1]. However, ossification of the tentorium cerebelli over the trigeminal notch is rare and may cause compression of the trigeminal nerve, leading to trigeminal neuralgia (TN) [2]. We report a case of TN secondary to tentorial ossification over the trigeminal notch depicted on magnetic resonance imaging (MRI) and computed tomography (CT).

2. Case Description

A 35-year-old woman visited the hospital with a chief complaint of left facial pain that had lasted one week. She had experienced three episodes of the pain over the past four years. Each pain attack lasted three or four months, with a pain-free period. The pain affected the left maxillary and temporal regions and the inside of the ear. The nature of the pain was electric-shock-like, paroxysmal, and lancinating. The intensity of the pain was 10 on the visual analogue scale (no pain is 0; imaginary maximal pain is 10). The pain was aggravated or precipitated by talking, swallowing, opening

the mouth, and eating. Neurologic examination was negative including sensory deficits. The clinical diagnosis was TN in the left maxillary and mandibular distribution. A brain MRI was performed to rule out other causes of the patient's facial pain. The MRI scan was obtained using a 1.5 Tesla MRI scanner (Signa HDxt, GE Healthcare Systems, Wauwatosa, WI, USA). Axial MR images with 3D fast imaging with steady-state acquisition (3D FIESTA) sequence (TR, 5.1 ms; TE, 2.0 ms; slice thickness, 1.0 mm; FOV, 22 × 22 cm; matrix, 320 × 320; and NEX, 1) showed nodular lesions with dark signal intensity adjacent to the porus trigeminus. The lesions were impinging upon the cisternal segment of the left trigeminal nerve (Figure 1). There was no evidence of vascular contact or compression of the cisternal segment of the left trigeminal nerve. The radiological diagnosis was ossification of the tentorium cerebelli over the trigeminal notch. A pain intervention doctor performed a diagnostic block of the left mandibular nerve with local anesthetics (Figure 2) and the patient's pain disappeared for about one hour. A brain CT (Brivo CT385, GE Healthcare Systems) obtained after the diagnostic block showed dense plaque-like ossification of the tentorium cerebelli over the trigeminal notch and an air bubble adjacent to left Meckel's cave (Figure 3). The patient was unable to eat meals or talk even after medications. Informed

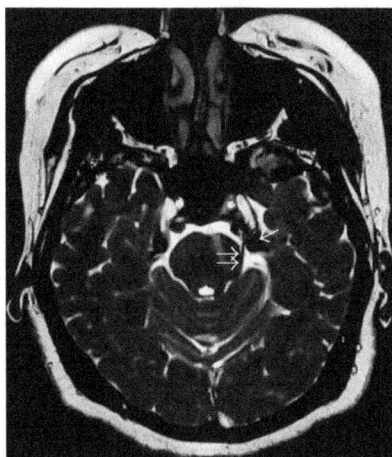

FIGURE 1: Axial 3D FIESTA MR image shows nodular lesions (arrow) with dark signal intensity adjacent to the porus trigeminus bilaterally. The cisternal segment of the left trigeminal nerve (double arrows) is impinged by nodular lesions.

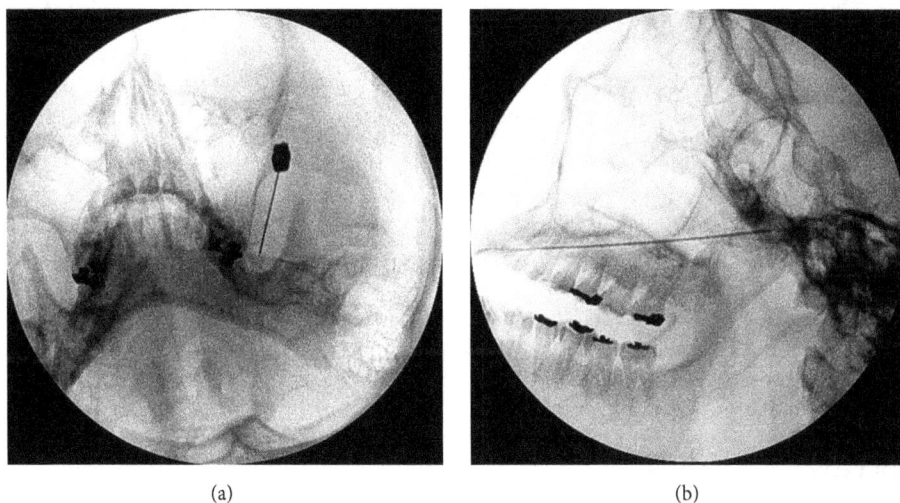

(a)   (b)

FIGURE 2: Fluoroscopy-guided diagnostic block of the left mandibular nerve. Anteroposterior (a) and lateral (b) views show the needle tip directed toward the left foramen ovale.

consent was obtained for a left mandibular nerve block with alcohol. Under fluoroscopic guidance, a left mandibular nerve block was performed with 0.5 mL of alcohol, and the patient's pain was completely relieved.

3. Discussion

The tentorium cerebelli is one of the most common sites of intracranial physiologic calcification [1]. In fact, the mineralization of the tentorium as visualized on radiographs is ossification rather than calcification [2]. Intracranial physiologic ossifications are generally unaccompanied by any evidence of disease and have no demonstrable pathologic cause. Ossifications of the falx, dura mater, or tentorium cerebelli occur in about 10% of the elderly population. Dural and tentorial ossifications usually have a laminar pattern and can occur anywhere within the cranium [1]. However, ossification of the tentorium cerebelli over the trigeminal notch is rare and is

a possible cause of TN [2]. Anatomically, the porus trigeminus, the opening of Meckel's cave, is bounded superiorly by the tentorium cerebelli and inferiorly by the trigeminal notch [2]. Standefer et al. reported a clinical case of TN secondary to tentorial ossification. However, the site of ossification was near the tentorial notch, somewhat apart from the trigeminal notch. Furthermore, there was no description of radiological evaluation such as by MRI and CT of the tentorial ossification; there was merely an artist's depiction of the operative procedure [3]. According to the International Classification of Headache Disorders, the etiology of TN is divided into classical TN, caused by vascular compression of the trigeminal root entry zone, and symptomatic TN, caused by tumors, demyelination, and vascular disorders [4]. Routine brain MRI reveals structural causes in up to 15% of TN patients [5]. The most common causes of symptomatic TN are cerebellopontine angle tumors and multiple sclerosis. As we know, typical ossification of the tentorium cerebelli shows laminar

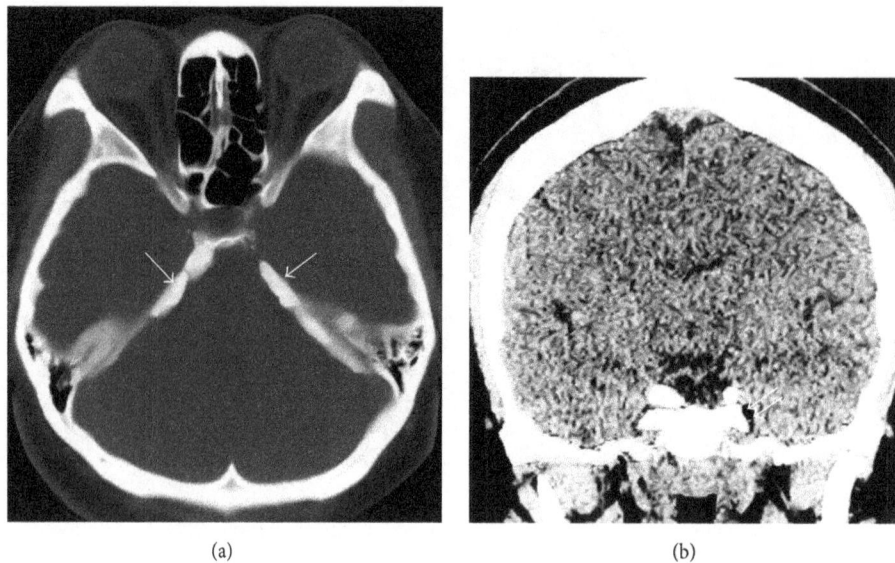

(a)   (b)

FIGURE 3: Brain CT image shows plaque-like tentorial ossification (arrow) on bone window (a) and an air bubble (double arrows) adjacent to left Meckel's cave on brain window (b).

or mildly nodular patterns and is a clinically insignificant finding [1]. But if the ossification is prominent, as observed in our case, compression of the cisternal segment of the trigeminal nerve is possible and symptomatic TN may develop.

On initial examination, the patient in this case presented with paroxysmal pain in the temporal area and inner ear triggered by swallowing and the authors considered that the most likely diagnosis would be trigeminal neuralgia combined with glossopharyngeal neuralgia. However, diagnostic mandibular nerve block produced complete pain relief for the duration of action of the local anesthetic, and a subsequently performed neurolytic mandibular nerve block led the patient to be pain-free.

We have described a case of TN caused by unusually prominent ossification of the tentorium cerebelli over the trigeminal notch that was depicted on MRI and CT.

References

[1] Y. Kıroğlu, C. Çallı, N. Karabulut, and C. Öncel, "Intracranial calcifications on CT," *Diagnostic and Interventional Radiology*, vol. 16, pp. 263–269, 2010.

[2] A. Perumal and M. Gayathri, "Anatomical study on ossification of tentorium cerebelli over the trigeminal notch," *International Journal of Health Sciences and Research*, vol. 4, no. 6, pp. 52–55, 2014.

[3] M. Standefer, J. W. Bay, and D. F. Dohn, "Trigeminal neuralgia secondary to a tentorial ossification: a case report," *Neurosurgery*, vol. 11, no. 4, pp. 527–529, 1982.

[4] Headache Classification Committee of the International Headache Society (IHS), "The International Classification of Headache Disorders, 3rd edition (beta version)," *Cephalalgia*, vol. 33, no. 9, pp. 629–808, 2013.

[5] M. Obermann and Z. Katsarava, "Update on trigeminal neuralgia," *Expert Review of Neurotherapeutics*, vol. 9, no. 3, pp. 323–329, 2009.

24

"High Frequency/Small Tidal Volume Differential Lung Ventilation": A Technique of Ventilating the Nondependent Lung of One Lung Ventilation for Robotically Assisted Thoracic Surgery

Bassam M. Shoman, Hany O. Ragab, Ammar Mustafa, and Rashid Mazhar

Cardiothoracic Anesthesia Department, Heart Hospital, Hamad Medical Corporation, P.O. Box 3050, Doha, Qatar

Correspondence should be addressed to Bassam M. Shoman; baskalito@hotmail.com

Academic Editor: Maria Jose C. Carmona

With the introduction of new techniques and advances in the thoracic surgery fields, challenges to the anesthesia techniques had became increasingly exponential. One of the great improvements that took place in the thoracic surgical field was the use of the robotically assisted thoracic surgical procedure and minimally invasive endoscopic thoracic surgery. One lung ventilation technique represents the core anesthetic management for the success of those surgical procedures. Even with the use of effective one lung ventilation, the patient hemodynamics and respiratory parameters could be deranged and could not be tolerating the procedure that could compromise the end result of surgery. We are presenting our experience in managing one patient who suffered persistent hypoxia and hemodynamic instability with one lung ventilation for robotically assisted thymectomy procedure and how it was managed till the completion of the surgery successfully.

1. Introduction

The development of lung isolation and one lung ventilation (OLV) accelerated the evolution of thoracic surgery as a subspecialty. Before the introduction of endotracheal tube and the cuffed endotracheal tube, only select few intrathoracic procedures were feasible. Rapid lung movement and quickly developing respiratory distress made the surgical procedures difficult and risky. Selective ventilation of one lung changed this scenario. It was first described in 1931 by Gale and Water and quickly led to increasingly complex lung resection surgery, with the first published pneumonectomy for cancer in 1933 [1]. Techniques and apparatus used for OLV have changed significantly in recent years. These changes have come largely in response to an increased use of OLV during lung surgery and the advent of newer, minimally invasive surgical procedures, whereas OLV in the operating room or intensive care unit was once viewed as a complex endeavor largely managed by experts in academic institutions. The introduction of newer limited access thoracic and cardiac procedures has made it necessary as anesthesia staff members to master lung isolation techniques. Modification of OLV technique is sometimes needed during the procedure to face the potential problems that could change the plans and covert the procedure to conventional lung ventilation. The well-known methods of increasing FIO_2, applying PEEP to the ventilated lung, use of CPAP to the nonventilated lung, or intermittent reinflation of the collapsed lung may not work to improve hypoxia and hypercarbia associated with OLV.

In this case report we are presenting a modification of the differential lung ventilation technique for managing hypoxia and hypercarbia during robotic assisted thymectomy using OLV [2].

2. Case Report

A 35-year-old female Asian patient who is known to be nonsmoker and nonalcoholic referred by the infection control department to the cardiothoracic surgery team after being treated from military tuberculosis by short-term anti-tuberculous regimen for 4 months. She had no neurological signs or symptoms of note. Her physical examination was unremarkable. She was a small-sized person with a body weight of 42 Kg and height of 142 cm.

Routine laboratory works were within normal limits; sputum microscopy was negative for acid-fast bacilli and no mycobacterium was isolated with culture and sensitivity tests. Also serology tests are negative for HbsAg, HCV, and HIV.

CT scan of chest had shown an anterior mediastinal mass, which measured 1.8 cm in its maximum anteroposterior diameter and 4.8 cm in its side-to-side dimensions with multiple peripherally located reticulonodular opacities suggesting tuberculous infection. Chest X-ray showed multiple faint nodular opacities noted in the right apical region with midprominence of the right hilar vascular shadows. The left lung field and both costophrenic angles were clear.

Patient was scheduled for robotic assisted thymus tumor excision with a working diagnosis of Thymic TB versus Thymoma.

On the day of the operation, her vital signs were HR 120/min, sinus rhythm, BP 150/80 mmHg, and SpO_2 98% on room air.

In the operation theater, patient was prepared by applying left peripheral venous cannula and right radial artery cannula. Monitoring intraoperatively consists of 5 leads ECG, pulse oximetry, invasive and noninvasive blood pressure, nasopharyngeal temperature, urine output, and bispectral index. Respiratory parameters' monitoring consisted of peak inspiratory pressure, gas analyzer, and O_2 monitor.

Anesthesia was induced by intravenous injection of propofol 2.5 mg/kg, fentanyl 1.5 mcg/kg, and cisatracurium 0.2 mg/kg followed by endotracheal intubation by double lumen Rusch Robertshaw Endobronchial Tubes Left Bronchus of 35F size and secured at 30 cm at lip level. Position is confirmed by routine breath sound auscultation algorithm. Tube position could not be checked by fiberoptic bronchoscopy only in this instance, as it was not available in theatre on the day of surgery for logistic reason of repair and disinfection. Two anesthetists reconfirm the position by auscultating all chest quadrants and again after port access of the thoracoscope with visual examination of proper lung ventilation during single lung ventilation.

Anesthesia was maintained by intermittent doses of muscle relaxants and fentanyl with inhalational sevoflurane anesthesia.

Patient was placed in supine position with a 30-degree leftward tilt. The endotracheal tube position was reconfirmed after position by auscultating all chest quadrants for effective OLV. The dependent lung was ventilated at respiratory rate of 14/minute, tidal volume of 350 mL, and PEEP of 5 cm H_2O.

Surgery was performed using a da Vinci Si Robotic system, with four portals. A 7 × 5 cm bulky highly vascular Thymus was excised clearing the region between phrenic to phrenic nerves and vertically from innominate vein till diaphragm.

After starting OLV the patient developed desaturation up to 87% with gradually rising up of $ETCO_2$ to 45 mmHg. To solve the problem, FIO_2 was first increased to 0.1 and then 6 cm H_2O PEEP applied to the ventilated lung and 5 cm H_2O CPAP applied to the nonventilated lung but patients' condition unfortunately did not improve. Intermittent reinflation of the collapsed lung by manual ventilation was done to overcome the desaturation problem with marked improvement of SpO_2 to 100% immediately. Again right lung was collapsed to resume the procedure with trial of pressure-controlled ventilation to the ventilated lung but again this maneuver did not improve the condition. We noticed that ventilating the collapsed lung manually with very small tidal volume and at a high rate of 35 to 40 breath per minute (i.e., pediatric mode of ventilation) through the CPAP circuit did not interfere with the surgical field exposure. In fact, the maneuver maintained SpO_2 saturation to 99-100% and $ETCO_2$ remained below 40 mmHg. ABG done after 10 minutes of this method of ventilation showed PaO_2 of 217 mmHg and $PaCO_2$ of 44 mmHg. Portable ventilation is connected to the nonventilated lung double lumen tube limb with pediatric mode of ventilation of tidal volume of 60 mL, respiratory rate of 35/minute, PEEP of 2 cm H_2O in order not to interfere with the surgical field, and I : E ratio range from 1 : 2 to 1 : 3. Patient maintained SpO_2 of 99-100% and $ETCO_2$ of 35–38 mmHg all through the procedure. The dependent lung was continued to be ventilated through the anesthesia machine ventilator at the same starting parameters. Surgery was accomplished robotically with complete excision of the tumor without any interfering effect of this mode of ventilation to the collapsed right lung.

At the end of the procedure, patient was extubated on the operating table and transferred to the recovery room for 2 hours monitoring and then transferred to wardroom. Patient was discharged from the hospital on the 5th postoperative day and followed up in the thoracic surgery clinic with normal postprocedure course.

3. Discussion

Differential lung ventilation is a well-known technique for ventilating patient with unilateral lung disease in the critical care settings in the ICU [3]. However, using this technique intraoperatively in the operative suite setting is rarely applied. Conventional one lung ventilation technique provides satisfactory gas exchange in the majority of cases. However, in some cases hypoxemia may occur secondary to the obligatory right to left transpulmonary shunt through the nonventilated, nondependent lung [4]. Another factor which could be added to the presented case is the past history of miliary pulmonary tuberculosis 6 months prior to the procedure. These factors will result in a much larger alveolar arterial oxygen difference and lower PaO_2 than does OLV. However, blood flow to the nonventilated lung is usually reduced by gravity in the complete lateral decubitus position, active hypoxic pulmonary vasoconstriction in the nonventilated lung, and nondependent lung collapse [5]. Watanabe et al. had investigated the effect of gravity as a major determinate of shunt and perfusion during thoracotomy procedures. Patients undergoing right thoracotomy were divided into three groups. One group was supine, one group was placed in the left semilateral decubitus position, and the third group was placed in the left full-lateral position. All patients were ventilated with 100% oxygen, and arterial blood gas samples were analyzed every 5 min after intentional collapse of the right lung. PaO_2 progressively decreased in all groups after two-lung ventilation (TLV) was discontinued. Nine out of 11 patients in the supine group experienced arterial oxyhemoglobin saturation (SaO_2) of less than 90% and had to have TLV reinstituted. Only one out of nine patients in the semilateral group and one out of 13 patients in the full-lateral group experienced that degree of hypoxemia. The time for PaO_2 to decrease to 200 mmHg after the start of SLV was very rapid: 354 s in the supine group compared with 583 s in the semilateral group and 794 s in the full-lateral group [6].

Bardoczky et al. compared the effects of position and fraction of inspired oxygen (FiO_2) during thoracic surgery. Randomly assigned patients were ventilated with a FiO_2 of 0.4, 0.6, or 1.0 during periods of TLV and SLV in the supine and lateral positions. PaO_2 decreased more during SLV compared with TLV in all groups in both positions. In all three groups PaO_2 was significantly higher during SLV in the lateral than in the supine position [7]. Those studies demonstrated that, during SLV with a patient in the full-lateral position, gravity augments the redistribution of perfusion to the ventilated lung, resulting in a better V/Q match and a higher PaO_2.

As a result of these factors, the degree of shunt and hence conventional ventilation with 100% oxygen is usually associated with accepted PaO_2 values. As in robotic thoracic surgery, partial lateral decubitus position with 30–45 degree surgery side up is utilized; blood flow to the nondependent lung is not completely reduced to decrease the shunt fraction, attributing to patient hypoxia as another added factor. As we had CPAP breathing circuit applied to the nondependent limb of the double lumen tube, the main advantage of this breathing circuit is that it has small reservoir bag that can be utilized for manually ventilating the collapsed lung with small pediatric tidal volumes simulating baby lung ventilation. Manually ventilating the lung all throughout the whole length of the procedure is not practically feasible in all situations and subjected to personal variations. Mechanically ventilating the nondependent lung with portable ventilator utilizing the pediatric mode of ventilation can replace this manual technique. We find it very effective in improving the oxygenation of the patient with decreased FIO_2 of the ventilated lung to 0.8 and at the same time, not disturbing the operative field.

Differential lung ventilation can be used during thoracotomy, VATS procedure, or robotically assisted thoracoscopic cardiac or thoracic surgery whenever OLV is followed by hypoxemia despite adequate ventilation of the dependent lung with 100% oxygen and failed other techniques to maintain oxygen saturation [8].

References

[1] J. Lohser, "Evidence-based management of one-lung ventilation," *Anesthesiology Clinics*, vol. 26, no. 2, pp. 241–272, 2008.

[2] W. Karzai and K. Schwarzkopf, "Hypoxemia during one-lung ventilation: prediction, prevention, and treatment," *Anesthesiology*, vol. 110, no. 6, pp. 1402–1411, 2009.

[3] D. Anantham, R. Jagadesan, and P. E. C. Tiew, "Clinical review: independent lung ventilation in critical care," *Critical Care*, vol. 9, no. 6, pp. 594–600, 2005.

[4] A. Baraka, "Differential lung ventilation as an alternative to one-lung ventilation during thoracotomy. Report of three cases," *Anaesthesia*, vol. 49, no. 10, pp. 881–882, 1994.

[5] S. Ishikawa, K. Nakazawa, and K. Makita, "Progressive changes in arterial oxygenation during one-lung anaesthesia are related to the response to compression of the non-dependent lung," *British Journal of Anaesthesia*, vol. 90, no. 1, pp. 21–26, 2003.

[6] S. Watanabe, E. Noguchi, S. Yamada, N. Hamada, and T. Kano, "Sequential changes of arterial oxygen tension in the supine position during one-lung ventilation," *Anesthesia and Analgesia*, vol. 90, no. 1, pp. 28–34, 2000.

[7] G. I. Bardoczky, L. L. Szegedi, A. A. d'Hollander, J.-M. Moures, P. De Francquen, and J.-C. Yernault, "Two-lung and one-lung ventilation in patients with chronic obstructive pulmonary disease: the effects of position and FiO_2," *Anesthesia and Analgesia*, vol. 90, no. 1, pp. 35–41, 2000.

[8] S. Cho, J. Lee, and M. Kim, "New method for reexpansion pulmonary edema: differential lung ventilation," *The Annals of Thoracic Surgery*, vol. 80, pp. 1933–1934, 2005.

25

Intraoperatively Diagnosed Tracheal Tear after Using an NIM EMG ETT with Previously Undiagnosed Tracheomalacia

Minal Joshi,[1] Simon Mardakh,[1] Joel Yarmush,[1] H. Kamath,[1] Joseph Schianodicola,[1] and Ernesto Mendoza[2]

[1] *Department of Anesthesiology, New York Methodist Hospital, 506 6th street, Brooklyn, NY 11215, USA*
[2] *Department of Surgery, New York Methodist Hospital, 506 6th Street, Brooklyn, NY 11215, USA*

Correspondence should be addressed to Minal Joshi; minuday2000@gmail.com

Academic Editors: M. J. C. Carmona and L. Hebbar

Tracheal rupture is a rare complication of endotracheal intubation. We present a case of tracheal rupture that was diagnosed intraoperatively after the use of an NIM EMG endotracheal tube. A 66-year-old female with a recurrent multinodular goiter was scheduled for total thyroidectomy. Induction of anesthesia was uncomplicated. Intubation was atraumatic using a 6 mm NIM EMG endotracheal tube (ETT). Approximately 90 minutes into the surgery, a tracheal tear was suspected. After confirming the diagnosis, conservative treatment with antibiotic coverage was favored. The patient made a full recovery with no complications. Diagnosis of the tracheal tear was made intraoperatively, prompting early management.

1. Introduction

Tracheal rupture is a rare iatrogenic complication, most commonly due to blunt trauma outside the hospital setting. It is occasionally a complication of surgical manipulation of the trachea. It can also complicate orotracheal intubation due to the tip of endotracheal tube (ETT) getting caught in the fold of posterior trachea during insertion. Diagnosis usually waits until after extubation based on clinical suspicion and confirmed by bronchoscopy. If not properly managed, severe respiratory distress and even death may result. We present a case of tracheal rupture that was diagnosed intraoperatively via bronchoscopy and managed conservatively.

2. Case Presentation

A 66-year-old female with a history of a subtotal thyroidectomy 20 years ago was scheduled for a total thyroidectomy due to a recurrent symptomatic multinodular goiter. She presented with increasing dysphagia, dyspnea, and a nontender neck mass. Preoperative fine-needle aspiration showed benign follicular hyperplasia. CT scan revealed an enlarged thyroid nodule on the left lobe measuring 4.7 × 3.1 cm with deviation of the trachea to the right (Figure 1). Other significant medical history included diabetes, hypertension, and hyperlipidemia.

After induction of anesthesia with propofol and succinylcholine, a 6 mm Medtronic nerve integrity monitor (NIM) EMG ETT was inserted over a stylet for an uneventful intubation.

Approximately 90 minutes into the surgery, a gurgling noise was perceived from the operative site. This was followed by an increase in inspiratory peak pressure and desaturation to 85%. Tube placement was confirmed by laryngoscopy, and the cuff was further inflated with 2 mL of air to minimize leaks. Fiber optic bronchoscopy revealed blood around the ETT, which was suctioned resulting in improved respiratory parameters.

After removal of the thyroid gland, the anterolateral aspect of the trachea was examined and palpated. No anterolateral tear was found. A repeat flexible bronchoscopy revealed a 5 cm tracheal tear on the posterior wall approximately 2 cm above the carina (Figure 2). Tracheomalacia was noted distal to the ETT. Flexible endoscopy performed at this time to rule out esophageal tear was unrevealing. The surgical incision was closed 4 hours after the start of the procedure.

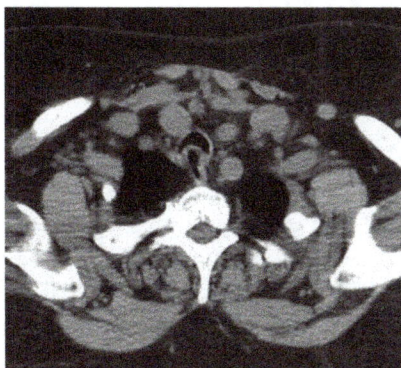

FIGURE 1: Preoperative CT scan showing deviation and compression of trachea.

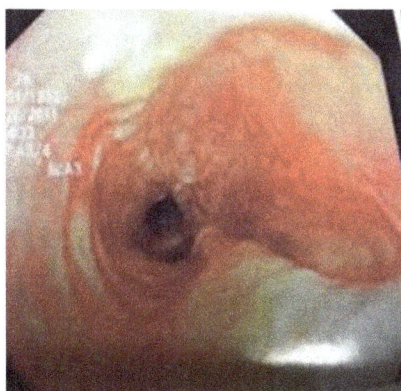

FIGURE 2: Tracheal tear on posterior wall on intraoperative flexible bronchoscopy.

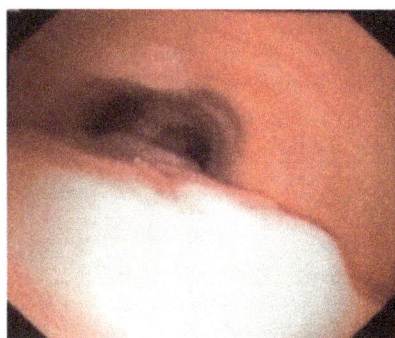

FIGURE 3: Healing with evidence of granulation tissue on POD 8.

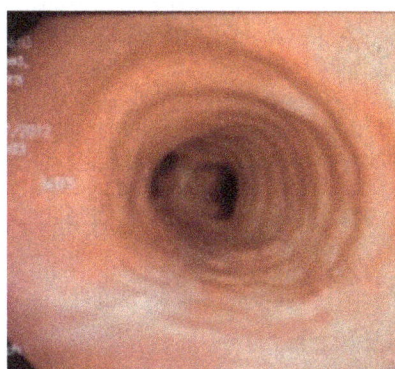

FIGURE 4: Bronchoscopy showing tracheomalacia on postoperative week no. 17. (note: complete healing).

The NIM EMG ETT was exchanged for a regular ETT. The patient was then transferred to the ICU.

On CMV (PIP of 25 cm H_2O, FiO_2 100%), the ABG showed pH 7.32, pCO_2 40, pO_2 96, and O_2 saturation 96%. A chest X-ray revealed no evidence of pneumomediastinum or subcutaneous emphysema. In the SICU, she was started on IV antibiotics and was monitored for respiratory distress. On postoperative day (POD) 1, she was put on CPAP trials and a flexible bronchoscopy confirmed the intraoperative findings. Subsequently, she was extubated and placed on supplemental oxygen via face mask. A chest X-ray was unchanged other than a new mild pleural effusion. A flexible bronchoscopy done on POD 5 showed the tracheal rupture in the initial healing phase. She was transferred to the general floor on POD 6. A flexible bronchoscopy done on POD 8 showed further healing of the tracheal rupture (Figure 3). The remainder of her hospital course was uneventful, and she was discharged on POD 12. Followup as an outpatient (week 17) revealed a fully healed tracheal tear with evidence of tracheomalacia (Figure 4).

3. Discussion

One of the rare complications of intubations is a tracheal tear. Estimates of its incidence in the last decade have ranged from approximately 0.05% to 0.37% of all orotracheal intubations [1]. A variety of risk factors both mechanical and anatomical predispose a patient to such an injury. Notable risk factors include a difficult intubation, the use of a stylet, prolonged intubation, and over inflation of the cuff. Patient risk factors include advanced age, female sex, tracheal anomalies, history of chronic obstructive pulmonary disease, and congenital tracheal anomalies such as tracheomalacia [2–4].

It presents more frequently in women owing to a weaker pars membranosa and the use of endotracheal tubes of a larger size than appropriate for women [5]. Usually diagnosed postoperatively, common symptoms include subcutaneous emphysema, mediastinal emphysema [6], pneumothorax, and hemoptysis. Tears under 2 cm are often asymptomatic [3]. Chest X-ray and CT scan show pneumomediastinum and/or pneumopericardium [3, 6]. Ventilation studies can show a persistent air leak. Bronchoscopy is needed for definitive diagnosis and to evaluate the extent of the tear.

Current management options for tracheal rupture are divided into conservative and surgical therapy. In most iatrogenic cases, the wound is limited, and the airway is maintained, allowing for conservative management. In traumatic injuries with loss of continuity in the proximal and distal part of the trachea, surgical intervention is required [3]. Surgical intervention is also recommended for complicated cases with rupture that extends into the main bronchi [4]. A study done by Cuesta et al. showed that conservative management is effective regardless of causation, size, or site of injury [7]. Conservative therapy includes orotracheal intubation, IV antibiotics, and parenteral nutrition. The cuff pressure of the ETT must be kept low and the tidal volume 5-6 mL/kg to expedite healing of the tear [6]. Extubation must be performed as soon as possible. Bronchoscopy should be utilized to monitor healing of the tear.

In this patient, the tracheal wall may have been compromised because of her undiagnosed tracheomalacia. The tracheomalacia, in turn, may have been a sequela of the original surgery and her long-standing goiter. Although in this case intubation was atraumatic, the use of an NIM EMG ETT in conjunction with undiagnosed tracheomalacia may have precipitated the tear. The NIM EMG tube uses a silicone elastomer cuff to allow better tracheal conformity and minimal tissue trauma. The designed elasticity may predispose the silicone-based cuff to asymmetrically inflate at very high cuff pressure [8].

Diagnosis of tracheobronchial injury can be made in a wide range of time periods. However, a delay in the diagnosis has been shown to have poor outcomes [4]. In our patient, the diagnosis of the tear was made intraoperatively, allowing a focused early management.

Authors' Contribution

M. Joshi, S. Mardakh, J. Yarmush, H. Kamath, J. Schianodicola, and E. Mendoza, hold the MD degree, helped write the paper and approved the final paper.

Acknowledgment

This work was funded by the Department of Anesthesiology, New York Methodist Hospital.

References

[1] E. Minambres, J. Buron, M. A. Ballesteros et al., "Tracheal rupture after endotracheal intubation: a literature systematic review," *European Journal of Cardio-Thoracic Surgery*, vol. 35, pp. 1056–1062, 2009.

[2] G. Cardillo, L. Carbone, F. Carleo et al., "Tracheal lacerations after endotracheal intubation: a proposed morphological classification to guide non-surgical treatment," *European Journal of Cardio-Thoracic Surgery*, vol. 37, no. 3, pp. 581–587, 2010.

[3] M. Conti, M. Pougeoise, A. Wurtz et al., "Management of postintubation tracheobronchial ruptures," *Chest*, vol. 130, no. 2, pp. 412–418, 2006.

[4] A. Zlotnik, S. Gruenbaum, B. Gruenbaum, M. Dubilet, and E. Cherniavsky, "Iatrogenic tracheobronchial rupture: a case report and review of literature," *International Journal of Case Reports and Images*, vol. 2, no. 3, pp. 12–16, 2011.

[5] H. Kaloud, F. M. Smolle-Juettner, G. Prause, and W. F. List, "Iatrogenic ruptures of the tracheobronchial tree," *Chest*, vol. 112, no. 3, pp. 774–778, 1997.

[6] B. Prunet, G. Lacroix, Y. Asencio, O. Cathelinaud, J. P. Avaro, and P. Goutorbe, "Iatrogenic post-intubation tracheal rupture treated conservatively without intubation: a case report," *Cases Journal*, vol. 1, pp. 259–262, 2008.

[7] P. Cuesta, R. Cantos, M. J. Sanchez, M. Geronimo, and R. Company, "Non-surgical treatment in iatrogenic tracheal rupture," *European Journal of Anaesthesiology*, vol. 27, no. 47, p. 188, 2010.

[8] G. G. Capra, A. N. Shah, J. D. Moore, W. S. Halsey, and E. Lujan, "Silicone-based endotracheal tube causing airway obstruction and pneumothorax," *Archives of Otolaryngology—Head & Neck Surgery*, vol. 138, no. 6, pp. 588–591, 2012.

26

Multifactorial Model and Treatment Approaches of Refractory Hypotension in a Patient Who Took an ACE Inhibitor the Day of Surgery

Karan Srivastava,[1] Vikas Y. Sacher,[1] Craig T. Nelson,[2] and John I. Lew[1,3]

[1] Department of Surgery, University of Miami Miller School of Medicine, Miami, FL 33136, USA

[2] Department of Anesthesiology, University of Miami Miller School of Medicine, Miami, FL 33136, USA

[3] University of Miami Leonard M. Miller School of Medicine and DeWitt Daughtry Family Department of Surgery, Division of Endocrine Surgery, University of Miami and Jackson Memorial Hospitals, 1120 NW 14th Street, CRB-Room 410P (M-875), Miami, FL 33136, USA

Correspondence should be addressed to John I. Lew; jlew@med.miami.edu

Academic Editors: D. Lee and J.-J. Yang

In the field of anesthesiology, there is wide debate on discontinuing angiotensin-converting enzyme inhibitor (ACEI) and angiotensin receptor blocker (ARB) therapy the day of noncardiac surgery. Although there have been many studies attributing perioperative hypotension to same-day ACEI and ARB use, there are many additional variables that play a role in perioperative hypotension. Additionally, restoring blood pressure in these patients presents a unique challenge to anesthesiologists. A case report is presented in which a patient took her ACEI the day of surgery and developed refractory hypotension during surgery. The evidence of ACEI use on the day of surgery and development of hypotension is reviewed, and additional variables that contributed to this hypotensive episode are discussed. Lastly, current challenges in restoring blood pressure are presented, and a basic model on treatment approaches for refractory hypotension in the setting of perioperative ACEI use is proposed.

1. Introduction

Approximately 65 million Americans actively receive antihypertensive agents for elevated blood pressure [1]. During surgery, beta-adrenergic blockers and alpha 2 agonists are routinely continued perioperatively because of their role in protecting the myocardium [2–5]. Additionally, calcium channel blockers are used in the perioperative period because of their reduction in myocardial ischemia, infarction, arrhythmias, and overall mortality [6, 7]. Since angiotensin-converting enzyme inhibitor (ACEI) attenuates the adrenergic response to stressful stimuli in cardiac, vascular, and cerebrovascular patients, ACEI is strongly recommended prior to and during these specific surgeries [8–11].

However, the use of ACEI and angiotensin receptor blocker (ARB) therapy in the preoperative period in noncardiac patients has been controversial because of its potential role in causing hemodynamic instability. Patients on chronic

ACEI or ARB therapy have a dampened sympathetic response [8]. Additionally, surgical patients can be volume depleted because of preoperative fasting, and this condition can cause additional stress during surgery. These combining factors result in reduced vascular capacitance and venous return, leading to decreased cardiac output and subsequent hypotension. To compensate for this hypotension, angiotensin II (ANG2) plays an important role in maintaining blood pressure through vasoconstriction. This vasoconstriction shunts blood away from the kidneys, bowels, and spleen [12, 13]. ANG2's short-term effect is to maintain blood pressure through vasoconstriction whereas its long-term effect, which takes hours to days, is volume regulation through sodium and water retention. Figure 1 explains the renin-angiotensin system.

Patients who have recently taken ACEI or ARB prior to surgery are unable to use ANG2 effects to counterbalance this

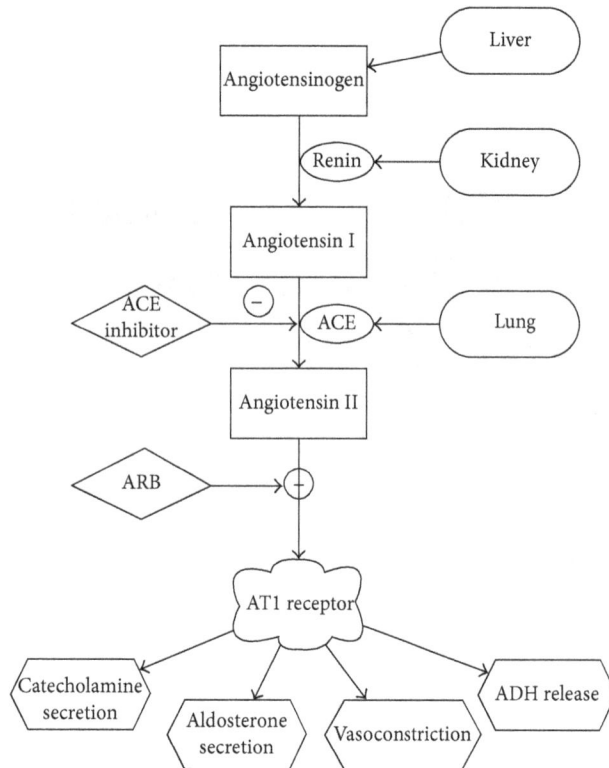

FIGURE 1: Physiology of the renin-angiotensin system and how angiotensin-converting enzyme inhibitors and angiotensin receptor blockers reduce blood pressure.

hypotension [12]. Compounding this problem is that anesthetic agents have been shown to competitively inhibit ANG2 in rat models [14]. Since there are multiple factors dampening the physiologic response to hypotension in surgical patients who chronically use ACEI therapy, there is a wide discussion as to whether to continue this medication on the day of surgery.

2. Case Report

A 70-year-old African American female with a left thyroid nodule with an indeterminate FNA result presented for left thyroid lobectomy with isthmusectomy. Her past medical history was significant for hypertension and dyslipidemia. The patient's past surgical history was significant for hysterectomy with no history of anesthesia complications during her prior surgery. Her medication use included lisinopril 40 mg and hydrochlorothiazide 25 mg. She only took lisinopril 40 mg on the day of the surgery. The patient's admission blood pressure was 157/79.

In the premedication stage of general anesthesia, the patient was given midazolam 2 mg. Noninvasive blood pressure, heart rate, and O_2 saturation were continuously monitored prior to surgery and during surgery. Ten minutes prior to induction, her blood pressure was 150/75. In the induction stage of general anesthesia, the patient was given fentanyl 125 mcg, lidocaine 100 mg, propofol 180 mg, and succinylcholine 100 mg. There were no complications in

establishing oral endotracheal intubation. Anesthesia was maintained with sevoflurane. Hypotension (92/54) was first noted 6 minutes after induction. Patient was subsequently given 100 mcg of phenylephrine. She remained hypotensive for the next 120 minutes, despite receiving a total of 1250 mcg of phenylephrine and 90 mg of ephedrine. During her hypotensive episode, the patient's pulse fluctuated from 57 to 95, and she was noted to have a very weak radial pulse bilaterally. At 70 minutes after induction, patient's blood pressure reached its nadir of 63/42 and surgery was halted. When the blood pressure improved slightly with systolic blood pressure in the 70s, surgery was subsequently restarted and completed. The patient's blood pressure was restored to 120/80s in the recovery room. V/Q scan obtained ruled out pulmonary embolism. The patient's lisinopril was withheld postoperative day 1 and her blood pressure was monitored. She spent a day in the surgical ICU and made an uneventful recovery.

3. Discussion

In this case report, the patient continued her ACEI therapy the day of the surgery, while withholding all other medications. Many studies confirm the relationship between hypotension in patients who receive ACEI the same day as surgery. Coriat et al. found that the incidence of induction-induced hypotension necessitating administration of ephedrine was higher in patients who received ACEI the day of surgery compared to patients who had ACEI withdrawn the day prior [15]. Comfere et al. studied the incidence of hypotension in patients who took their last dose of ACEI or ARB less than 10 hours prior to induction, and in patients who took their last dose of ACEI or ARB more than 10 hours prior to induction [16]. Moderate hypotension was defined as systolic blood pressure less than 85 mmHg and severe hypotension as less than 65 mmHg. Patients who received ACEI or ARB less than 10 hours prior to anesthesia had an increased likelihood of developing moderate hypotension only during the first 30 minutes. There was no significant difference in the development of severe hypotension in either group. Rosenman et al. conducted a meta-analysis studying the effect of continuing ACEI and ARB up to the morning of nonemergent surgery [17]. The data selection consisted of 5 studies totaling 434 patients. The meta-analysis found that patients who received the morning dose of ACEI/ARB had a statistically significant increased incidence of perioperative hypotension requiring vasopressors.

Although ACEI played a role in the development of hypotension in this patient, there are other factors that contributed to her hypotension. Although previous studies have indicated a link between intraoperative hypotension and same-day ACEI therapy, there are other variables confounding these results.Da Costa et al. published a case control retrospective study that found an association between ACEI and hypotension after induction using univariate analysis [18]. However, stratified analysis did not find a statistical significance for an association between ACEI and hypotension. The study showed that when parameters such as age and

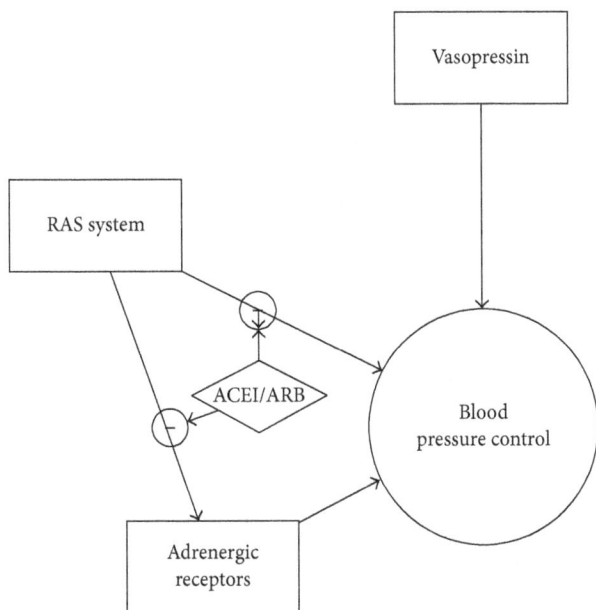

FIGURE 2: A Description of how ACEI/ARB block the RAS system and adrenergic pathway allowing only vasopressin to regulate blood pressure. (angiotensin-converting enzyme inhibitor) ACEI; (angiotensin receptor blocker) ARB.

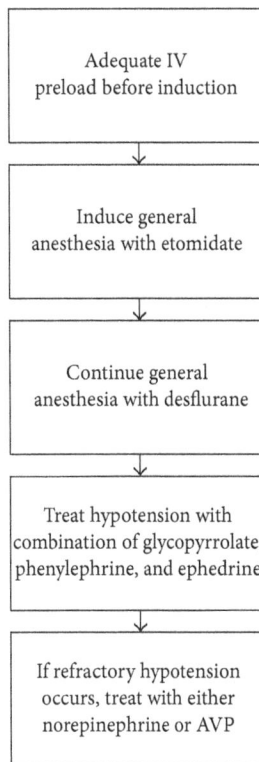

FIGURE 3: Protocol for refractory hypotension.

patient size were controlled for, the use of ACEI was not found to be a dominant risk factor in development of hypotension whereas age was found to be a significant risk factor.

Other studies have tried to address the role of polypharmacy and the development of hypotension perioperatively. Kheterpal et al. performed a prospective, observational study that showed a synergistic hemodynamic effect in patients who are taking ACEI and diuretic therapy. Patients on chronic ACEI/ARB and diuretic therapy had more episodes of hypotension and required vasopressor boluses more often than the patient solely on chronic diuretic therapy [19]. The study also identified 3 groups of patients on chronic ACEI/ARB therapy who did not have a statistically significant increase in the number of hypotensive episodes. These groups included patients who were on chronic ACEI/ARB but were not taking diuretics or calcium-channel blockers patients who were on chronic ACEI and taking both diuretics and calcium-channel blockers, and patients who were taking chronic ACEI along with calcium-channel blockers. There was no explanation as to why these 3 groups of patients did not have increased incidence of hypotensive episodes. The analysis of polypharmacy interactions of antihypertensive agents is still in the nascent stages. As more pharmacology research is performed and more sophisticated models are developed, physicians answer on whether to continue antihypertensive agents the day of the surgery.

Anesthetic agents also alter a patient's ability to compensate for hemodynamic instability [20]. Weisenberg et al. did a prospective randomized trial that studied the relationship between the dosage of propofol and the degree of hypotension in patients chronically taking ACEI [21]. Patients were randomly assigned to different propofol dose groups: 1.3, 1.6, 2.0, or 2.3 (mg/kg). A multivariable negative binomial regression

model indicated that for each propofol dose increase of 0.3 mg/kg there was an associated 31% increase in mean number of hypotensive/bradycardic episodes. The study also found that the propofol dose of 1.3 mg/kg required the least number of interventions for hypotension or bradycardia during the first 10 minutes after induction. Lastly, the study suggested that adjustments to propofol dose might be effective in reducing perioperative hemodynamic disturbances in patients who chronically take ACEI.

Although many variables may have contributed to the patient's hypotension, what is most puzzling about this case is that the patient's hypotension was refractory despite administration of phenylephrine and ephedrine. There is no standard treatment protocol for perioperative hypotension. Nevertheless, the most common treatment approach is the following. First, the depth of anesthesia is reduced and IV fluid is administered. If hypotension persists, phenylephrine, ephedrine, or epinephrine is administered [22]. Wheeler et al. described a case in which a patient on chronic ARB remained hypotensive during surgery despite aggressive administration of phenylephrine, ephedrine, and epinephrine. Eventually, vasopressin was successful in restoring the patient's blood pressure. The authors describe the phenomenon of catecholamine resistance resulting in refractory hypotension in a patient on chronic ACEI therapy. Rat models have further corroborated this possibility. Godínez-Hernández et al. found that ACEI treatment leads to a reduction in alpha-adrenergic receptors density in rats. Even when phenylephrine was administered, there was a 60% decrease in aortic contractility compared to rats not treated with an

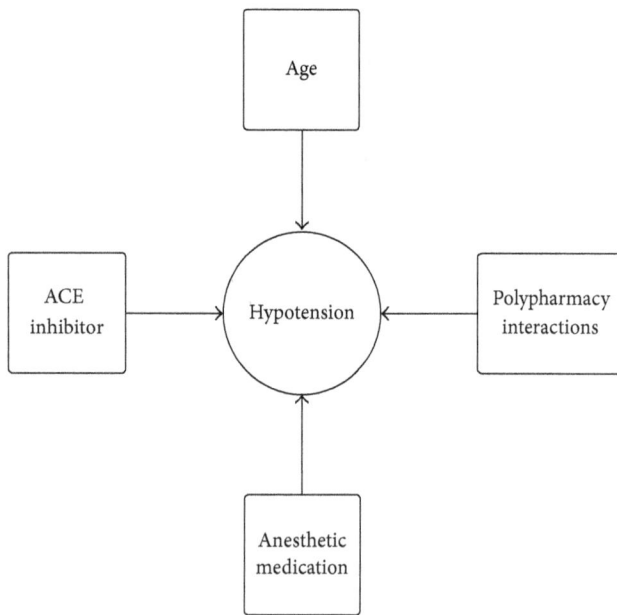

FIGURE 4: Multiple variables causing hypotension in this case. These models provide a paradigm on how to evaluate patients with perioperative hypotension.

ACE inhibitor [23]. Since blocking the RAS system disrupts adrenergic receptors, studies have indicated that a possible treatment for refractory hypotension is vasopressin. The vasopressin pathway remains intact even with ACEI or ARB therapy [22, 23]. Figure 2 explains the physiology behind the treatment model for refractory hypotension. The most recent suggested treatment protocol for hypotension in patients on chronic ACEI or ARB therapy is shown in Figure 3 [24]. Thus, there are multiple factors that contribute to the development of refractory hypotension in this patient including age, use of ACEI on the day of surgery, chronic use of ACEI and diuretic therapy as antihypertensives, and the dose of propofol administered at the time of induction. Furthermore, this case suggests and emphasizes that management of refractory hypotension in the setting of ACEI use on the day of surgery should also include the use of vasopressin.

Although this report initially appears to be a simple case of hypotension caused by ACEI treatment on the same day as surgery, there are many additional variables that possibly contributed to hypotension. In this case, the patient was a 71-year-old female on chronic ACEI and diuretic therapy. The patient took her ACEI therapy the day of the surgery. During induction, she was given a total of 180 mg of propofol, which amounts to 2.5 mg/Kg. Figure 4 is a dynamic model describing the numerous variables that have an effect on blood pressure. These models help illustrate the multifactorial causes of perioperative hypotension. Using such models will be beneficial as more detailed studies describe the precise pharmacology causing perioperative hypotension.

References

[1] J. D. Wright, J. P. Hughes, Y. Ostchega, S. S. Yoon, and T. Nwankwo, "Mean systolic and diastolic blood pressure in adults aged 18 and over in the United States, 2001–2008," *National Health Statistics Reports*, no. 35, pp. 1–22, 2011.

[2] D. T. Mangano, E. L. Layug, A. Wallace, and I. Tateo, "Effect of atenolol on mortality and cardiovascular morbidity after noncardiac surgery. Multicenter Study of Perioperative Ischemia Research Group," *New England Journal of Medicine*, vol. 335, no. 23, pp. 1713–1720, 1996.

[3] A. Wallace and D. T. Mangano, "Use of β-blockade to prevent death after noncardiac surgery," *Western Journal of Medicine*, vol. 166, no. 3, pp. 203–204, 1997.

[4] A. Wallace, B. Layug, I. Tateo et al., "Prophylactic atenolol reduces postoperative myocardial ischemia. McSPI Research Group," *Anesthesiology*, vol. 88, no. 1, pp. 2–17, 1998.

[5] R. D. Stevens, H. Burri, and M. R. Tramer, "Pharmacologic myocardial protection in patients undergoing noncardiac surgery: a quan-titative systematic review," *Anesthesia & Analgesia*, vol. 97, no. 3, pp. 623–633, 2003.

[6] D. N. Wijeysundera and W. S. Beattie, "Calcium channel blockers for reducing cardiac morbidity after noncardiac surgery: a meta-analysis," *Anesthesia & Analgesia*, vol. 97, no. 3, pp. 634–641, 2003.

[7] J. Butterworth and C. D. Furberg, "Improving cardiac outcomes after noncardiac surgery," *Anesthesia & Analgesia*, vol. 97, no. 3, pp. 613–615, 2003.

[8] M. Licker, P. Neidhart, S. Lustenberger et al., "Long-term angiotensin-converting enzyme inhibitor treatment attenuates adrenergic responsiveness without altering hemodynamic control in patients undergoing cardiac surgery," *Anesthesiology*, vol. 84, no. 4, pp. 789–800, 1996.

[9] M. Licker, M. Bednarkiewicz, P. Neidhart et al., "Preoperative inhibition of angiotensin-converting enzyme improves systemic and renal haemodynamic changes during aortic abdominal surgery," *British Journal of Anaesthesia*, vol. 76, no. 5, pp. 632–639, 1996.

[10] H. Tohmo, M. Karanko, M. Scheinin, O. Viinamaki, M. Salonen, and V. Nieminen, "Enalapril premedication attenuates the blood pressure response to tracheal intubation and stabilizes postoperative blood pressure after controlled hypotension with sodium nitroprusside in neurovascular patients," *Journal of Neurosurgical Anesthesiology*, vol. 5, no. 1, pp. 13–21, 1993.

[11] F. Ryckwaert and P. Colson, "Hemodynamic effects of anesthesia in patients with ischemic heart failure chronically treated with angiotensin-converting enzyme inhibitors," *Anesthesia & Analgesia*, vol. 84, no. 5, pp. 945–949, 1997.

[12] R. Behnia, A. Molteni, and R. Igić, "Angiotensin-converting enzyme inhibitors: mechanisms of action and implications in anesthesia practice," *Current Pharmaceutical Design*, vol. 9, no. 9, pp. 763–776, 2003.

[13] J. A. Herd, "Cardiovascular response to stress," *Physiological Reviews*, vol. 71, no. 1, pp. 305–330, 1991.

[14] E. D. Miller, D. E. Longnecker, and M. J. Peach, "The regulatory function of the renin-angiotensin system during general anesthesia," *Anesthesiology*, vol. 48, no. 6, pp. 399–403, 1978.

[15] P. Coriat, C. Richer, T. Douraki et al., "Influence of chronic angiotensin-converting enzyme inhibition on anesthetic induction," *Anesthesiology*, vol. 81, no. 2, pp. 299–307, 1994.

[16] T. Comfere, J. Sprung, M. M. Kumar et al., "Angiotensin system inhibitors in a general surgical population," *Anesthesia & Analgesia*, vol. 100, no. 3, pp. 636–644, 2005.

[17] D. J. Rosenman, F. S. McDonald, J. O. Ebbert, P. J. Erwin, M. LaBella, and V. M. Montori, "Clinical consequences of withholding versus administering renin-angiotensin-aldosterone system antagonists in the preoperative period," *Journal of Hospital Medicine*, vol. 3, no. 4, pp. 319–325, 2008.

[18] V. V. Da Costa, A. C. Caldas, L. G. Nunes, P. S. Beraldo, and R. A. Saraiva, "Influence of angiotensin-converting enzyme inhibitors on hypotension after anesthetic induction: is the preoperative discontinuation of this drug necessary?" *Revista Brasileira de Anestesiologia*, vol. 59, no. 6, pp. 704–715, 2009.

[19] S. Kheterpal, O. Khodaparast, A. Shanks, M. O'Reilly, and K. K. Tremper, "Chronic angiotensin-converting enzyme inhibitor or angiotensin receptor blocker therapy combined with diuretic therapy is associated with increased episodes of hypotension in noncardiac surgery," *Journal of Cardiothoracic and Vascular Anesthesia*, vol. 22, no. 2, pp. 180–186, 2008.

[20] T. J. Ebert, D. D. Kanitz, and J. P. Kampine, "Inhibition of sympathetic neural outflow during thiopental anesthesia in humans," *Anesthesia & Analgesia*, vol. 71, no. 4, pp. 319–326, 1990.

[21] M. Weisenberg, D. I. Sessler, M. Tavdi et al., "Dose-dependent hemodynamic effects of propofol induction following brotizolam premedication in hypertensive patients taking angiotensin-converting enzyme inhibitors," *Journal of Clinical Anesthesia*, vol. 22, no. 3, pp. 190–195, 2010.

[22] A. D. Wheeler, J. Turchiano, and J. D. Tobias, "A case of refractory intraoperative hypotension treated with vasopressin infusion," *Journal of Clinical Anesthesia*, vol. 20, no. 2, pp. 139–142, 2008.

[23] D. Godínez-Hernández, I. A. Gallardo-Ortíz, P. López-Sánchez, and R. Villalobos-Molina, "Captopril therapy decreases both expression and function of alpha-adrenoceptors in pre-hypertensive rat aorta," *Autonomic and Autacoid Pharmacology*, vol. 26, no. 1, pp. 21–29, 2006.

[24] B. Mets, "Management of hypotension associated with Angiotensin-axis blockade and general anesthesia administration," *Journal of Cardiothoracic and Vascular Anesthesia*, vol. 27, no. 1, pp. 156–167, 2013.

27

Spinal Anaesthesia for Emergency Caesarean Section in a Morbid Obese Woman with Severe Preeclampsia

Ebirim N. Longinus, Lagiri Benjamin, and Buowari Yvonne Omiepirisa

Department of Anaesthesiology, University of Port Harcourt Teaching Hospital, Port Harcourt, 6173 Rivers State, Nigeria

Correspondence should be addressed to Ebirim N. Longinus, ginebirim@yahoo.com

Academic Editors: A. Apan, M. R. Chakravarthy, and E. A. Vandermeersch

Background. Morbid obesity in a pregnancy is a great challenge to medical practice especially when the patient requires caesarean section. *Case Summary*. A 38-year-old unbooked gravida 3 Para 2^{+0} weight 195 kg, height 1.7 m with a blood pressure of 210/160 mmhg had spinal anaesthesia for emergency caesarean section which was technically difficult for severe preeclampsia at 32-week gestation. She had poor wound healing and spent 18 days postoperatively on hospital admission. *Conclusion*. Morbid obesity is a challenge to both obstetric and anaesthetic practice. Antenatal care is necessary in reducing both maternal morbidity and mortality.

1. Introduction

Pre-eclampsia is a disorder that occurs in pregnancy after twenty weeks of gestation which manifests as hypertension and proteinuria, may progress to eclampsia and may regress following delivery [1–4]. Hypertension without proteinuria arising after twenty weeks gestation is referred to as pregnancy-induced hypertension [5]. Proteinuria is defined as at least 300 mg protein in a 24-hour urine collection or ++ dipstick 30 mg/dL in single urine sample [2]. The precise aetiology of preeclampsia is still unknown [1, 6], and multifactorial [7]. Preeclampsia is a disorder unique to human pregnancy [6], may involve the maternal cardiovascular, renal, coagulation, and hepatic system, and is associated with increased maternal and fatal morbidity and mortality [3, 8]. It occurs in 5–10% of all pregnancies [3, 5, 6]. Most definitions of hypertension in pregnancy are based on a diastolic blood pressure greater than 90 mmhg on two occasions or diastolic blood pressure greater than or equal to 110 mmhg on one occasion [4]. Four million women worldwide will develop preeclampsia annually and a further 100,000 will have eclampsia [7]. However, it remains a major cause of maternal and perinatal morbidity and mortality worldwide [6]. The incidence of preeclampsia varies according to the population studied and the criteria used for establishing the diagnosis [6]. Obesity is on the increase and carries increased morbidity and mortality in pregnancy [9]. Morbidly obese patients should be seen as high risk [9]. Obesity is a growing problem worldwide [10]. A subject is described as morbidly obese if the body mass index (BMI) is greater than 40 kg/m^2 [11]. A case of a morbidly obese parturient that had a technically difficult spinal anaesthesia for emergency caesarean section for severe preeclampsia is presented.

2. Case Presentation

A 38-year-old unbooked gravida 3 Para 2^{+0} two alive woman with no formal education was booked at the antenatal clinic for elective caesarean section at 32 weeks for severe preeclampsia. Blood pressure at booking was 220/160 mmhg. Patient later went into spontaneous labour on the same day and developed cord prolapse for which she was booked for emergency caesarean section. On examination, she was in painful distress, anasarca, sacral oedema, bilateral pitting pedal oedema up to the knee joint, and periorbital oedema. Weight was 195 kg, height 1.7 m, pulse rate 100 beats per minute, and blood pressure 210/160 mmhg after receiving three doses of 5 mg diazepam, 10 mg hydralazine, and 25 mg magnesium sulphate. Auscultation of the chest was vesicular breath sounds. She was pale, anicteric, and febrile to touch. Urinalysis showed protein ++ and glucose +. Radom blood sugar was 6 mmol/dL. The temporomandibular joint was mobile with mallampati IV. Packed cell volume was 34%. An assessment of ASA IIIE with severe preeclampsia and prematurity in morbidly obese obstetric patient was made. The patient was counselled for surgery and informed consent obtained. Spinal anaesthesia was administered after several attempts with 2 mLs of hypobaric bupivacaine and L4, L5 interspace. The height of block was T4. She was given oxygen by facemask. During surgery, a male baby was extracted birth weight 2.1 kg, Apgar score [5, 7]. Blood pressure at the end of surgery was 200/160 mmhg. She spent several days in hospital because of poor wound healing and the blood pressure was persistently high despite administration of antihypertensive. She was discharged home 18 days postoperative due to industrial action by the hospital medical staff.

3. Discussion

Both severe preeclampsia and eclampsia can seriously endanger the life of both mother and foetus and may account for up to 80% of maternal deaths in some parts of the developing world [3]. Preeclampsia and eclampsia remain among the most rewarding challenges in practice as a wide range of pathophysiological changes require an individualized approached to each case [12]. The incidence of preeclampsia is significantly increased in nulliparous women, in women with multiple gestations, in those with previous pre-eclampsia/eclampsia, and in women with underlying vascular or renal disease [6]. This patient was multiparous with a singleton pregnancy. Her two previous pregnancies were unsupervised, therefore, it cannot be deduced if there is a history of previous pre-eclampsia. She spent more days in hospital because she was morbidly obese and had pre-eclampsia. There are a number of potential problems relating to preeclampsia [13]. The choice of anaesthetic technique in severely pre-eclamptic women requiring caesarean section has been controversial for a number of years, but clinical experience has demonstrated the relative safety and value of well-managed incremental epidural anaesthesia [14]. The patient was given subarachnoid block (spinal anaesthesia) with hypobaric bupivacaine although it was technically difficult because of the patient's body size and subcutaneous fat. It was given in the sitting position. The benefits of spinal anaesthesia include rapid onset of reliable, high quality surgical anaesthesia, and avoidance of complications related to emergency general anaesthesia. The hazards of general anaesthesia in severe preeclampsia are well recognised. The anaesthetist often prefers the use of the sitting position in the obese patient since it is simpler to identify the midline and the obese patient prefers this position [15]. An obese patient poses a challenge to the anaesthetist. The obese patient is one of the anaesthetist nightmares as it carries a high morbidity and mortality [10]. In the obese parturient, there is increased oxygen consumption, abdominal weight that restricts the diaphragm and reduces chest wall compliance, difficult subarachnoid block, and wound infection [9]. The anaesthetic problems presented by the morbidly obese obstetric patient have risks and problems of a regional anaesthetic technique, particularly the technical difficulties. High spread can result in respiratory insufficiency and cardiovascular collapse [16]. The benefits of spinal anaesthesia include provision of a rapid, sense, and predictable block suitable for surgery while avoiding the risks of general anaesthesia. Caesarean section under general anaesthesia in severe preeclampsia is a high-risk procedure. The factors, which make general anaesthesia in preeclampsia particularly hazardous, include the increased risk of difficult airway and intubation and marked pressor response at laryngoscopy, intubation and extubation resulting in dangerous surges in blood pressure. There is a significant risk of intracranial haemorrhage secondary to uncontrolled severe hypertension at induction of general anaesthesia [4]. Generally, the decision when to deliver remains a clinical one based on gestation and foetal and maternal condition with the mother always taking priority if there is significant increase in maternal risk [7]. The benefits of antenatal care cannot be over emphasized most especially in the reduction of maternal and perinatal morbidity and mortality [17].

4. Conclusion

Morbid obesity is a challenge to anaesthetic and obstetric practice as its problems of transportation of the patient from the ward to the operating room, wound healing, and difficulties in establishing regional blocks because of difficulties in identifying landmarks. Longer needles are required, which are not readily available in developing countries like Nigeria.

References

[1] E. I. Agaba and A. N. Odili, "Pre-eclampsia presenting as nephrotic syndrome: a case report," *Nigerian Journal of Medicine*, vol. 13, no. 1, pp. 62–63, 2004.

[2] K. S. Adedapa, O. Olayemi, A. A. Odukogbe, C. O. Aimakhu, A. O. Kehinde, and B. L. Salako, "Relationship between oxidative stress and pre-eclamspia in Nigerian women," *Tropical Journal of Obstetrics and Gynaecology*, vol. 26, no. 2, pp. 102–107, 2009.

[3] U. V. Okafor and O. Okezie, "Maternal and fetal outcome of anaesthesia for caesarean delivery in preeclampsia/eclampsia in Enugu, Nigeria: a retrospective observational study," *International Journal of Obstetric Anesthesia*, vol. 14, no. 2, pp. 108–113, 2005.

[4] J. Hull and M. Rucklidge, "Management of severe preeclampsia and eclampsia," *Update in Anaesthesia*, vol. 25, no. 2, pp. 50–54, 2009.

[5] G. Sharwood-Smith, V. Clark, and E. Watson, "Regional anaesthesia for caesarean section in severe preeclampsia: spinal anaesthesia is the preferred choice," *International Journal of Obstetric Anesthesia*, vol. 8, no. 2, pp. 85–89, 1999.

[6] "The case for magnesium sulphate in pre-eclampsia-eclampsia," *International Journal of Obstetric Anesthesia*, vol. 1, pp. 167–175, 1992.

[7] K. Hinshaw, "Pre-eclampsia revisited. Obstetric issues. Three-day course on obstetric anaesthesia and analgesia," pp. 117–120, 2008.

[8] T. Engelhardt and F. M. MacLennan, "Fluid management in pre-eclampsia," *International Journal of Obstetric Anesthesia*, vol. 8, no. 4, pp. 253–259, 1999.

[9] V. Clark, "The obese parturient. Intercurrent illness. Three-day course on obstetric anaesthesia and analgesia," p. 101, 2008.

[10] H. K. Baddoo, F. K. Boni, and E. Lamptey, "Body mass index (BMI) in patients attending the anaesthesia clinic: implications for anaesthesia," *African Journal of Anaesthesia and Intensive Care*, vol. 9, no. 2, pp. 10–13, 2009.

[11] R. J. Whitty, C. V. Maxwell, and J. C. A. Carvalho, "Complications of neuraxial anesthesia in an extreme morbidly obese patient for cesarean section," *International Journal of Obstetric Anesthesia*, vol. 16, no. 2, pp. 139–144, 2007.

[12] M. G. Mörtl and M. C. Schneider, "Key issues in assessing, managing and treating patients presenting with severe preeclampsia," *International Journal of Obstetric Anesthesia*, vol. 9, no. 1, pp. 39–44, 2000.

[13] S. Galloway and G. Lyons, "Preeclampsia complicated by placental abruption, HELLP, coagulopathy and renal failure—further lessons," *International Journal of Obstetric Anesthesia*, vol. 12, no. 1, pp. 35–39, 2003.

[14] P. Howell, "Spinal anaesthesia in severe preeclampsia: time for reappraisal, or time for caution?" *International Journal of Obstetric Anesthesia*, vol. 7, no. 4, pp. 217–219, 1998.

[15] K. R. Milligan, P. Cramp, L. Schatz, D. Johnston, and H. Carp, "The effect of patient position and obesity on the spread of epidural analgesia," *International Journal of Obstetric Anesthesia*, vol. 2, no. 3, pp. 134–136, 1993.

[16] K. R. Milligan and H. Carp, "Continuous spinal anaesthesia for caesarean section in the morbidly obese," *International Journal of Obstetric Anesthesia*, vol. 1, no. 2, pp. 111–113, 1992.

[17] M. A. Lamina, A. O. Sule-Odu, and E. O. Jagun, "Factors militating against delivery among patients booked in Olabisi Onabanjo University Teaching Hospital, Sagamu," *Nigerian Journal of Medicine*, vol. 13, no. 1, pp. 52–55, 2004.

28

Submental Intubation Including Extubation: Airway Complications of Maxillomandibular Fixation

Santosh Kumar Yadav[1] and Gopendra Deo[2]

[1] *Department of Oral and Maxillofacial Surgery, Chitwan Medical College, P.O. Box 42, Bharatpur-10, Chitwan, Nepal*
[2] *Department of Anesthesiology, Chitwan Medical College, P.O. Box 42, Bharatpur-10, Chitwan, Nepal*

Correspondence should be addressed to Gopendra Deo, sonikadeepti@yahoo.co.in

Academic Editors: R. Riley and D. A. Story

Hernandez first described the submental route for endotracheal intubation in 1986 as an alternative airway maneuver for maxillofacial procedures. Since that time, several case studies have been performed demonstrating the efficacy of the submental approach. This method was recently implemented in the case of a patient with altered nasal anatomy who sustained a mandibular fracture necessitating maxillomandibular fixation. Unlike most of the cases described in the literature, this patient's operative course was confounded by the need to extubate through the submental tunnel. The patient tolerated the procedure well and was able to avoid other forms of surgical airway.

1. Introduction

Several procedures exist in which the surgeon requires access to areas that would otherwise be obscured by an endotracheal tube. Means of securing a patient's airway other than the conventional oral intubation include nasotracheal intubation and surgical airways such as tracheostomy. In 1986, Hernandez described submental intubation as an alternative to the classic methods [1]. His technique consisted of passing the endotracheal tube through the anterior floor of the mouth to allow free intraoperative access to the dental occlusion and to the nasal pyramid without endangering patients with skull base trauma [2]. This technique allows for the avoidance of tracheal dissection and eliminates the risks associated with nasotracheal intubation in the setting of facial trauma.

As described in a paper by Caubi et al., the surgeon performs the procedure by creating a small incision just medial to the lower border of the mandible. The subcutaneous tissues and the tissues of the floor of the mouth are bluntly dissected through with Kelly forceps to the point of entering the oral cavity just anterior to the sublingual caruncle. Care is taken to avoid nerves, vessels, and salivary structures. The endotracheal tube is then disconnected from the ventilatory circuit and is pulled through the submental tunnel, along with the pilot balloon, using the forceps [3]. The circuit is then quickly reconnected and tube positioning is confirmed by comparing the position of the tube with regard to the teeth before and after submental positioning as well as confirming bilateral breath sounds. At the end of the operation, the tube is disconnected, pulled back into the oral cavity and reconnected. The submental incision is sutured and the patient is extubated in the usual fashion [2, 4].

Several case studies have been performed since the introduction of the procedure in 1986. These reports consistently show no motor or sensory deficit, normal healing of the mucosal floor, and preservation of the salivary ducts and saliva production [2, 5]. Of the complications experienced, one report by Meyer et al. found an 8% occurrence of oral floor abscesses and a 4% occurrence of hypertrophic scar formation. However, the patient population in this series was rather small ($n = 25$) [2]. Caubi et al. describe an intraoperative complication in only one of their study patients in which high pressures where observed due to compression of the endotracheal tube as a result of the acute angle the tube takes in the oropharynx [3]. Despite long-term airway support and maintenance being listed as a contraindication to submental intubation in the MacInnis and Baig trial, they did observe one patient who remained intubated in the ICU for 3 days and found that delayed extubation had been uncomplicated in all cases where it was required [6].

The consensus among the various reports all concludes that the complications are minimal and that patients are overall very satisfied with the lack of scarring. In addition to the obvious benefits of submental endotracheal intubation in maxillofacial trauma procedures, elective use of this maneuver has been described as efficacious in procedures where an unobstructed oral or nasal cavity is beneficial to the surgeons, such as orthognathic surgery and even transfacial cranial base surgery [4, 7].

2. Case Report

The patient was a 30-year-old, 60 kg male who presented several days after sustaining blunt trauma to the left side of his jaw. The patient was playing football and was elbowed in this area. He immediately had swelling and pain in the left mandibular area adjacent to his ear. He had limited jaw mobility, which greatly exacerbated his pain and was only able to tolerate eating soft foods. On admission, the patient had obvious facial swelling to the left side of his face and dental misalignment was noted. A maxillofacial CT scan was obtained which showed an acute left mandibular fracture just inferior to the condyles. The remaining facial bones were intact without acute fracture. Also observed on the CT scan were narrow nasal passages and a leftward deviated nasal septum. Otolaryngology scheduled surgical intervention for fracture reduction and maxillomandibular fixation.

Evaluation preoperatively showed poor mouth opening secondary to pain. He was appointed a Mallampati score of II and was estimated to have a thyromental distance greater than 6 cm. Nasotracheal intubation was the proposed means of airway control due to the necessity of maxillomandibular fixation thus precluding orotracheal intubation. The patient demonstrated patency of both nares and provided no history of nasal trauma or knowledge of any nasal septal deviation. The patient was premedicated with midazolam 2 mg intravenously and fentanyl 100 mcg intravenously. All standard monitors were applied. The patient received 3 sprays of oxymetazoline to each naris. Anesthesia was induced with propofol 200 mg intravenously and fentanyl 150 mcg intravenously. After successful mask ventilation, succinylcholine 100 mg was administered intravenously. Easy mask ventilation was achieved with confirmation of end-tidal CO_2 and adequate oxygenation. A nasal RAE endotracheal tube was then introduced into the right naris with immediate resistance. Repositioning of the angle of entry did not overcome the difficult passage, nor did downsizing to a smaller nasal RAE endotracheal tube. Intubation via the right naris was aborted and intubation through the left naris was attempted. However, immediate resistance was again experienced and it was felt at this time that nasotracheal intubation was not going to be possible. The patient was mask ventilated again and was then intubated orally with an 8.0 endotracheal tube. On direct laryngoscopy, miniscule amounts of blood were noted in the patient's pharynx from

the nasal trauma sustained during the initial intubation attempts. Bilateral breath sounds and end-tidal CO_2 were confirmed. The surgeon then made a small, approximately 2 cm incision in the right submental region and bluntly dissected through the floor of the mouth with Kelly forceps. The ventilator was then briefly disconnected and the endotracheal tube and pilot balloon were pulled through the submental tunnel via the Kelly forceps. The circuit was reconnected, end-tidal CO_2 and bilateral breath sounds were confirmed, and direct laryngoscopy was repeated to confirm tube placement. The supraglottic and oropharyngeal areas were adequately suctioned and the surgeons proceeded with the case. Anesthesia was successfully maintained with inhaled isoflurane. The patient's initial airway pressures while orotracheally intubated were consistently 15-16 cm H_2O. However, after tunneling the endotracheal tube through the floor of the mouth, peak pressures increased to 25–30 cm H_2O. These increased pressures were felt to be secondary to the acute bend that the tube was required to make in the oropharynx. No other issues with ventilation or oxygenation were encountered throughout the case. The surgical team inserted four, 8 mm self-drilling screws into the patient's maxilla and mandible and used 26-gauge wire to achieve properly aligned dental occlusion. The submental incision was then infiltrated with lidocaine and epinephrine. A soft suction catheter was used to attempt to remove as much secretions as possible from the patient's pharynx. The inhalational agent was turned off and the patient awakened. The surgical team was standing by with wire cutters in hand should airway compromise had been encountered. It was felt that the patient was adequately awake when he was able to generate sufficient and consistent tidal volumes, follow commands to squeeze fingers and maintain a head lift when asked. At this time the cuff was deflated and the endotracheal tube was slowly removed through the submental tunnel. The surgical team closed the submental incision, first with 4-0 Vicryl for the subcutaneous plane and a 5-0 fast absorbable suture for the skin. The patient maintained excellent ventilation and oxygenation and at no time experienced any airway compromise or oxygen desaturation. He was taken to the postanesthesia care unit in excellent condition.

3. Discussion

Submental intubation has been heralded as a simple, secure, and effective procedure for operative airway control in major maxillofacial traumas. It allows practitioners to avoid the risk of epistaxis, iatrogenic meningitis, or trauma of the anterior skull base after nasotracheal intubation, as well as complications, such as tracheal stenosis, injury to cervical vessels or the thyroid gland, subcutaneous emphysema, or recurrent laryngeal nerve injury related to tracheostomy [3, 8]. The scar from the submental incision is thought to be less visible than a tracheostomy scar and has been well tolerated by patients [2]. In addition to possible hypertrophy of the submental scar, other complications include accidental extubation, accidental advancement of the endotracheal tube into a mainstem bronchus, bleeding, infection, mucocele formation, and damage to salivary ducts and glands. However, these complications have proven to be quite rare according to data from various trials over the past 24 years. In our particular case, the submental intubation approach allowed for appropriate alignment and maxillomandibular fixation, all while maintaining a secure airway. We did experience an increase in peak airway pressures, which were attributed to the compression of the endotracheal tube as it acutely bends in its path through the oropharynx and into the larynx. However, the increase in pressure was not significant enough to warrant us attempting to exchange the endotracheal tube for a reinforced endotracheal tube with the included risk of possibly losing control of the airway. In addition, unlike the great majority of cases reported in the literature, we were not afforded the luxury of being able to reverse the submental intubation into a regular oral intubation at the end of the case due to the surgical fixation. Therefore, absolute assurance of the patient's ability to protect his airway was necessary prior to submental extubation. Any complications occurring after submental extubation, such as emesis with aspiration or laryngospasm, would have proven disastrous, as the patient had undergone fixation of his mandible and was unable to open his mouth. The importance of communication and cooperation between the anesthesia and surgical teams cannot be overemphasized in this situation, as the surgical team was ready to immediately clip the fixation wires to allow for jaw opening, suction, and emergent reintubation if needed. Only after the patient had as much of his oropharyngeal secretions suctioned as possible and was completely and purposefully following commands, he was extubated with immediate suturing of his submental incision.

Alternative routes of management for this patient included not performing the procedure at all, repeated attempts at nasotracheal intubation with a smaller endotracheal tube and fiber optic laryngoscopy, or tracheostomy. Not performing the procedure would have caused the patient great morbidity in terms of pain, trismus, possible malunion, and permanent defects in mastication secondary to poor healing. Therefore it was felt that the procedure must be performed. Repeated attempts at nasotracheal intubation could have been performed, but not without the risks of further nasal mucosal trauma and increased bleeding. Again, as the patient was to have maxillomandibular fixation, any increased amount of blood in the glottic area would put the patient at higher risk for laryngospasm, and thus, no further attempts were felt to be in the patient's best interest. Tracheostomy is another form of a surgical airway, but carries the risk of possible tracheal stenosis and damage to surrounding tissues, vessels, and nerves. Also, the scar of tracheostomy is more visible than that of the submental incision, which is hidden on the underside of the mandible. After all of the above alternatives had their risks and benefits weighed, we felt that submental intubation was properly indicated for this particular case.

Our patient, like those described in the existing literature, tolerated the procedure well and had completely successful management of his airway, as well as uncomplicated extubation, with the submental endotracheal airway management approach.

What lacks in the current literature are any large-scale case series or prospective trials comparing the efficacy of submental intubation to that of other types of surgical airway. This type or airway management is even being used electively for certain types of procedures including skull base surgery. It is difficult to truly assess the overall incidence of complications that occur with submental intubation when most case series are only reporting on 8–10 cases. The current data must be interpreted with caution and much more research into this area of airway management is warranted.

References

[1] A. Hernandez, "The submental route for endotracheal intubation," *Journal of Oral and Maxillofacial Surgery*, vol. 14, p. 645, 1986.

[2] C. Meyer, J. Valfrey, T. Kjartansdottir, A. Wilk, and P. Barrière, "Indication for and technical refinements of submental intubation in oral and maxillofacial surgery," *Journal of Cranio-Maxillofacial Surgery*, vol. 31, no. 6, pp. 383–388, 2003.

[3] A. F. Caubi, B. C. D. E. Vasconcelos, R. J. D. H. Vasconcellos, H. H. A. De Morais, and N. S. Rocha, "Submental intubation in oral maxillofacial surgery: review of the literature and analysis of 13 cases," *Medicina Oral, Patologia Oral y Cirugia Bucal*, vol. 13, no. 3, pp. 197–200, 2008.

[4] Z. Nyárády, F. Sári, L. Olasz, and J. Nyárády, "Submental endotracheal intubation in concurrent orthognathic surgery: a technical note," *Journal of Cranio-Maxillofacial Surgery*, vol. 34, no. 6, pp. 362–365, 2006.

[5] C. Davis, "Submental intubation in complex craniomaxillofacial trauma," *ANZ Journal of Surgery*, vol. 74, no. 5, pp. 379–381, 2004.

[6] E. MacInnis and M. Baig, "A modified submental approach for oral endotracheal intubation," *International Journal of Oral and Maxillofacial Surgery*, vol. 28, no. 5, pp. 344–346, 1999.

[7] F. Biglioli, P. Mortini, M. Goisis, A. Bardazzi, and N. Boari, "Submental orotracheal intubation: an alternative to tracheotomy in transfacial cranial base surgery," *Skull Base*, vol. 13, no. 4, pp. 189–195, 2003.

[8] M. Amin, P. Dill-Russell, M. Manisali, R. Lee, and I. Sinton, "Facial fractures and submental tracheal intubation," *Anaesthesia*, vol. 57, no. 12, pp. 1195–1212, 2002.

29

Discharge against Medical Advice in Surgical Patients with Posttraumatic Stress Disorder: A Case Report Series Illustrating Unique Challenges

Marek Brzezinski,[1,2] **Maren Gregersen,**[1,2] **Luiz Gustavo Schuch,**[1,2] **Ricarda Sawatzki,**[1,2] **Joy W. Chen,**[1,2] **Grant Gauger,**[3,4] **Jasleen Kukreja,**[5,6] **and Brian Cason**[1,2]

[1]*VA Medical Center, Anesthesia Services, 4150 Clement Street, San Francisco, CA 94121, USA*

[2]*Department of Anesthesia and Perioperative Care, University of California, San Francisco, 521 Parnassus Avenue Room C-450, San Francisco, CA 94143-0648, USA*

[3]*VA Medical Center, Neurosurgery Services, 4150 Clement Street, San Francisco, CA 94121, USA*

[4]*Department of Neurosurgery, University of California, San Francisco, 400 Parnassus Ave., San Francisco, CA 94143, USA*

[5]*VA Medical Center, Surgery Services, 4150 Clement Street, San Francisco, CA 94121, USA*

[6]*Department of Surgery, University of California, San Francisco, 400 Parnassus Ave., San Francisco, CA 94143, USA*

Correspondence should be addressed to Marek Brzezinski; brzezinm@anesthesia.ucsf.edu

Academic Editor: Kuang-I Cheng

Discharge against medical advice (DAMA) can have detrimental effects on patient outcomes. Recently, the diagnosis of posttraumatic stress disorder (PTSD) has been linked with DAMA in the *mental health* setting. However, PTSD as a risk factor for DAMA in *surgical* patients has not received much consideration, although such patients may be at risk for triggering or amplification of PTSD symptoms perioperatively. We present the first case report series of three surgical patients with PTSD who left the hospital AMA. These cases differ markedly from DAMA in non-PTSD patients. In all three subjects, the stress of feeling misunderstood by clinicians and the distress of public detainment by hospital security in the setting of chronic PTSD led to aggressive and risky behavior. All three subjects represented a risk to themselves and to others at the time of DAMA. Finally, all three subjects were difficult to contact for follow-up or medical care and missed appointments.

1. Introduction

Up to 2% of inpatients in the US leave the hospital against medical advice (AMA) [1, 2]. Discharge AMA (DAMA) has been associated with poor compliance, increased mortality and morbidity, higher readmission rates, longer subsequent hospital stays, increased health care costs, and increased risk of suicide [1, 2]. Furthermore, DAMA can lead to long-term patient stigmatization in health care settings, compounding the aforementioned problems [1].

Psychiatric comorbidities are frequently associated with DAMA [3, 4]. The rate of DAMA in psychiatric patients in mental health settings has been reported to be between 6% and 35% [4]. Recently, diagnosis of posttraumatic stress disorder (PTSD) in *psychiatric hospitalized* patients was reported to be associated with hostile behavior at the time of discharge and increased likelihood of DAMA [5]. PTSD as a risk factor for DAMA in *surgical* patients, however, has not received much consideration, although *surgical patients with PTSD* may be at particularly high risk for triggering or amplifying PTSD symptoms as a result of perioperative pain and stress. Disconcertingly, DAMA could have more detrimental sequelae in patients with PTSD, as they are already at high risk for poor compliance, loss to follow-up, suicide, and increased health care costs [6–9].

Herein, we present three surgical patients with PTSD diagnosis who left AMA, focusing on patient behavior and challenges to health care providers. These cases differ markedly from DAMA in non-PTSD patients. With steadily increasing numbers of patients with PTSD requiring surgical procedures, health care providers must be familiar with the unique challenges these patients present in the perioperative period.

2. Case Reports

2.1. Case 1. A 61-year-old man underwent placement of a left superficial femoral artery stent without complications. His past medical history included war-related PTSD, diabetes, hypertension, and heavy smoking. Medications included aspirin, lisinopril, glyburide, metformin, and fentanyl patch. Shortly after his surgical procedure, the patient threatened to leave AMA unless he was allowed to *"roll around"* in a wheelchair *"as he pleased."* He was permitted to briefly leave the ward with his peripheral intravenous (IV) catheter left in place. The next morning, the patient was awake, alert, and fully oriented. About two hours later, he was increasingly lethargic with apneic episodes and oxygen saturation 80–85%. Other vital signs were unremarkable. His glucose was 246 mg/dL and was treated accordingly. After he was given Narcan (0.2 mg IV), the patient became markedly more alert and was transferred to the Intensive Care Unit (ICU). He denied self-administration of medication. A urine toxicology test was positive for benzodiazepines (received during anesthesia the day before). His arterial blood gases demonstrated a hypercarbic respiratory acidosis with pH 7.32, P_aCO_2 68.3 mmHg, and P_aO_2 99 mmHg. After he received a second dose of Narcan (0.2 mg), he became agitated and wheeled himself out of the unit and eventually the hospital with IV still in place and his care team in pursuit. He got in his car and drove until he encountered a barricade set up by hospital police officers to stop him as he presented a potential danger to himself and to others. The patient agreed to return to the ICU but refused all tests. The next morning, despite his systolic blood pressure being 231 mmHg, the patient left the hospital AMA after removal of his peripheral IV catheter. He never returned to our facility for follow-up or medical care.

2.2. Case 2. A 60-year-old man underwent an elective video-assisted thoracoscopic surgery for lung biopsy. His past medical history was significant for heavy smoking with chronic dyspnea and war-related PTSD. His medications included inhalers and prazosin. His surgery and postoperative course were unremarkable. Around 5:00 a.m. on the morning of postoperative day 2, the patient declared that he would be leaving the hospital at 7:00 a.m. and demanded removal of the peripheral IV catheter. Upon being informed that the removal can only occur with a written order by his doctor, the patient left the ward. The grounds were searched but he was unable to be located. Shortly thereafter, the patient returned to the unit and stated, *"I want this IV out and I am leaving at 0700."* After the risks associated with leaving AMA were discussed (e.g., tension pneumothorax) and understood by the patient, his peripheral IV was removed, and he left the hospital AMA for a long distance drive home alone. Subsequently, he missed follow-up appointments and refused emergency treatment when he developed cardiac chest pain at home (unrelated to surgery).

2.3. Case 3. A 57-year-old man was admitted to the hospital after being found at home lethargic and minimally responsive after a fall. The noncontrast computer tomography (CT) of the head showed a large, acute-on-chronic right subdural hematoma measuring up to 1.7 cm, with a 6 mm right-to-left midline shift and subfalcine herniation. The patient was admitted to ICU for assessment and urgent treatment. His past medical history was significant for diabetes, polysubstance abuse, war-related PTSD, and heavy smoking. The patient had a history of noncompliance. His medications on admission included metformin, trazodone, and methadone. Given the clinical presentation and head-CT findings, the neurosurgical team recommended proceeding emergently with evacuation of the subdural hematoma. However, the patient refused to consent stating that he would rather die than have surgery, stating *"It would be fine [if he died]; it would relieve me of my pain"*, but that he *"will not die,"* because he was a Navy Seal. Psychiatric consultation found the patient lacking in decision-making capacity. Given the danger to self and the potential threat he posed to others, they recommended holding the patient in the ICU and restarting his home medications. Psychiatric reassessment a day later determined that the patient had regained his decision-making capacity. His vital signs, mental status, and neurological exam results were stable. Following thorough presentation and discussion of the risks associated with leaving AMA and assertion by the patient that he understood, he left the hospital. Subsequently, he was difficult to contact and missed appointments.

3. Discussion

DAMA represents a well-recognized problem with approximately 500,000 cases estimated every year in the US [1, 2] and results in adverse patient outcomes [1, 13–15]. Patients leaving AMA have higher mortality and hospital readmission rate, increased risk of suicide, and higher overall healthcare costs [1, 3, 16]. Moreover, DAMA is likely to impair the doctor-patient relationship and reduce patient adherence to medical treatments [1, 2]. Known predictors of DAMA include male gender, younger age, lower socioeconomic class, history of substance abuse, lack of health insurance, and previous history of leaving AMA [1, 3, 10, 11, 17, 18].

Recently, the diagnosis of PTSD was shown to be associated with hostile behavior at hospital discharge and more than a sixfold increase in risk of DAMA in the mental health setting [5]. The lifetime prevalence of PTSD is estimated to be 8% among US citizens [6] and 10–18% among military veterans [7], yet PTSD as a risk factor for leaving AMA in surgical inpatients has not received much consideration. PTSD [6, 8, 9, 19] and DAMA [1, 13, 14] are independently associated with poor compliance, loss to follow-up, suicide, and high costs of health care. Some aspects of PTSD, such as physical and cognitive deficits, behavioral issues, and anger and aggression problems, can interfere with decision-making

TABLE 1: Interventions for consideration in surgical patients with PTSD [1, 2, 10–12].

Consideration	Intervention
Be proactive.	Identify history of AMA, poor compliance, or violence to better assess current risk.
	Provide social and psychological support.
	Provide realistic information about the postoperative period.
	Maintain open patient-doctor communication.
	Ensure the continuation of medication for PTSD while being in the hospital.
Be aware and prepared.	Develop collaborative approaches and effective rescue strategies that could be implemented as soon as the patient wishes to leave AMA.
	Handle aggressive and hostile behaviors in a productive and constructive way.
	Avoid getting upset or frustrated; instead, be positive and encouraging.
	Try to reduce the danger of losing the patient's trust by utilizing communication that emphasizes understanding of their unique issues with cultural sensitivity.
Decrease stigma.	Actively maintain the patient-doctor-relationship, ensuring proper follow-up.

Note. AMA = against medical advice; PTSD = posttraumatic stress disorder.

abilities [1]. Therefore, DAMA in surgical patients with PTSD could amplify the negative effects leading to worse outcome than in patients without PTSD [6–9]. We present the first case series of DAMA demonstrating unique challenges in surgical patients with PTSD who left AMA either before or after scheduled surgery.

Caring for such patients can be challenging. Aggression at the time of discharge was expressed by all three patients and required the use of hospital security. Such interactions negatively impact the patient-doctor relationship and alienate the patient. Conversely, aggressive behavior by the patient could also distress the health care providers and damage their perception of the patient or potentially any patient with PTSD, compounding the problem further.

Such patients pose risk to themselves and others. Two patients disappeared from the ward with a functioning peripheral IV catheter in place (Cases 1 and 2). Leaving with an IV in situ poses the risk of self-administration of drugs and driving under the influence. In fact, one patient attempted to drive away until the hospital police intervened.

Stress of attempting to leave the hospital AMA, the perception of being misunderstood, and emotionally charged interactions with staff and police could exacerbate PTSD symptoms. While the severity of PTSD was not explicitly measured at the time of DAMA, at least one patient made comments related to war.

All three patients showed decreased compliance following DAMA and either were difficult to contact, missed appointments, or never returned to our facility for any follow-ups. Abrupt DAMA makes the preparation for future follow-up almost impossible. Decreased compliance has long-term impact on PTSD surgical care and PTSD care, exacerbating PTSD symptoms. The issues summarized above highlight the

potential risk of increased long-term health care costs in the surgical population with PTSD.

The link between PTSD and DAMA needs to be examined more rigorously in a perioperative context. Meanwhile, clinicians should focus on establishing strong patient-physician relationship, communicating effectively with the patient, and constructively addressing patient's concerns [1, 2, 10–12, 20]. These interventions should be complemented with PTSD-unique considerations (Table 1) that focus on maintaining the therapeutic bond by ensuring a safe discharge and supporting the patient through follow-ups [1, 2, 10–12].

In conclusion, this series highlights how the acute stress of feeling misunderstood by clinicians and the distress of public detainment by hospital security—in addition to the chronic stress of PTSD—can lead to more aggressive and risky behavior in the perioperative period. Patients with PTSD leaving AMA represent a risk to themselves and to others and may suffer from more negative long-term sequelae. Consequently, DAMA could have more detrimental effects on patients with PTSD than those without. With increasing numbers of surgical patients with preexistent PTSD, health care providers should be familiar with the unique challenges these patients present in the perioperative period.

Acknowledgments

The authors appreciate the administrative and editorial assistance of John Rukkila, ELS.

References

[1] D. Alfandre, "Reconsidering against medical advice discharges: embracing patient-centeredness to promote high quality care and a renewed research agenda," *Journal of General Internal Medicine*, vol. 28, no. 12, pp. 1657–1662, 2013.

[2] D. J. Alfandre, ""I'm going home": discharges against medical advice," *Mayo Clinic Proceedings*, vol. 84, no. 3, pp. 255–260, 2009.

[3] M. Choi, H. Kim, H. Qian, and A. Palepu, "Readmission rates of patients discharged against medical advice: a matched cohort study," *PLoS ONE*, vol. 6, no. 9, Article ID e24459, 2011.

[4] A. J. Dalrymple and M. Fata, "Cross-validating factors associated with discharges against medical advice," *Canadian Journal of Psychiatry*, vol. 38, no. 4, pp. 285–289, 1993.

[5] P. E. Holtzheimer, J. Russo, D. Zatzick, C. Bundy, and P. P. Roy-Byrne, "The impact of comorbid posttraumatic stress disorder on short-term clinical outcome in hospitalized patients with depression," *American Journal of Psychiatry*, vol. 162, no. 5, pp. 970–976, 2005.

[6] W. V. R. Vieweg, D. A. Julius, A. Fernandez, M. Beatty-Brooks, J. M. Hettema, and A. K. Pandurangi, "Posttraumatic stress disorder: clinical features, pathophysiology, and treatment," *American Journal of Medicine*, vol. 119, no. 5, pp. 383–390, 2006.

[7] C. W. Hoge, C. A. Castro, and S. C. Messer, "Combat duty in Iraq and Afghanistan, mental health problems and barriers to care," *U.S. Army Medical Department Journal*, pp. 7–17, 2008.

[8] D. F. Zatzick, C. R. Marmar, D. S. Weiss, and etal., "Posttraumatic stress disorder and functioning and quality of life outcomes in a nationally representative sample of male Vietnam veterans," *The American journal of psychiatry*, vol. 154, pp. 1690–1695, 1997.

[9] J. Sareen, "Posttraumatic stress disorder in adults: impact, comorbidity, risk factors, and treatment," *Canadian Journal of Psychiatry*, vol. 59, no. 9, pp. 460–467, 2014.

[10] M. A. Clark, J. T. Abbott, and T. Adyanthaya, "Ethics Seminars: a best-practice approach to navigating the against-medical-advice discharge," *Academic Emergency Medicine*, vol. 21, no. 9, pp. 1050–1057, 2014.

[11] M. E. Menendez, C. N. van Dijk, and D. Ring, "Who leaves the hospital against medical advice in the orthopaedic setting?" *Clinical Orthopaedics and Related Research*, vol. 473, no. 3, pp. 1140–1149, 2015.

[12] J. T. Berger, "Discharge against medical advice: ethical considerations and professional obligations," *Journal of Hospital Medicine*, vol. 3, no. 5, pp. 403–408, 2008.

[13] A. Garland, C. D. Ramsey, R. Fransoo et al., "Rates of readmission and death associated with leaving hospital against medical advice: a population-based study," *CMAJ*, vol. 185, no. 14, pp. 1207–1214, 2013.

[14] Z. Y. Aliyu, "Discharge against medical advice: sociodemographic, clinical and financial perspectives," *International Journal of Clinical Practice*, vol. 56, pp. 325–327, 2002.

[15] S. W. Hwang, J. Li, R. Gupta, V. Chien, and R. E. Martin, "What happens to patients who leave hospital against medical advice?" *Canadian Medical Association Journal*, vol. 168, no. 4, pp. 417–420, 2003.

[16] J. M. Glasgow, M. Vaughn-Sarrazin, and P. J. Kaboli, "Leaving against medical advice (AMA): risk of 30-day mortality and hospital readmission," *Journal of General Internal Medicine*, vol. 25, no. 9, pp. 926–929, 2010.

[17] D. Alfandre, "Reconsidering against medical advice discharges," *Journal of General Internal Medicine*, vol. 29, no. 5, p. 706, 2014.

[18] D. Alfandre and J. H. Schumann, "What is wrong with discharges against medical advice (and how to fix them)," *Journal of the American Medical Association*, vol. 310, no. 22, pp. 2393–2394, 2013.

[19] L. Amaya-Jackson, J. R. Davidson, D. C. Hughes et al., "Functional impairment and utilization of services associated with posttraumatic stress in the community," *Journal of Traumatic Stress*, vol. 12, no. 4, pp. 709–724, 1999.

[20] D. M. Windish and N. Ratanawongsa, "Providers' perceptions of relationships and professional roles when caring for patients who leave the hospital against medical advice," *Journal of General Internal Medicine*, vol. 23, no. 10, pp. 1698–1707, 2008.

30

Use of Peripheral Nerve Blocks with Sedation for Total Knee Arthroplasty in a Patient with Contraindication for General Anesthesia

Eric Kamenetsky,[1] **Antoun Nader,**[2] **and Mark C. Kendall**[2]

[1] *McGaw Medical Center of Northwestern University, Chicago, IL 60611, USA*
[2] *Feinberg School of Medicine, Northwestern University, Chicago, IL 60611, USA*

Correspondence should be addressed to Mark C. Kendall; m-kendall@northwestern.edu

Academic Editor: Richard Riley

Although peripheral nerve blocks are commonly used to provide postoperative analgesia after total knee arthroplasty (TKA) and other lower extremity procedures, these blocks are rarely used for intraoperative anesthesia. Most TKAs are performed under general anesthesia (GA) or neuraxial anesthesia (NA). The knee has a complex sensory innervation that makes surgical anesthesia difficult with peripheral nerve blocks alone. Rarely are both GA and NA relatively contraindicated and alternatives are considered. We present a patient who underwent TKA performed under peripheral nerve block and sedation alone.

1. Introduction

Although peripheral nerve blocks are commonly used to provide postoperative analgesia after total knee arthroplasty (TKA) and other lower extremity procedures, these blocks are rarely used as the sole anesthetic. The majority of TKAs are performed under general anesthesia (GA) in the United States (57.9%), with most other cases utilizing neuraxial anesthesia (NA) [1]. The knee has a complex sensory innervation that makes surgical anesthesia difficult with peripheral nerve blocks (PNBs) alone. The knee is innervated by the lumbosacral plexus. Few publications exist about lumbar plexus block in combination with sciatic nerve block.

Innervation of the anterior knee joint is primarily supplied by the femoral nerve. The posterior knee joint is supplied by the genicular branches of the sciatic nerve, with contribution from the obturator nerve supplying the medial portion of the knee joint. The cutaneous innervation of the thigh and knee involves multiple nerve distributions [2]. The lateral femoral cutaneous nerve (LFCN) supplies portions of the anterior and lateral thigh, extending to the knee. The posterior femoral cutaneous nerve (PFCN) is a pure sensory nerve that, in a majority of cases, emerges from the greater

sciatic foramen beneath the piriformis muscle. The PFCN then travels medial to the sciatic nerve and lies directly on the deep surface of the gluteus maximus muscle. Here, the PFCN has been described to divide into many branches which continue inferiorly, supplying sensation to the posterior thigh, popliteal region, and calf area and occasionally extending to the calcaneal region. The anterior femoral cutaneous nerves (AFCNs), which include the intermediate femoral and medial femoral cutaneous nerves, are reported to be branches of the anterior division of the femoral nerve. The intermediate femoral cutaneous nerve supplies the anterior thigh as far distal as the knee, with the medical cutaneous branches supplying the adjacent medial portions of the thigh, not covered by the obturator nerve. Collectively, the sensory nerve branches that terminate at the knee are commonly referred to as the patellar plexus [3, 4].

At our institution, neuraxial blocks are performed as the primary anesthetic for more than 95 percent of TKAs. For the vast majority of cases where NA is contraindicated, a general anesthetic is performed. It is uncommon that both GA and NA are contraindicated and alternatives should be considered. We present a patient who underwent TKA using multiple PNBs with local anesthetic and sedation alone. Written consent for publication was obtained from the patient.

2. Case Description

A sixty-one-year old Caucasian female is scheduled for a left TKA. The patient had a history of pulmonary fibrosis requiring 4 L supplemental O_2 with exercise, OSA, idiopathic thrombocytopenic purpura, gastroesophageal reflux disease, and obesity. She also had a recent history of pulmonary embolism (PE) necessitating early, postoperative anticoagulation for deep venous thrombosis and PE prevention. Preoperative platelet count was 88,000/μL, which was stable for the preceding two years. During a formal six-minute walk test, the patient desaturated to 85% on room air and required 5 L O_2 to keep $SpO_2 > 88\%$. Decision was made to proceed with TKA under PNBs and minimal sedation. Complete surgical anesthesia was achieved and patient underwent TKA without complications.

3. Block Descriptions

An ultrasound-guided infragluteal-parabiceps approach was used for sciatic nerve blockade (SNB) [5]. Ten mL of 0.5% bupivacaine with 1 : 300,000 epinephrine was administered deep to the common investing extraneural layer around the sciatic nerve (Figure 1).

The PFCN was identified deep to the gluteus maximus muscle, lateral to the biceps femoris, and posterior to the sciatic nerve. Here, 3 mL of 0.5% bupivacaine with 1 : 300,000 epinephrine was injected (Figure 1). With the patient supine, the LFCN was identified lateral to the sartorius muscle, anterior to the iliotibial tract, and below fascia lata. Five mL of 0.5% bupivacaine with 1 : 300,000 epinephrine was administered at this location (Figure 2).

The distal divisions of the obturator nerve were identified between the adductor longus and brevis muscles (anterior division) and between adductor brevis and magnus (posterior division). A total of 10 mL of 0.5% bupivacaine with 1 : 300,000 epinephrine was used for the obturator nerve block, 5 mL for each division (Figure 3).

The anterior femoral cutaneous nerve was identified at the level of the inguinal crease in a plane superficial to fascia lata and adjacent to a superficial arterial branch of the femoral artery. Here, 2 mL of 0.5% bupivacaine with 1 : 300,000 epinephrine was administered (Figure 4).

Finally, a femoral nerve catheter (FNC) was placed using a sterile technique. A 4 cm 18-gauge stimulating Tuohy needle, connected to the negative lead of a constant voltage nerve stimulator (Stimuplex DIG; B-Braun/McGaw Medical, Bethlehem, PA), was inserted at the inguinal crease using ultrasound guidance (Figure 4). With quadriceps evoked motor response (EMR) at 0.5 mA, a 20 G stimulating catheter (StimuCath; Arrow International, Reading, PA, USA) was advanced while maintaining the evoked motor response of the quadriceps muscle throughout catheter advancement. The femoral catheter was advanced 11 cm beyond the needle tip. A total of 15 mL of 0.5% ropivacaine with 1 : 300,000 epinephrine was administered through the catheter after

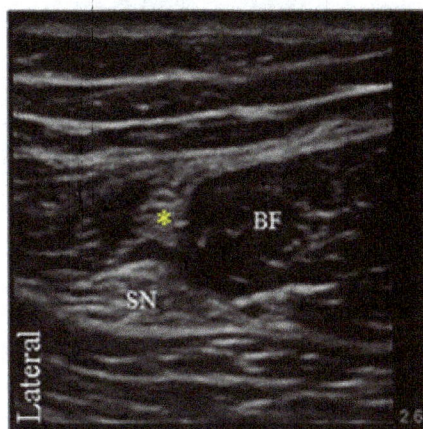

FIGURE 1: Transverse ultrasound image of the posterior femoral cutaneous nerve (asterisk) located deep to the gluteus maximus muscle and lateral to the biceps femoris muscle (BF). Sciatic nerve (SN).

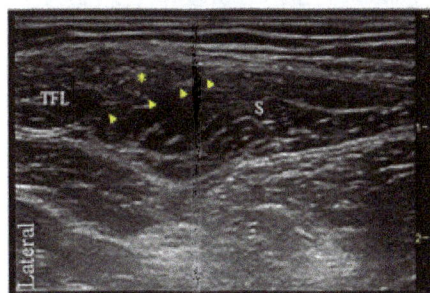

FIGURE 2: Transverse ultrasound image of the lateral femoral cutaneous nerve (asterisk) lying below fascia lata and lateral to the sartorius muscle (S) and medial to the tensor fasciae latae muscle (TFL). Arrow heads point to the fascia that separates the sartorius muscle from the LFCN.

placement. A 2.5 cm broadband linear array transducer (7–13 MHz probe, Sonosite, M Turbo, Bothell, WA, USA) was used for all PNBs. For the single-shot PNBs, a 21 G echogenic stimulating needle was used (Pajunk, Medizintechnologie, Geisingen, Germany).

4. Discussion

Over the last decade, various anesthetic techniques have been used to care for patients undergoing TKA. Regional and neuraxial techniques are often chosen to improve postoperative analgesia and to minimize adverse effects from systemic opioids.

There are several reports of lower extremity surgery performed utilizing a lumbar plexus block (LPB) in combination with a sciatic nerve block. Luber et al. evaluated the efficacy of lumbar plexus block techniques for TKA [6]. Although no complications related to the LBP were reported in this study group of patients, there are several known risks. Retroperitoneal hematomas and other hemorrhagic complications have been reported in case studies [7, 8]. American Society of Regional Anesthesia (ASRA) guidelines state, for

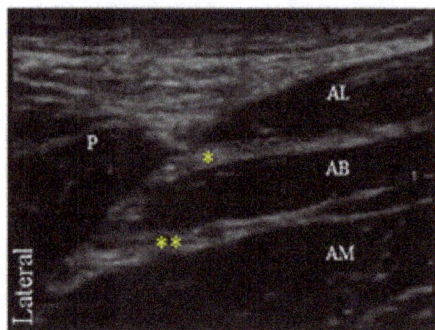

FIGURE 3: Transverse ultrasound image of the obturator nerve. The distal portion of the obturator nerve divides into an anterior division (single asterisk), identified between the adductor longus (AL) and brevis muscles (AB) and a posterior division (double asterisks) located between adductor brevis and magnus (AM) muscles. Pectineus muscle (P).

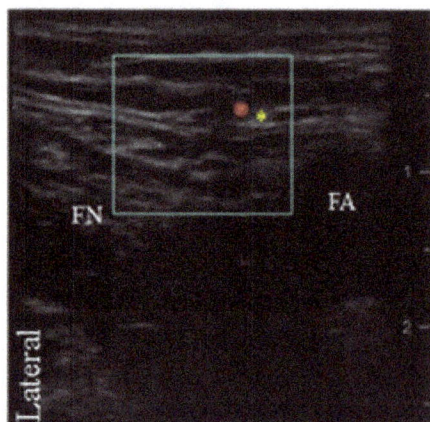

FIGURE 4: Transverse ultrasound image of the femoral nerve (FN) and femoral artery (FA). The anterior femoral cutaneous nerve of the thigh with its accompanying artery is also shown (asterisk).

patients undergoing deep plexus block, recommendations for neuraxial techniques should be similarly applied to minimize the risk of hemorrhagic complications [9].

Regional techniques specifically targeting the intermediate cutaneous nerve of the thigh with ultrasound guidance are not well described in the literature. A cadaveric study evaluating the fascicular anatomy of the femoral nerve showed that the distance from the inguinal ligament to the first branching point of the femoral nerve was 1.50 ± 0.47 cm [10]. Anterior and medial thigh cutaneous coverage may be partially missed if a FNB is performed distal to its cutaneous branching points, thus resulting in inadequate cutaneous anesthesia of the thigh and knee.

It has been shown that PFCN blockade during SNB is likely consequence of local anesthetic diffusion [11, 12]. A targeted block of the PFCN was performed in our case to ensure anesthesia of the posterior thigh for a thigh tourniquet and to provide cutaneous anesthesia of the posterior knee in an effort to minimize patient appreciation of knee manipulation during TKA.

Using peripheral nerve blocks alone to perform TKA may have several limitations and considerations. First, the total dose of local anesthetic used in this case approaches the maximum recommended dose of local anesthetic. We chose to use ropivacaine when dosing through the FNC for this reason. Also, the technique we describe requires multiple separate needle entry points and perineural injections. Transient postoperative neurologic symptoms after PNBs have been reported to occur at rates from 0 to 15%, with a rate of ~8% seen after nerve-stimulation assisted sciatic nerve blockade [13, 14]. No studies have evaluated the incidence of neurologic sequelae after performing femoral, sciatic, and multiple cutaneous PNBs, similar to the technique used in this case. The innervation of the knee is highly variable, particularly cutaneous innervation, which makes complete surgical anesthesia a challenge using PNBs alone. The techniques we describe achieved complete anesthesia of the knee joint, as well as cutaneous anesthesia. Any small, unidentified gaps in cutaneous coverage were likely compensated by small doses of sedation given intraoperatively.

The techniques we describe may help other anesthesiologists when encountering patients with contraindications for both GA and NA. With the growing demand for TKA, anesthesiologists will likely encounter an increasing number of patients similar to those presented in this case [15].

References

[1] P. M. Fleischut, J. M. Eskreis-Winkler, L. K. Gaber-Baylis et al., "Variability in anesthetic care for total knee arthroplasty: an analysis from the anesthesia quality institute," *American Journal of Medical Quality*, vol. 30, no. 2, pp. 172–179, 2015.

[2] R. C. Wasielewski, "Surgical anatomy of the knee," in *The Adult Knee*, J. J. Callaghan, A. G. Rosenberg, H. E. Rubash, P. T. Simonian, and T. L. Wickiewicz, Eds., p. 77, Lippincott Williams & Wilkins, Philadelphia, Pa, USA, 1st edition, 2003.

[3] H. Gray and C. D. Clemente, *Anatomy of the Human Body*, Lea & Febiger, Philadelphia, Pa, USA, 30th edition, 1985.

[4] F. H. Netter, *Atlas of Human Anatomy*, Saunders Elsevier, Philadelphia, Pa, USA, 4th edition, 2006.

[5] A. Nader, M. C. Kendall, G. S. De Oliveira et al., "A dose-ranging study of 0.5% bupivacaine or ropivacaine on the success and duration of the ultrasound-guided, nerve-stimulator-assisted sciatic nerve block: a double-blind, randomized clinical trial," *Regional Anesthesia and Pain Medicine*, vol. 38, no. 6, pp. 492–502, 2013.

[6] M. J. Luber, R. Greengrass, and T. P. Vail, "Patient satisfaction and effectiveness of lumbar plexus and sciatic nerve block for total knee arthroplasty," *The Journal of Arthroplasty*, vol. 16, no. 1, pp. 17–21, 2001.

[7] R. S. Weller, J. C. Gerancher, J. C. Crews, and K. L. Wade, "Extensive retroperitoneal hematoma without neurologic deficit in two patients who underwent lumbar plexus block and were later anticoagulated," *Anesthesiology*, vol. 98, no. 2, pp. 581–585, 2003.

[8] C. Aveline and F. Bonnet, "Delayed retroperitoneal haematoma after failed lumbar plexus block," *British Journal of Anaesthesia*, vol. 93, no. 4, pp. 589–591, 2004.

[9] T. T. Horlocker, D. J. Wedel, J. C. Rowlingson et al., "Regional anesthesia in the patient receiving antithrombotic or thrombolytic therapy: American Society of Regional Anesthesia and Pain Medicine Evidence-Based Guidelines (third edition)," *Regional Anesthesia & Pain Medicine*, vol. 35, no. 1, pp. 64–101, 2010.

[10] K. J. Gustafson, G. C. J. Pinault, J. J. Neville et al., "Fascicular anatomy of human femoral nerve: implications for neural prostheses using nerve cuff electrodes," *Journal of Rehabilitation Research and Development*, vol. 46, no. 7, pp. 973–984, 2009.

[11] C. Barbero, R. Fuzier, and K. Samii, "Anterior approach to the sciatic nerve block: adaptation to the patient's height," *Anesthesia and Analgesia*, vol. 98, no. 6, pp. 1785–1788, 2004.

[12] J. E. Chelly and L. Delaunay, "A new anterior approach to the sciatic nerve block," *Anesthesiology*, vol. 91, no. 6, pp. 1655–1660, 1999.

[13] R. Brull, C. J. L. McCartney, V. W. S. Chan, and H. El-Beheiry, "Neurological complications after regional anesthesia: contemporary estimates of risk," *Anesthesia and Analgesia*, vol. 104, no. 4, pp. 965–974, 2007.

[14] A. Nader, M. C. Kendall, R. Doty Jr. et al., "Nerve stimulator-guided supplemental popliteal sciatic nerve block after a failed sciatic block does not increase the incidence of transient postoperative neurologic sequelae," *Anesthesiology*, vol. 115, no. 3, pp. 596–603, 2011.

[15] S. Kurtz, K. Ong, E. Lau, F. Mowat, and M. Halpern, "Projections of primary and revision hip and knee arthroplasty in the United States from 2005 to 2030," *Journal of Bone and Joint Surgery A*, vol. 89, no. 4, pp. 780–785, 2007.

31

Perioperative Management of Interscalene Block in Patients with Lung Disease

Eric S. Schwenk, Kishor Gandhi, and Eugene R. Viscusi

Department of Anesthesiology, Jefferson Medical College, Suite 8490, 111 South 11th Street, Philadelphia, PA 19107, USA

Correspondence should be addressed to Eric S. Schwenk; eric.schwenk@jefferson.edu

Academic Editors: R. S. Gomez and J. G. Jakobsson

Interscalene nerve block impairs ipsilateral lung function and is relatively contraindicated for patients with lung impairment. We present a case of an 89-year-old female smoker with prior left lung lower lobectomy and mild to moderate lung disease who presented for right shoulder arthroplasty and insisted on regional anesthesia. The patient received a multimodal perioperative regimen that consisted of a continuous interscalene block, acetaminophen, ketorolac, and opioids. Surgery proceeded uneventfully and postoperative analgesia was excellent. Pulmonary physiology and management of these patients will be discussed. A risk/benefit discussion should occur with patients having impaired lung function before performance of interscalene blocks. In this particular patient with mild to moderate disease, analgesia was well managed through a multimodal approach including a continuous interscalene block, and close monitoring of respiratory status took place throughout the perioperative period, leading to a successful outcome.

1. Introduction

Impaired lung function has traditionally been considered a relative contraindication to interscalene plexus block (ISB). ISB has been shown to cause ipsilateral hemidiaphragmatic paresis virtually 100% of the time [1, 2] with significant decreases in several pulmonary measurements [1]. Knowledge of the potential complications is critical, even if they occur rarely. At the same time, opioids impair respiratory function and should be minimized if lung function is tenuous [3]. The elderly in particular are sensitive to the depressant effects of anesthetics and medications that cause muscle weakness [4], especially opioids. Excellent postoperative analgesia, therefore, is a key component in the prevention of postoperative pulmonary complications in this population.

2. Case Description

The patient was an 89-year-old woman, American Society of Anesthesiologists Physical Status 3, with hypertension, hypothyroidism, and a 58-pack-year history of smoking who five years prior had undergone a left lung lower lobectomy for cancer. She was scheduled to undergo a right total shoulder replacement for worsening degenerative disease and pain. Pulmonary function testing performed 17 months prior to surgery revealed a FEV_1/FVC ratio of 0.68, indicating mild obstructive disease, and a diffusion capacity (DLCO) of 9.5 mL/mm Hg/min, indicating a moderate gas transfer defect. Physical examination revealed clear lung fields bilaterally and a short hyomental distance on airway exam. Preoperative pulse oximetry on room air revealed an oxygen saturation of 100%. The patient and her family wished to proceed with surgery only under regional anesthesia after consulting with her primary care physician. After discussion of the risks and benefits of regional anesthesia, including the possibility of impaired lung function, pneumothorax on the operative side postoperatively, and mechanical ventilation postoperatively, the patient agreed to perform surgery under a continuous interscalene nerve block (CISB) with light sedation.

The block was performed using continuous ultrasound guidance (GE Logic E, Wauwatosa, WI) and nerve stimulation (B. Braun, Bethlehem, PA). An in-plane, posterior approach technique was utilized for needle insertion and visualization based on the preference of the anesthesiologist performing the procedure (Figure 1). A total of 30 mL of

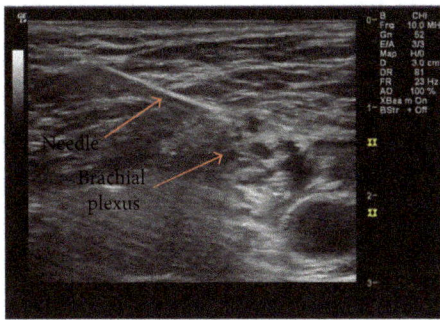

FIGURE 1: Ultrasound image of low interscalene block.

ropivacaine 0.5% was injected incrementally after negative aspiration to the area adjacent to the C5 and C6 nerve roots and a 20 g multiorifice peripheral nerve catheter (B. Braun Medical Inc., Bethlehem, PA) was inserted 5 cm beyond the needle tip. Sensory block was confirmed with decreased pinprick sensation in the C5 and C6 dermatomes. The patient was given a propofol infusion of 15–25 mcg/kg/min for sedation with oxygen via nasal cannula and surgery proceeded uneventfully.

In the postoperative anesthesia care unit (PACU) the patient had excellent analgesia. Intravenous fentanyl and morphine were available but she requested no rescue opioids or other medications. Close postoperative monitoring was continued on a surgical ward with frequent pulse oximetry measurements. Analgesia consisted of a multimodal regimen including CISB with ropivacaine 0.2% running at 8 mL/h without a demand function and ketorolac, aspirin, and pregabalin, with a morphine PCA for breakthrough pain. She consumed the equivalent of morphine 17.5 mg IV for breakthrough pain during the first 24 h postoperatively. She reported no side effects and denied significant dyspnea while the catheter was in place, receiving no more than 2 L/min of oxygen via nasal cannula as a precautionary measure during her admission. She used her incentive spirometer multiple times per day. She was discharged home on postoperative day no. 2 after the continuous interscalene catheter had been removed.

3. Discussion

3.1. Pulmonary Function Changes after ISB. Although ISB has traditionally been relatively contraindicated in those with decreased pulmonary function, we presented a case of an elderly woman with prior partial lung resection who experienced a successful outcome through minimizing opioids and close postoperative monitoring. Urmey and McDonald [1] demonstrated that multiple indices of lung function, including forced vital capacity (FVC), forced expiratory volume in one second (FEV_1), and midexpiratory flow rate, are depressed when an ISB is performed. These findings have been subsequently confirmed by others [2, 5, 6]. Such changes are mostly due to the ipsilateral hemidiaphragmatic paresis that occurs with ISB, which likely persists for greater than four hours [2] and in one study extended to beyond

eight hours after block [5]. The affected hemidiaphragm, in fact, will move in a paradoxical (i.e., cephalad) fashion after ISB in many patients [2]. There is some evidence that partial compensation by the contralateral hemidiaphragm may occur [6], however, which may explain why some patients with mild respiratory impairment can tolerate ISB without difficulty.

Phrenic nerve function is affected by the presence of a CISB, even after the primary block has been resolved. Pere and colleagues [5] demonstrated that some patients will have persistent impairment of diaphragm function for the duration of the continuous infusion. The implication is that sending an ambulatory patient with compromised respiratory function home with a continuous catheter could create a dangerous situation and should probably be avoided. The catheter for the patient described here was removed before discharge.

Pneumothorax following ISB is another consideration that should be discussed. Although many believe pneumothorax is less likely to follow ISB than supraclavicular block, and a recent prospective registry of more than 1,100 brachial plexus blocks (ISB and supraclavicular blocks) reported no pneumothoraces [7], caution must still be exercised. Several recent case reports document the occurrence of pneumothorax after ISB [8, 9]. Such a complication may go unnoticed in a healthy patient but could have serious consequences in someone with underlying lung disease or prior lung surgery. A pneumothorax could have been devastating for this patient, as it would have further decreased the lung area for gas exchange, potentially to a critical level, given her preexisting moderate gas exchange defect. Extra caution and discussion of this specific risk of ISB should precede its performance in a patient with prior lung resection or compromise for any other reason.

Finally, the long-term consequences of interscalene blocks are rarely discussed, but a recent case series [10] describing 14 patients who experienced long-term phrenic nerve paresis after ISB must be taken into context and factored into each case. These patients required surgical intervention to restore respiratory function. Unlike the patient in this case, all 14 patients were overweight or obese males.

3.2. Effects of Posterior versus Anterolateral Approach for the Interscalene Block. The anesthesiologist performing the block used an in-plane, posterior approach in which the entire needle is visualized, theoretically providing increased safety, more precise needle positioning, and avoidance of the surgical field [11]. This was chosen based on the preference of the anesthesiologist. However, the only prospective trial comparing the two approaches concluded that the anterolateral (out-of-plane) approach provided more pain-free time in the recovery room and easier catheter placement [12]. The issue remains unresolved, but, as it applies to this patient, evidence is lacking to support either technique reducing pulmonary complications.

3.3. Effects of Digital Pressure during Interscalene Block on Pulmonary Function. Digital pressure above the level of the

ISB has been studied as a technique used to decrease the spread of local anesthetic to the phrenic nerve. Despite initial enthusiasm, this has been shown repeatedly to be ineffective [13–15].

3.4. Effects of Reducing Local Anesthetic Volume or Concentration on Pulmonary Function. Several investigators have studied the effects of decreasing the local anesthetic volume on hemidiaphragmatic paresis and other respiratory parameters. The results have been inconclusive, with some reporting an improvement in pulmonary function [16–18] and others finding that the diaphragm remains impaired [2, 6].

Studies examining the effects of using dilute local anesthetic solutions suggest that doing so may decrease some of the unwanted respiratory side effects [19, 20]. However, duration of analgesia would likely be shorter and potentially require the addition of a continuous catheter to provide adequate analgesia.

3.5. Comparison of Risks and Benefits. It has been shown that FVC, FEV_1, and total lung capacity are reduced after lung lobectomy [21, 22], which for this patient resulted in mild obstructive disease and moderate gas exchange defect. Sengul et al. [23] found that pulmonary compensation after lower lobectomy in particular is achieved by expansion of the contralateral lung. A pneumothorax on the right (surgical) side for this patient, therefore, could have been especially deleterious. However, these concerns must be weighed against the pain and its detrimental effects on recovery. The benefits of adequate analgesia extend past the immediate postoperative period, as poorly controlled perioperative pain can lead to delayed hospital discharge and chronic pain syndromes [24].

Opioids remain an option but their unwanted side effects, in particular respiratory depression, limit their effectiveness in patients with compromised lung function. Specifically, opioids impair the diaphragm and thoracic muscles, decreasing functional residual capacity and leading to atelectasis [3]. A multimodal analgesic approach that includes regional analgesic techniques, nonsteroidal anti-inflammatory drugs (NSAIDs), acetaminophen, and opioids as rescue agents is ideal. The risks of ISB must be weighed against the potential respiratory effects of larger doses of opioids. For the intraoperative management, the decrease in functional residual capacity [25] and the atelectasis [26] that often occur under general anesthesia must be considered. Finally, some data have shown that regional anesthesia may reduce the risk of postoperative cognitive dysfunction in the elderly when compared to general anesthesia [27].

In summary, this 89-year-old woman was a motivated patient who understood the risks involved. Despite having mild to moderate lung disease, this patient was fairly well compensated and symptom-free on the day of surgery. Although this was reassuring, the potential for respiratory complications was nevertheless present. We believed that the benefits of regional anesthesia outweighed those of general anesthesia, taking the physiologic changes, patient preferences, and our own preferences into account. Through close observation in the PACU and continuing on the surgical ward, her respiratory status was maintained and clinically significant dyspnea and hypoxia were avoided. We believe this was a result of maximizing nonopioid agents and minimizing the consumption of opioids, encouraging incentive spirometer use, and close monitoring for any change in respiratory status.

Authors' Contribution

Eric S. Schwenk took care of the patient, conceived the idea for the case report, and helped write the paper. Kishor Gandhi took care of the patient and helped write the paper. Eugene R. Viscusi helped write the paper.

Funding

The authors received departmental funding.

References

[1] W. F. Urmey and M. McDonald, "Hemidiaphragmatic paresis during interscalene brachial plexus block: effects on pulmonary functin and chest wall mechanics," *Anesthesia and Analgesia*, vol. 74, no. 3, pp. 352–257, 1992.

[2] S. K. Sinha, J. H. Abrams, J. T. Barnett et al., "Decreasing the local anesthetic volume from 20 to 10 mL for ultrasound-guided interscalene block at the cricoid level does not reduce the incidence of hemidiaphragmatic paresis," *Regional Anesthesia and Pain Medicine*, vol. 36, no. 1, pp. 17–20, 2011.

[3] N. Sasaki, M. J. Meyer, and M. Eikermann, "Postoperative respiratory muscle dysfunction: pathophysiology and preventive strategies," *Anesthesiology*, vol. 118, pp. 961–978, 2013.

[4] J. Sprung, O. Gajic, and D. O. Warner, "Review article: age related alterations in respiratory function—anesthetic considerations," *Canadian Journal of Anesthesia*, vol. 53, no. 12, pp. 1244–1257, 2006.

[5] P. Pere, M. Pitkanen, P. H. Rosenberg et al., "Effect of continuous interscalene brachial plexus block on diaphragm motion and on ventilatory function," *Acta Anaesthesiologica Scandinavica*, vol. 36, no. 1, pp. 53–57, 1992.

[6] C. T. Hartrick, Y.-S. Tang, D. Siwek, R. Murray, D. Hunstad, and G. Smith, "The effect of initial local anesthetic dose with continuous interscalene analgesia on postoperative pain and diaphragmatic function in patients undergoing arthroscopic shoulder surgery: a double-blind, randomized controlled trial," *BMC Anesthesiology*, vol. 12, article 6, 2012.

[7] S. S. Liu, M. A. Gordon, P. M. Shaw, S. Wilfred, T. Shetty, and J. T. YaDeau, "A prospective clinical registry of ultrasound-guided regional anesthesia for ambulatory shoulder surgery," *Anesthesia and Analgesia*, vol. 111, no. 3, pp. 617–623, 2010.

[8] B. L. S. Mandim, R. R. Alves, R. Almeida, J. P. J. Pontes, L. J. Arantes, and F. P. Morais, "Pneumothorax post brachial plexus block guided by ultrasound: a case report," *Revista Brasileira de Anestesiologia*, vol. 62, pp. 741–747, 2012.

[9] E. Montoro, F. Ferre, H. Yonis, C. Gris, and V. Minville, "Pneumothorax as a complication of ultrasound-guided interscalene block for shoulder surgery," *European Journal of Anaesthesiology*, vol. 30, pp. 90–94, 2013.

[10] M. R. Kaufman, A. I. Elkwood, M. I. Rose et al., "Surgical treatment of permanent diaphragm paralysis after interscalene nerve block for shoulder surgery," *Anesthesiology*, vol. 119, pp. 484–487, 2013.

[11] E. R. Mariano, V. J. Loland, and B. M. Ilfeld, "Interscalene perineural catheter placement using an ultrasound-guided posterior approach," *Regional Anesthesia and Pain Medicine*, vol. 34, no. 1, pp. 60–63, 2009.

[12] M. J. Fredrickson, C. M. Ball, and A. J. Dalgleish, "Posterior versus anterolateral approach interscalene catheter placement: a prospective randomized trial," *Regional Anesthesia and Pain Medicine*, vol. 36, no. 2, pp. 125–133, 2011.

[13] W. F. Urmey, P. Grossi, N. E. Sharrock, J. Stanton, and P. J. Gloeggler, "Digital pressure during interscalene block is clinically ineffective in preventing anesthetic spread to the cervical plexus," *Anesthesia and Analgesia*, vol. 83, no. 2, pp. 366–370, 1996.

[14] S.-E. Bennani, F. Vandenabele-Teneur, J.-B. Nyarwaya, M. Delecroix, and R. Krivosic-Horber, "An attempt to prevent spread of local anaesthetic to the phrenic nerve by compression above the injection site during the interscalene brachial plexus block," *European Journal of Anaesthesiology*, vol. 15, no. 4, pp. 453–456, 1998.

[15] X. Sala-Blanch, J. R. Lázaro, J. Correa, and M. Gómez-Fernandez, "Phrenic nerve block caused by interscalene brachial plexus block: effects of digital pressure and a low volume of local anesthetic," *Regional Anesthesia and Pain Medicine*, vol. 24, no. 3, pp. 231–235, 1999.

[16] J.-H. Lee, S.-H. Cho, S.-H. Kim et al., "Ropivacaine for ultrasound-guided interscalene block: 5 mL provides similar analgesia but less phrenic nerve paralysis than 10 mL," *Canadian Journal of Anesthesia*, vol. 58, no. 11, pp. 1001–1006, 2011.

[17] S. H. Renes, H. C. Rettig, M. J. Gielen, O. H. Wilder-Smith, and G. J. Van Geffen, "Ultrasound-guided low-dose interscalene brachial plexus block reduces the incidence of hemidiaphragmatic paresis," *Regional Anesthesia and Pain Medicine*, vol. 34, no. 5, pp. 498–502, 2009.

[18] S. Riazi, N. Carmichael, I. Awad, R. M. Holtby, and C. J. L. McCartney, "Effect of local anaesthetic volume (20 vs 5 ml) on the efficacy and respiratory consequences of ultrasound-guided interscalene brachial plexus block," *British Journal of Anaesthesia*, vol. 101, no. 4, pp. 549–556, 2008.

[19] E. M. Thackeray, J. D. Swenson, M. C. Gertsch et al., "Diaphragm function after interscalene brachial plexus block: a double-blind, randomized comparison of 0. 25% and 0. 125% bupivacaine," *Journal of Shoulder and Elbow Surgery*, vol. 22, pp. 381–386, 2013.

[20] A. A. Al-Kaisy, V. W. S. Chan, and A. Perlas, "Respiratory effects of low-dose bupivacaine interscalene block," *British Journal of Anaesthesia*, vol. 82, no. 2, pp. 217–220, 1999.

[21] C. T. Bolliger, P. Jordan, M. Solèr et al., "Pulmonary function and exercise capacity after lung resection," *European Respiratory Journal*, vol. 9, no. 3, pp. 415–421, 1996.

[22] C. Pelletier, L. Lapointe, and P. LeBlanc, "Effects of lung resection on pulmonary function and exercise capacity," *Thorax*, vol. 45, no. 7, pp. 497–502, 1990.

[23] A. T. Sengul, B. Sahin, C. Celenk, and A. Basoglu, "Postoperative lung volume change depending on the resected lobe," *The Journal of Thoracic and Cardiovascular Surgery*, vol. 61, pp. 131–137, 2013.

[24] G. P. Joshi and B. O. Ogunnaike, "Consequences of inadequate postoperative pain relief and chronic persistent postoperative pain," *Anesthesiology Clinics of North America*, vol. 23, no. 1, pp. 21–36, 2005.

[25] G. Hedenstierna, A. Strandberg, and B. Brismar, "Functional residual capacity, thoracoabdominal dimensions, and central blood volume during general anesthesia with muscle paralysis and mechanical ventilation," *Anesthesiology*, vol. 62, no. 3, pp. 247–254, 1985.

[26] A. Strandberg, L. Tokics, and B. Brismar, "Atelectasis during anaesthesia and in the postoperative period," *Acta Anaesthesiologica Scandinavica*, vol. 30, no. 2, pp. 154–158, 1986.

[27] S. E. Mason, A. Noel-Storr, and C. W. Ritchie, "The impact of general and regional anesthesia on the incidence of postoperative cognitive dysfunction and post-operative delirium: a systematic review with meta-analysis," *Journal of Alzheimer's Disease*, vol. 22, no. 3, pp. S67–S79, 2010.

32

Can ACE-I Be a Silent Killer While Normal Renal Functions Falsely Secure Us?

Ahmed Abdelaal Ahmed Mahmoud ⓘ, Mark Campbell, and Margarita Blajeva

Department of Anaesthesia and Intensive Care Medicine, Tallaght University Hospital (Adelaide and Meath Incorporating National Children's Hospital), Ireland

Correspondence should be addressed to Ahmed Abdelaal Ahmed Mahmoud; dr.ahmedabdelaalmahmoud@gmail.com

Academic Editor: Stefano Faenza

The current case report represents a warning against serious hyperkalaemia and acidosis induced by ACE-I during surgical stress while normal renal function could deceive the attending anaesthetist. Arterial gas analysis for follow-up of haemoglobin loss accidentally discovered hyperkalaemia and acidosis. Glucose-insulin and furosemide successfully corrected hyperkalaemia after 25 minutes and acidosis after 3 hours. These complications could be explained by a deficient steroid stress response to surgery secondary to suppression by ACE-I. Event analysis and database search found that ACE-I induced aldosterone deficiency aggravated by surgical stress response with an inadequate increase in aldosterone secretion due to angiotensin II deficiency as a sequel of ACE-I leading to defective secretion of H+ and K+. Furosemide is recommended to secrete H+ and K+ compensating for aldosterone deficiency in addition to other antihyperkalaemia measures. Anaesthetising an ACE-I treated patient requires considering ACE-I as a potential cause of hyperkalaemia and acidosis.

1. Introduction

We present a case of accidentally discovered, unexpected intraoperative acidosis and hyperkalaemia in an ACE-I treated patient with no renal impairment or diabetes. Written consent was obtained from the patient for publication.

It is not uncommon for the anaesthetists to manage a hypertensive patient treated with Angiotensin Converting Enzyme Inhibitors (ACE-I) scheduled for either elective or emergency surgery. ACE-I are well known to be associated with a potential risk of perioperative side effects and complications as intraoperative hypotension and need for vasopressors, preoperative hyperkalaemia, perioperative drug-induced angioedema, and possible postoperative hypertension [1].

The risk of hyperkalaemia in ACE-I treated patients is higher in patients with type II diabetes or renal insufficiency. At least 10% of patients treated with ACE-I will experience even mild hyperkalaemia during their course of treatment with ACE-I [2]. The mechanism of ACE-I associated hyperkalaemia is mainly due to aldosterone deficiency with resultant decreased effect of aldosterone on collecting tubules leading to reduced excretion of potassium and decreased sodium reabsorption [2, 3].

2. Case Description

A 59-year-old male was scheduled for elective open retropubic prostatectomy for a benign enlarged prostate weighing approximately 65 grams. The patient's weight was 89 kg, ASA physical status II, diagnosed with essential hypertension two years ago, and controlled with ACE-I, Ramipril 10 mg once daily. No other morbidities were associated and no other medications were taken by the patient. The preoperative assessment did not reveal any other abnormality related to anaesthesia with normal vital signs, omitting Ramipril for 48 hours before the operation and normal baseline laboratory results including renal profile (creatinine 87 micromole/L, urea 7.9 mmol/L, Na 140 mmol/L, and K 4.1 mmol/L).

Following discussion with the patient and the surgical team, the anaesthetic plan was general anesthesia (GA) with postoperative patient-controlled analgesia (PCA) with

TABLE 1: Arterial blood gases following induction of anaesthesia and till discharge from the recovery unit.

ABG	11:20	13:14	13:39	14:20	14:51	15:37	17:16
pH	7.38	7.32	7.33	7.31	7.30	7.31	7.37
PCO2 (kPa)	5.5	6.2	6	5.9	6.1	6.2	5.5
PO2 (kPa)	12.5	20.8	22.3	26	20.8	15.5	11.7
sO2 (%)	95	97	98	98	98	98	95
Base Excess(mmol/L)	0	-2	-2	-4	-4	-3	-1
Standard Bicarbonate (mmol/L)	24	23	23	21	21	22	23
Actual Bicarbonate (mmo/L)	25	24	24	22	22	23	24
Total haemoglobin (g/dl)	12.9	13	12.9	11	9.8	10.4	10.5
Carboxyhaemoglobin (%)	0.2	0.1	0.2	0.5	0.6	1.2	0.7
Whole blood glucose (mmol/L)	5.9	7.1	8	16.9	9.2	7.2	8.9
Methaemoglobin (%)	1.5	1.5	1.6	1.6	1.8	1.9	1.8
Sodium (mmol/L)	139	137	136	133	138	138	138
Potassium (mmol/L)	4.2	6.1	6.5	4.6	4.0	4.1	3.8
Lactate (mmol/L)	0.7	0.8	1.0	1.5	1.8	2.0	0.7

TABLE 2: Renal function tests of the patient.

Renal function test	Preoperative	Day 1 postoperative	Day 2 postoperative
Sodium (mmol/L)	140	141	140
Potassium (mmol/L)	4.1	4.4	3.9
Creatinine (umol/L)	87	99	85
Urea (mmol/L)	7.9	6.6	5.4
$_e$GFR	80	69	82

$_e$GFR: estimated glomerular filtration rate, calculated by Cockcroft and Gault modified equation.

morphine. Relatively uneventful induction of GA by propofol (2mg/kg), fentanyl (100 micrograms), and rocuronium (0.6 mg/kg) with endotracheal intubation, radial arterial cannulation for IBP monitoring, and two wide-bore peripheral cannulas (18G) were inserted. Induction was accompanied by hypotension (BP dropped from 112/68 to 73/46) and bradycardia (HR dropped from 78/min. to 38/min.) that required two successive doses of ephedrine each 6 mg were followed by restoration of BP and HR. Baseline arterial blood gas (ABG) after positioning was normal (Table 1). At 2 hours after the start of surgery, the estimated blood was about 350 ml and the urinary output (UOP) was 120 ml (over 2 hours) with mean arterial pressure (MAP) being maintained above 70 mmHg without further vasopressors required other than the initial 12 mg of ephedrine required immediately after induction. An arterial blood gas (2 hours after start of surgery) was initially performed for monitoring haemoglobin level showed hyperkalaemia (6.1 mmol/L) with acidosis (pH 7.33 and PCo2 6.2 kPa). The initial explanation was respiratory acidosis, and ventilation parameters were increased. Twenty-five minutes later ABG showed a decrease of PCo2 to normal with normal anion gap acidosis and increasing potassium to 6.5 mmol/L. Hyperkalaemia was treated with glucose-insulin (10 units of insulin added to 1 litre of glucose 10%) and mild hyperventilation and furosemide (20 mg bolus) with a change of the maintenance fluid from compound lactate solution to normal saline with the same rate (225ml/h). Forty minutes later, these measures had reduced potassium from 6.5 mmol/L to 4.1 mmol/L.

Despite normalization of potassium level (k 4.1 mmol/L) following the measures mentioned above, the acidosis persisted with maintained normal bicarbonate level and normal PCo2 (Table 1). From the time of normalized potassium, the acidosis required three hours to normalize which was two hours after recovery from GA. The presence of acidosis did not affect emergence from anaesthesia or recovery of the patient.

Postoperative follow-up of the renal function tests and electrolytes (Table 2) revealed normalization over a period of two days postoperatively with the patient restored intake of ACE-I on day one postoperatively with no effect on potassium level.

At the end of surgery, the estimated blood loss was about 635 ml, UOP was 700 ml (over an operative time of 4 hours), and the infused fluids included 450 ml of Hartman's solution (over the first 2 hours), 950 ml of 0.9% normal saline, and 500 ml of Gelofusine 4% (over the second 2 hours) in addition to 1 litre of glucose 10% with insulin. No blood transfusion was required and no MAP <70 mmHg was recorded.

3. Discussion

Systematic analysis of the event did not reveal any cause for the hyperkalaemia and acidosis except the history of treatment with ACE-I that may be associated with renal tubular acidosis (RTA), normal anion gap acidosis, and hyperkalaemia [2–13]; this explanation was supported by results from database search [1–15] including the effect of furosemide in hyperkalaemic RTA [11].

Glucocorticoid (Cortisol)	Mineralocorticoid (Aldosterone)
Increases K excretion	Increases K excretion
Increases Na excretion	Increases Na excretion
No effect on H^+ excretion	Increases H^+ excretion

Stress response → Increased cortisol and aldosterone →
- Increases serum Na (Hypernatremia)
- Decreases serum K (hypokalemia)
- Decreases serum H+ (metabolic alkalosis)

ACE-I →
Decreased Aldosterone
Decreased stress response→ Decreased Cortisol and
→ Hyperkalemia and acidosis

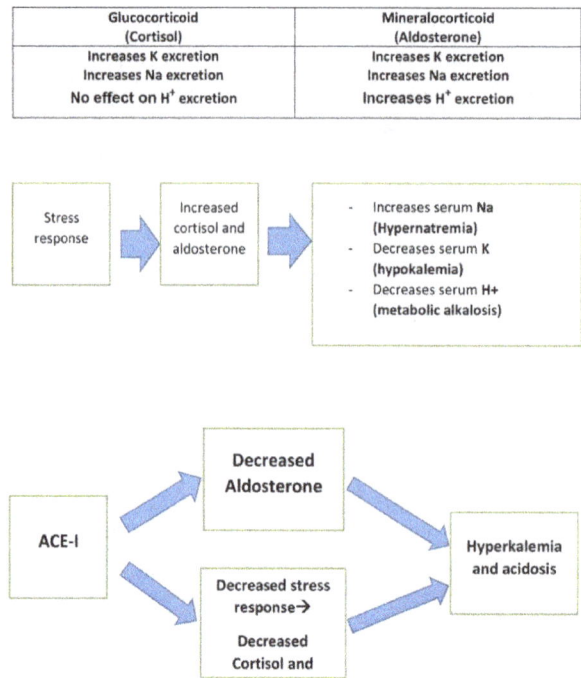

FIGURE 1: Pathophysiology of ACE-I induced hyperkalaemia and acidosis. ACE-I: Angiotensin Converting Enzyme Inhibitor.

The patient did not receive blood transfusion and did not experience hypotensive events apart from a single induction related hypotension event that was corrected by a small dose of ephedrine; this excludes the possibility of either transfusion related or acute kidney injury due to hypotension as possible causes of hyperkalaemia. A single dose of propofol was used for induction of anaesthesia making the possibility of propofol infusion syndrome extremely unlikely.

The steroid hormone aldosterone acts on a mineralo-corticoid receptor in the renal collecting ducts through a protein kinase mechanism leading to stimulation of Na+ reabsorption and active secretion of both H+ and K with potential risk for hyperkalaemia and acidosis in case of aldosterone deficiency [4, 5].

Angiotensin II is essential for the secretion of aldosterone [5] with ACE-I can produce a variable degree of hyporenine-mic hypoaldosteronism or type IV renal tubular acidosis [6–10] characterized by metabolic acidosis and hyperkalaemia due to aldosterone deficiency.

Furosemide can be beneficial in type IV renal tubular acidosis by stimulation of K+ and H+ secretion from distal collecting tubules in case of hypoaldosteronism [11].

Typically, surgical induced stress response is associated with increased secretion of cortisol and aldosterone through stimulation of the hypothalamic-pituitary-adrenocortical axis (HPA-axis) with subsequent electrolyte changes including salt and water retention with hypokalaemia [12].

Experimental research demonstrated that angiotensin II and ACE could intervene with the pituitary hormones secretion like corticotropin (ACTH) and enhances the stimulatory effects of corticotropin-releasing hormone (CRH), thus contributing to the stress-related activation of the

hypothalamic-pituitary-adrenocortical (HPA) axis [13, 14]. Subsequently the inhibition of ACE with ACE-I will be associated decreased stress response, and with reduced cortisol secretion, this can aggravate the risk of hyperkalaemia and acidosis in ACE-I treated patients when exposed to surgical stress response (**Figure 1**).

Although, our patient stopped ACE-I 48 hours before surgery, it has been proved that aldosterone level does not change up to 15 days after cessation of Ramipril [16]. This augments the explanation that the hyperkalaemia can be due to the residual effect of ACE-I on aldosterone level.

It is known that renal impairment and diabetes can be associated with increased risk of hyperkalaemia and acidosis in ACE-I treated patients who may warn the anaesthetists to suspect, monitor, and detect such complication; however, we reported a case of unexpected hyperkalaemia and acidosis in a surgical patient treated with ACE-I with normal baseline renal function, with adequate response to dextrose insulin and furosemide and correction of both hyperkalaemia and acidosis. This event in our case report may be triggered by surgical stress response with deficient steroid secretion especially aldosterone; this is supported by the ability of furosemide to reverse the effects of aldosterone deficiency by secreting hydrogen ion and potassium.

Although the lactate level increased during the surgery, this cannot be explained by increased production as no haemodynamic instability was recorded but may be related to impaired excretion of lactate as a part of renal tubular acidosis.

The current patient experienced a mild increase in creatinine level and a mild drop in in glomerular filtration rate. The derangement in renal function postoperatively may be due to the use of furosemide intraoperatively, which has been recorded before to produce drop GFR [17].

Acidosis persisted despite potassium normalization with insulin, until successful correction was achieved with the diuretic effect of furosemide. Insulin administration produced correction of potassium but not acidosis as insulin may participate to acidosis [18] and this supports the fact that acidosis in our case was most probably due to the fact that renal tubular acidosis was induced by the preoperative use of ACE-I.

The possibility that catecholamines may shifted potassium intracellularly is not possible as catecholamines are also suppressed with ACE-I [19]

Patients on ACE-I are recommended for perioperative monitoring of potassium for early detection and management of such possible complications especially with unexplained ECG signs of hyperkalaemia and haemodynamic instability. In case of developing hyperkalaemia and acidosis, furosemide is recommended to secrete H+ and K+ compensating for aldosterone deficiency in addition to other antihyperkalaemia measures.

A limitation in our case report is that we did not measure the aldosterone level after the event.

4. Future Research

No previous studies [15] examined the effect of ACE-I on potassium and hydrogen ion during the surgical stress response; additionally, no information is available if ACE-I treated patients have a normal cortisol stress response or not in the perioperative period.

A future research study can assess the risk of hyperkalaemia and acidosis during the operative period in patients treated with ACE-I in addition to assessment of cortisol stress response in this category of patients.

Authors' Contributions

Ahmed Abdelaal Ahmed Mahmoud contributed to writing the manuscript. Mark Campbell revised the final manuscript. Margarita Blajeva collected data of the patient. All the three authors were involved in the clinical management of the case described.

References

[1] B. Mets, "To stop or not?" *Anesthesia & Analgesia*, vol. 120, no. 6, pp. 1413–1419, 2015.

[2] M. A. Raebel, "Hyperkalemia Associated with Use of Angiotensin-Converting Enzyme Inhibitors and Angiotensin Receptor Blockers," *Cardiovascular Therapeutics*, vol. 30, no. 3, pp. e156–e166, 2012.

[3] L. C. Reardon and D. S. Macpherson, "Hyperkalemia in outpatients using angiotensin-converting enzyme inhibitors: How much should we worry?" *JAMA Internal Medicine*, vol. 158, no. 1, pp. 26–32, 1998.

[4] W. Thomas and B. J. Harvey, "Mechanisms Underlying Rapid Aldosterone Effects in the Kidney," *Annual Review of Physiology*, vol. 73, no. 1, pp. 335–357, 2011.

[5] J. H. Pratt, J. K. Rothrock, and J. H. Dominguez, "Evidence that angiotensin-II and potassium collaborate to increase cytosolic calcium and stimulate the secretion of aldosterone," *Endocrinology*, vol. 125, no. 5, pp. 2463–2469, 1989.

[6] F. E. Karet, "Mechanisms in hyperkalemic renal tubular acidosis," *Journal of the American Society of Nephrology*, vol. 20, no. 2, pp. 251–254, 2009.

[7] M. Schambelan, A. Sebastian, and E. G. Biglieri, "Prevalence, pathogenesis, and functional significance of aldosterone deficiency in hyperkalemic patients with chronic renal insufficiency," *Kidney International*, vol. 17, no. 1, pp. 89–101, 1980.

[8] A. G. Sousa, J. V. Cabral, W. B. El-Feghaly, L. S. Sousa, and A. B. Nunes, "Hyporeninemic hypoaldosteronism and diabetes mellitus: Pathophysiology assumptions, clinical aspects and implications for management," *World Journal of Diabetes*, vol. 7, no. 5, p. 101, 2016.

[9] R. Düsing and F. Sellers, "ACE inhibitors, angiotensin receptor blockers and direct renin inhibitors in combination: A review of their role after the ONTARGET trial," *Current Medical Research and Opinion*, vol. 25, no. 9, pp. 2287–2301, 2009.

[10] C. S. Haas, I. Pohlenz, U. Lindner et al., "Renal tubular acidosis type IV in hyperkalaemic patients - A fairy tale or reality?" *Clinical Endocrinology*, vol. 78, no. 5, pp. 706–711, 2013.

[11] S. Rastogi, J. M. Bayliss, L. Nascimento, and J. A. L. Arruda, "Hyperkalemic renal tubular acidosis: Effect of furosemide in humans and in rats," *Kidney International*, vol. 28, no. 5, pp. 801–807, 1985.

[12] D. Burton, G. Nicholson, and G. M. Hall, "Endocrine and metabolic response to surgery," *Continuing Education in Anaesthesia, Critical Care and Pain*, vol. 4, no. 5, pp. 144–147, 2004.

[13] I. Armando, S. Volpi, G. Aguilera, and J. M. Saavedra, "Angiotensin II AT1 receptor blockade prevents the hypothalamic corticotropin-releasing factor response to isolation stress," *Brain Research*, vol. 1142, no. 1, pp. 92–99, 2007.

[14] M. G. Pavlatou, G. Mastorakos, I. Lekakis et al., "Chronic administration of an angiotensin II receptor antagonist resets the hypothalamic-pituitary-adrenal (HPA) axis and improves the affect of patients with diabetes mellitus type 2: Preliminary results," *Stress*, vol. 11, no. 1, pp. 62–72, 2008.

[15] Z. Zou, H. B. Yuan, B. Yang et al., "Perioperative angiotensin-converting enzyme inhibitors or angiotensin II type 1 receptor blockers for preventing mortality and morbidity in adults," *Cochrane Database of Systematic Reviews*.

[16] D. Stephan, M. Grima, M. Welsch, M. Barthelmebs, D. Vasmant, and J. Imbs, "Interruption of prolonged ramipril treatment in hypertensive patients: Effects on the renin-angiotensin system," *Fundamental & Clinical Pharmacology*, vol. 10, no. 5, pp. 474–483, 1996.

[17] H. Trivedi, T. Dresser, and K. Aggarwal, "Acute effect of furosemide on glomerular filtration rate in diastolic dysfunction," *Renal Failure*, vol. 29, no. 8, pp. 985–989, 2007.

[18] J. M. Goguen and M. L. Halperin, "Can insulin administration cause an acute metabolic acidosis in vivo? - An experimental study in dogs," *Diabetologia*, vol. 36, no. 9, pp. 813–816, 1993.

[19] A. V. Sidorov and M. M. J. Fateev, "Effect of angiotensin-converting enzyme inhibitors, beta-adrenoblockers and their combinations on survival and blood plasma catecholamine levels in rats with chronic heart failure with induced exacerbations," *Journal of Evolutionary Biochemistry and Physiology*, vol. 49, 330 pages, 2013.

33

Transient Femoral Nerve Palsy Complicating "Blind" Transversus Abdominis Plane Block

Dimitrios K. Manatakis,[1] **Nikolaos Stamos,**[1] **Christos Agalianos,**[1]
Michail Athanasios Karvelis,[2] **Michael Gkiaourakis,**[2] **and Demetrios Davides**[1]

[1] *1st Surgical Department, Athens Naval and Veterans Hospital, 70 Dinokratous Street, 11521 Athens, Greece*
[2] *Department of Anesthesiology, Athens Naval and Veterans Hospital, 70 Dinokratous Street, 11521 Athens, Greece*

Correspondence should be addressed to Dimitrios K. Manatakis; dmanatak@yahoo.gr

Academic Editors: A. Apan and U. Buyukkocak

We present two cases of patients who reported quadriceps femoris weakness and hypoesthesia over the anterior thigh after an inguinal hernia repair under transversus abdominis plane (TAP) block. Transient femoral nerve palsy is the result of local anesthetic incorrectly injected between transversus abdominis muscle and transversalis fascia and pooling around the femoral nerve. Although it is a minor and self-limiting complication, it requires overnight hospital stay and observation of the patients. Performing the block under ultrasound guidance and injecting the least volume of local anesthetic required are ways of minimizing its incidence.

1. Introduction

Transient femoral nerve palsy (TFNP) occurs in 5–8% of ilioinguinal/iliohypogastric nerve (IIN/IHN) blocks [1, 2]. To the best of our knowledge it has been reported only once following a transversus abdominis plane (TAP) block [3].

We present our experience with 2 cases of TFNP complicating "blind" TAP blocks for inguinal herniorrhaphy, investigate its mechanism, and discuss possible ways of prevention.

2. Case 1

An otherwise healthy, 26-year-old, nonobese, male patient was scheduled to undergo right inguinal hernia plug-and-patch repair as a day case, under TAP block anesthesia and conscious sedation. Twenty mL of 0,5% ropivacaine were administered by an experienced anesthesiologist, using the landmark-based "two-pop" technique as described by McDonnell et al. [4]. Surgery was uneventful, with a duration of 45 minutes.

At the postoperative ward round, the patient was disturbed and reported inability to extend the ipsilateral knee joint. Clinical examination revealed quadriceps femoris paresis, hypoesthesia over the anterior aspect of the thigh, and absent patellar reflex. The patient and his family were reassured, and the self-limiting nature of the complication was explained. He was admitted overnight for observation. On the following morning, symptoms had completely remitted, and he was discharged.

3. Case 2

A 62-year-old, nonobese, male patient, with an unremarkable past medical history, was scheduled to undergo left inguinal hernia plug-and-patch repair as a day case, under TAP block anesthesia and conscious sedation. Twenty mL of 0,5% ropivacaine were injected into the TAP by the same anesthesiologist. Surgery was uneventful, with a duration of 50 minutes.

Two hours postoperatively he suffered from a minor orthopedic injury (ankle sprain) on his attempt to stand up from bed. On clinical examination he was found to have quadriceps femoris muscle weakness (grade 1/5 according to Louisiana State University Health Services Center grading system) and hypoesthesia of the anterior thigh. Symptoms lasted for 8 hours. The patient was admitted overnight, recovered fully, and was discharged on the following morning.

4. Discussion

Transversus abdominis plane (TAP) is the anatomic space between the transversus abdominis and internal oblique muscles. Its clinical significance lies in the fact that it is traversed by the nerves that provide sensory supply to the anterolateral abdominal wall (T7-T11 intercostal, subcostal, iliohypogastric, and ilioinguinal nerves) [5, 6].

TAP is approached traditionally through the lumbar triangle of Petit by a "blind" landmark-based technique or in the midaxillary line under ultrasound guidance [4, 7, 8]. TAP block provides regional lower abdominal anesthesia and is mainly used as a component of multimodal postoperative analgesia regimens [9].

It is generally considered a safe procedure with only few cases of complications found in the literature [10, 11]. A thorough search of the English-speaking literature revealed only one case of TFNP following a TAP block. In a letter to the editor, Dr. Walker briefly described a case of a patient fracturing their ankle, when trying to mobilize from bed [3].

In their cadaveric study Rosario et al. found that at the level of the anterior superior iliac spine the femoral nerve lies in the groove formed by the psoas major and the iliacus muscles, covered by the iliacus fascia. The authors demonstrated that the iliacus fascia is the posterolateral continuation of the transversalis fascia, meaning that the femoral nerve lies in the same tissue plane as the space deep to the transversus abdominis muscle [12]. Therefore advancement of the needle and injection of local anesthetic into the wrong tissue plane, that is, between the transversus abdominis muscle and the transversalis fascia (instead of the plane between the internal oblique and transversus abdominis muscles), lead to the injectate tracking along the transversalis fascia and eventually accumulating around the femoral nerve.

The ensuing femoral nerve palsy results in quadriceps femoris paresis or weakness and hypoaesthesia over the anteromedial thigh that usually last for 6 to 8 hours (up to 36 hours in one case report [13]) and resolve spontaneously without permanent neurological deficit.

Another possible mechanism proposed by Rosario et al. is the direct injection of local anaesthetic around the femoral nerve, if the injection is performed 3-4 cm more medially than that recommended for IIN/IHN blocks [12]. Walker warns that injection point for blind TAP block is even more posterior and likely closer to the femoral nerve trunk [3]. Interestingly, the distance between needle point and femoral nerve was found longer in females than in males, making TFNP perhaps less likely to occur in female patients [12].

Kulacoglu et al. drew the same conclusions in their cadaveric study [14]. They further suggest that a step-by-step infiltration technique under direct surgical vision is safer than blind blocks. Ghani et al. however failed to show a difference in TFNP incidence between anaesthetists who performed blind blocks preoperatively and surgeons who performed blocks under direct vision intraoperatively [1]. McDermott et al. used ultrasound to assess needle position and administration of local anaesthetic. They found that the local anaesthetic was correctly delivered into the TAP only in

23,6% of patients, while in 30% it was injected deeper than required [15].

A second aspect of the mechanism of TFNP is the choice and dosage of local anaesthetic. Rosario et al., using methylene blue as injectate, demonstrated that as little as 1 mL of dye injected in the wrong tissue plane was sufficient to pool around the femoral nerve, while Kulacoglu et al. used a volume of 10 mL to better match a clinical scenario [12, 14]. Given the different tissue conditions in vivo, safe conclusions can not be drawn from cadaveric studies, as to the volume and concentration of local anaesthetic required to produce TFNP.

Epperson and Reese reported a case of TFNP, following a field block with 20 mL of 0,5% bupivacaine and 1 : 200000 epinephrine after inguinal herniorrhaphy, which led only to femoral sensory neuropraxia with preservation of normal motor function [16]. Similarly Wulf et al. reported consistent sensory blockade with all examined dosing schemes of ropivacaine but motor blockade only at higher dosages, implying use of the least amount and lowest concentration of local anaesthetic possible, to minimise TFNP incidence [17]. To date, there is insufficient evidence to support any particular local anaesthetic, and the ideal combination and dosage have yet to be determined [9, 18].

Essentially the majority of TAP block complications and failures is the result of wrong needle placement and local anaesthetic injection either too deep or too superficial [16, 19]. Performing the block under real-time ultrasound guidance is a valid option. Advancement of needle and injection of local anaesthetic are more accurate than those by "blind" techniques [6, 9, 20]. Ultrasound-guided infiltration has also been reported to achieve faster absorption and higher plasma concentrations of local anaesthetic, suggesting that smaller volumes may be required, for equal anaesthetic effect [21–23].

Hebbard and Shibata approach the TAP by placing the ultrasound probe transversely across the midaxillary line, where the layers of the abdominal wall can be more easily visualised [8, 24]. With this technique the needle is introduced more anteriorly than the triangle of Petit and further from the femoral nerve. Moreover, using a blunt-tipped needle and advancing it obliquely instead of perpendicularly increase the resistance of each aponeurotic layer, making the "pop" sensation of fascial piercing more discernible [25].

5. Conclusion

TFNP after TAP block is the result of local anaesthetic incorrectly injected between the transversus abdominis muscle and the transversalis fascia and accumulating around the femoral nerve. While it is not a major cause of postoperative morbidity, it may cause patient discomfort and anxiety as well as unexpected injuries due to falls. It is a self-limiting complication, but patients require overnight admittance for observation, thus increasing length of stay and hospital costs. Performing the TAP block under ultrasound guidance and injecting the least volume of local anaesthetic required are effective ways to reduce its occurrence.

References

[1] K. R. Ghani, R. McMillan, and S. Paterson-Brown, "Transient femoral nerve palsy following ilio-inguinal nerve blockade for day case inguinal hernia repair," *Journal of the Royal College of Surgeons of Edinburgh*, vol. 47, no. 4, pp. 626–629, 2002.

[2] A. K. Lipp, J. Woodcock, B. Hensman, and K. Wilkinson, "Leg weakness is a complication of ilio-inguinal nerve block in children," *British Journal of Anaesthesia*, vol. 92, no. 2, pp. 273–274, 2004.

[3] G. Walker, "Transversus abdominis plane block: a note of caution!," *British Journal of Anaesthesia*, vol. 104, no. 2, p. 265, 2010.

[4] J. G. McDonnell, B. O'Donnell, G. Curley, A. Heffernan, C. Power, and J. G. Laffey, "The analgesic efficacy of transversus abdominis plane block after abdominal surgery: a prospective randomized controlled trial," *Anesthesia and Analgesia*, vol. 104, no. 1, pp. 193–197, 2007.

[5] Z. Jankovic, "Transversus abdominis plane block: the Holy Grail of anaesthesia for (lower) abdominal surgery," *Periodicum Biologorum*, vol. 111, no. 2, pp. 203–208, 2009.

[6] T. M. N. Tran, J. J. Ivanusic, P. Hebbard, and M. J. Barrington, "Determination of spread of injectate after ultrasound-guided transversus abdominis plane block: a cadaveric study," *British Journal of Anaesthesia*, vol. 102, no. 1, pp. 123–127, 2009.

[7] A. N. Rafi, "Abdominal field block: a new approach via the lumbar triangle," *Anaesthesia*, vol. 56, no. 10, pp. 1024–1026, 2001.

[8] P. Hebbard, Y. Fujiwara, Y. Shibata, and C. Royse, "Ultrasound-guided transversus abdominis plane (TAP) block," *Anaesthesia and Intensive Care*, vol. 35, no. 4, pp. 616–617, 2007.

[9] M. J. Young, A. W. Gorlin, V. E. Modest, and S. A. Quraishi, "Clinical implications of the transversus abdominis plane block in adults," *Anesthesiology Research and Practice*, vol. 2012, Article ID 731645, 11 pages, 2012.

[10] M. Farooq and M. Carey, "A case of liver trauma with a blunt regional anesthesia needle while performing transversus abdominis plane block," *Regional Anesthesia and Pain Medicine*, vol. 33, no. 3, pp. 274–275, 2008.

[11] P. Lancaster and M. Chadwick, "Liver trauma secondary to ultrasound-guided transversus abdominis plane block," *British Journal of Anaesthesia*, vol. 104, no. 4, pp. 509–510, 2010.

[12] D. J. Rosario, S. Jacob, J. Luntley, P. P. Skinner, and A. T. Raftery, "Mechanism of femoral nerve palsy complicating percutaneous ilioinguinal field block," *British Journal of Anaesthesia*, vol. 78, no. 3, pp. 314–316, 1997.

[13] D. J. Rosario, P. P. Skinner, and A. T. Raftery, "Transient femoral nerve palsy complicating preoperative ilioinguinal nerve blockade for inguinal herniorrhaphy," *British Journal of Surgery*, vol. 81, no. 6, p. 897, 1994.

[14] H. Kulacoglu, Z. Ergul, A. F. Esmer, T. Sen, T. Akkaya, and A. Elhan, "Percutaneous ilioinguinal-iliohypogastric nerve block or step-by-step local infiltration anesthesia for inguinal hernia repair: what cadaveric dissection says?" *Journal of the Korean Surgical Society*, vol. 81, no. 6, pp. 408–413, 2011.

[15] G. McDermott, E. Korba, U. Mata et al., "Should we stop doing blind transversus abdominis plane blocks?" *British Journal of Anaesthesia*, vol. 108, no. 3, pp. 499–502, 2012.

[16] J. Epperson and A. Reese, "Transient femoral nerve palsy following field block for inguinal herniorraphy," *The Internet Journal of Anesthesiology*, vol. 11, no. 2, 2007.

[17] H. Wulf, F. Worthmann, H. Behnke, and A. S. Böhle, "Pharmacokinetics and pharmacodynamics of ropivacaine 2 mg/ml, 5 mg/ml, or 7.5 mg/mL after ilioinguinal blockade for inguinal hernia repair in adults," *Anesthesia and Analgesia*, vol. 89, no. 6, pp. 1471–1474, 1999.

[18] F. W. Abdallah, V. W. Chan, and R. Brull, "Transversus abdominis plane block: a systematic review," *Regional Anesthesia and Pain Medicine*, vol. 37, no. 2, pp. 193–209, 2012.

[19] R. Taylor Jr., J. V. Pergolizzi, A. Sinclair et al., "Transversus abdominis block: clinical uses, side effects, and future perspectives," *Pain Practice*, vol. 13, no. 4, pp. 332–344, 2013.

[20] M. Milone, M. N. D. Di Minno, and M. Musella, "Outpatient inguinal hernia repair under local anaesthesia: feasibility and efficacy of ultrasound-guided transversus abdominis plane block," *Hernia*, 2012.

[21] M. Weintraud, M. Lundblad, S. C. Kettner et al., "Ultrasound versus landmark-based technique for ilioinguinal-iliohypogastric nerve blockade in children: the implications on plasma levels of ropivacaine," *Anesthesia and Analgesia*, vol. 108, no. 5, pp. 1488–1492, 2009.

[22] N. Kato, Y. Fujiwara, M. Harato et al., "Serum concentration of lidocaine after transversus abdominis plane block," *Journal of Anesthesia*, vol. 23, no. 2, pp. 298–300, 2009.

[23] J. D. Griffiths, F. A. Barron, S. Grant, A. R. Bjorksten, P. Hebbard, and C. F. Royse, "Plasma ropivacaine concentrations after ultrasound-guided transversus abdominis plane block," *British Journal of Anaesthesia*, vol. 105, no. 6, pp. 853–856, 2010.

[24] Y. Shibata, Y. Sato, Y. Fujiwara, and T. Komatsu, "Transversus abdominis plane block," *Anesthesia and Analgesia*, vol. 105, no. 3, p. 883, 2007.

[25] Z. Jankovic, N. Ahmad, N. Ravishankar, and F. Archer, "Transversus abdominis plane block: how safe is it?" *Anesthesia and Analgesia*, vol. 107, no. 5, pp. 1758–1759, 2008.

34

Postoperative Airway Obstruction by a Bone Fragment

Patrick Schober,[1] **K. Hakki Karagozoglu,**[2] **Stephan A. Loer,**[1] **and Lothar A. Schwarte**[1]

[1]*Department of Anesthesiology, VU University Medical Center, De Boelelaan 1117, 1007 MB Amsterdam, Netherlands*
[2]*Academic Centre for Dentistry Amsterdam (ACTA) and Department of Oral and Maxillofacial Surgery/Oral Pathology,*
VU University Medical Center, De Boelelaan 1117, 1007 MB Amsterdam, Netherlands

Correspondence should be addressed to Lothar A. Schwarte; l.schwarte@vumc.nl

Academic Editor: Anjan Trikha

Postoperative airway obstructions are potentially life-threatening complications. These obstructions may be classified as *functional* (sagging tongue, laryngospasm, or bronchospasm), *pathoanatomical* (airway swelling or hematoma within the airways), or *foreign body-related*. Various cases of airway obstruction by foreign bodies have previously been reported, for example, by broken teeth or damaged airway instruments. Here we present the exceptional case of a postoperative airway obstruction due to a large fragment of the patient's maxillary bone, left accidentally in situ after transoral surgical tumor resection. Concerning this type of airway obstruction, we discuss possible causes, diagnosis, and treatment options. Although it is an exceptional case after surgery, clinicians should be aware of this potentially life-threatening complication. In summary, this case demonstrates that the differential diagnosis of postoperative airway obstructions should include foreign bodies derived from surgery, including tissue and bone fragments.

1. Introduction

Postoperative airway obstructions are potentially life-threatening complications. The obstruction can be classified as *functional* (sagging tongue, laryngospasm, or bronchospasm), *pathoanatomical* (airway swelling or hematoma within the airways), or *foreign body-related*. Various cases of airway obstruction by foreign bodies have been reported. Here we present a previously unreported case of postoperative airway obstruction due to an unrecognized fragment of the patient's maxillary bone.

2. Case Description

A 74-year-old, male ASA-III patient presented with an adenocarcinoma of the right palatomaxillary region (Figure 1) and was scheduled for maxillectomy for tumor excision and placement of an obturator prosthesis. Preoperative workup revealed a history of smoking, COPD (under therapy with fluticasone, tiotropium, and a budesonide-formoterol combination), mild aortic insufficiency, and an incomplete right bundle branch block on the ECG.

Premedication (oxazepam), induction (propofol, sufentanil, and rocuronium), and maintenance (sevoflurane, N_2O)

of anesthesia were uneventful. The airway was secured by endotracheal intubation via the nasal route to allow optimal transoral access to the posterior maxilla. The pharynx was packed with gauze using a Magill-type forceps to scavenge intraoperative blood and tissue debris, which otherwise could enter the larynx or esophagus.

At the end of surgery, the pharyngeal tamponade was removed and the surgeon rechecked the surgical site for adequate hemostasis. Thereafter, administration of sevoflurane and N_2O was stopped and the patient was allowed to awaken from anesthesia. With the surgical site being the upper airway, we extubated the patient only after complete return of protective airway reflexes, in particular after occurrence of effective coughing. After extubation, the patient was transferred to the postanesthesia care unit (PACU). When the patient was fully awake, he started to cough, accompanied by tachycardia and arterial hypertension. He was moderately agitated and reported dyspnea and intense pain in his throat, which was attributed to airway irritation following surgery, pharyngeal tamponade, and endotracheal intubation (Table 1). Treatment included administration of analgesia (piritramide i.v. in doses of 2.5 mg) and inhalational nebulizer therapy (with salbutamol and ipratropium bromide). To prevent rebleed in the coughing patient, he received tranexamic

TABLE 1

Parameter	Bone fragment in situ	Bone fragment expelled
Mental state	Agitated	Cooperative
Patient's position	Upright preferred	Regular
Respiration	Coughing	Normal breathing
O_2 flow [l/min]	9	3
RF [/min]	20	15
SpO_2 [%]	92%	97%
RR [mmHg]	151/79	121/70
HR [/min]	80 (136)	64

Key variables before (bone fragment in situ, left column) and after the bone fragment were expelled by the patient (right column) in the postoperative period. After expelling the bone fragment, all variables returned towards normal values. In parallel also the oxygen requirement could be markedly reduced. O_2 flow: oxygen flow via the face mask; RF: respiratory frequency; SpO_2: pulse oximetric arterial oxygen saturation; RR: arterial blood pressure; HR: heart rate. The heart rate in brackets indicates the peak heart rate recorded during this period.

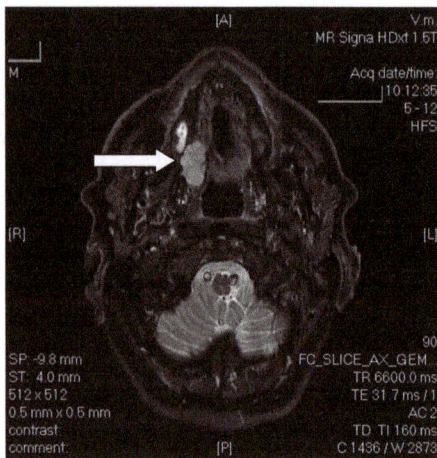

FIGURE 1: Preoperative horizontal MRI scan indicating the location (white arrow) of the adenocarcinoma of the right palatomaxillary region. [L]: left side; [R]: right side; [A]: anterior aspect; [P]: posterior aspect.

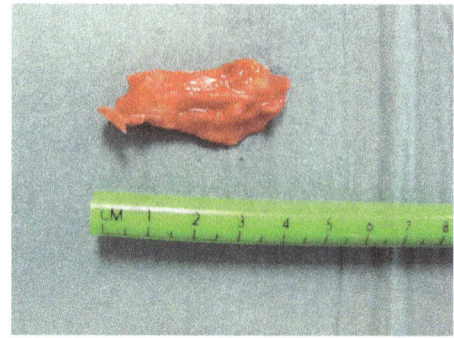

FIGURE 2: The expelled bone fragment and a cm-scale. The bone fragment has the dimension of 4×2 cm.

acid (500 mg loading dose, followed by 1500 mg i.v. over 15 min).

About 45 min after admittance to the PACU, the patient still presented regular series of coughing. During such a cough attack, the patient suddenly expelled a considerably large, bloody mass. Directly hereafter, frequency and intensity of coughing decreased and the feeling of dyspnea and throat pain disappeared. In parallel, the vegetative stress symptoms like tachycardia and hypertension diminished (Table 1). At closer inspection of the expelled bloody mass, we identified a clot-covered bone fragment of about 4×2 cm size (Figure 2). Analysis of the bone at the university pathology institute confirmed that the bone derived from the maxilla.

3. Discussion

Perioperative respiratory complications are relatively frequent, with a potentially life-threatening subgroup being postoperative airway obstructions [1], particularly in patients with surgery at the airways. Here we present the case of a foreign body resulting from surgery itself by an intraoperatively "separated" bone fragment. Airway obstruction by a bone fragment was not included in our primary differential diagnosis.

In our literature review on foreign body-induced postoperative airway obstruction, we found cases for various objects left in situ to cause airway problems in the postoperative period. From an anesthesiological perspective, teeth broken during intubation might remain in the airway and even migrate deeper into the tracheobronchial tree [2]. From the devices used intraoperatively, reported objects causing airway obstruction include damaged intubation aids [3], displaced airway packings [4], or forgotten gauze packs [5].

Pharyngeal tamponades with gauze packing are controversially discussed in their efficacy to scavenge intraoperative blood and debris from the surgical wound and thus in their efficacy to seal the esophagus (to prevent emesis) and the larynx (to prevent laryngospasm and airway obstruction) from blood and surgical debris. In the presented case, evidently, the pharyngeal tampon was an insufficient measure to scavenge the large bone fragment. On the other hand, forgetting to remove the pharyngeal tamponade after surgery may itself result in severe airway obstruction and even death.

We add the presented case of a large surgery-derived bone fragment to the list of foreign bodies causing postoperative airway obstruction. In contrast to the clearly defined, inventoried set of surgical instruments used or the known number of gauzes used intraoperatively, there is usually no registration regarding removed tissue and bone pieces intraoperatively. The amount of removed tissue is difficult to quantify and varies from operation to operation. This is of particular importance when tissue is intraorally separated from the patient.

Regarding postoperative airway management, the anesthesiologist should be aware of the different presentations of airway obstruction, for example, inspiratory or expiratory stridor, depending on the level of airway obstruction, to allow proper diagnosis and prompt therapy. In case that the predominant clinical symptom accompanying dyspnea is persistent coughing and (unexpected) airway related pain, the possibility of airway obstruction by a foreign body should be considered and checked by direct inspection or endoscopy, also in the immediate postoperative period. In contrast to prehospital choking, where the typical anamnestic setting (e.g., onset during a meal, or kids having played with small objects) and the sudden onset of coughing are directing towards the correct diagnosis of a foreign body airway obstruction, both aspects are not valid in the postoperative setting and thus the correct diagnosis may be more difficult.

Concerning the question of how such a large bone fragment could remain within the airway and not being scavenged by the pharynx tampon, we speculate that the bone fragment's shape allowed wedging in situ (explaining the initially frustrated coughing and throat pain of the patient) or that the bone stuck together with blood in situ (explaining the covering blood clot simultaneously expelled with the bone fragment).

Clearly, attempting removal of the foreign body is pivotal to relieve airway obstruction once the diagnosis appears likely, either after direct visualisation (e.g., by a Magill-type forceps) or indirectly, applying endoscopy. Alternative rescue methods to support removal of the obstructing foreign airway body, such as the Heimlich manoeuvre [6] or the Table manoeuvre [7], whereby external force is applied to the thorax, appear to be prone for complications and should be restricted to cases of severe airway obstruction where the patient is unable to breathe or cough and when an immediate direct removal appears impossible.

In summary, this case demonstrates that the differential diagnosis of postoperative airway obstructions should include foreign bodies derived from surgery, including tissue and bone fragments.

References

[1] J. M. Mhyre, M. N. Riesner, L. S. Polley, and N. N. Naughton, "A series of anesthesia-related maternal deaths in Michigan, 1985–2003," *Anesthesiology*, vol. 106, no. 6, pp. 1096–1104, 2007.

[2] Y. Ostrinsky and Z. Cohen, "Images in clinical medicine. Tooth aspiration," *The New England Journal of Medicine*, vol. 354, no. 24, article e25, 2006.

[3] P. Schober, S. A. Loer, and L. A. Schwarte, "Airway obstruction by an unexpected equipment damage," *Journal of Clinical Anesthesia*, vol. 32, pp. 59–61, 2016.

[4] E. Yanagisawa and R. Latorre, "Choking spells following septorhinoplasty secondary to displaced nasal packing," *Ear, Nose and Throat Journal*, vol. 74, no. 11, pp. 744–746, 1995.

[5] C. Ozer, F. Ozer, M. Sener, and H. Yavuz, "A forgotten gauze pack in the nasopharynx: an unfortunate complication of adenotonsillectomy," *American Journal of Otolaryngology—Head and Neck Medicine and Surgery*, vol. 28, no. 3, pp. 191–193, 2007.

[6] G. Cecchetto, G. Viel, A. Cecchetto, S. Kusstatscher, and M. Montisci, "Fatal splenic rupture following heimlich maneuver: case report and literature review," *American Journal of Forensic Medicine and Pathology*, vol. 32, no. 2, pp. 169–171, 2011.

[7] H. Blain, M. Bonnafous, N. Grovalet, O. Jonquet, and M. David, "The table maneuver: a procedure used with success in four cases of unconscious choking older subjects," *The American Journal of Medicine*, vol. 123, no. 12, pp. 1150.e7–1150.e9, 2010.

35

Unique Phrenic Nerve-Sparing Regional Anesthetic Technique for Pain Management after Shoulder Surgery

Jason K. Panchamia, David A. Olsen, and Adam W. Amundson

Department of Anesthesiology and Perioperative Medicine, Mayo Clinic, Rochester, MN, USA

Correspondence should be addressed to Jason K. Panchamia; panchamia.jason@mayo.edu

Academic Editor: Pavel Michalek

Background. Ipsilateral phrenic nerve blockade is a common adverse event after an interscalene brachial plexus block, which can result in respiratory deterioration in patients with preexisting pulmonary conditions. Diaphragm-sparing nerve block techniques are continuing to evolve, with the intention of providing satisfactory postoperative analgesia while minimizing hemidiaphragmatic paralysis after shoulder surgery. *Case Report.* We report the successful application of a combined ultrasound-guided infraclavicular brachial plexus block and suprascapular nerve block in a patient with a complicated pulmonary history undergoing a total shoulder replacement. *Conclusion.* This case report briefly reviews the important innervations to the shoulder joint and examines the utility of the infraclavicular brachial plexus block for postoperative pain management.

1. Introduction

Total shoulder arthroplasty is a major surgical procedure, with the potential for severe postoperative pain, especially in the first 48 hours after surgery [1]. The interscalene brachial plexus block is considered the optimal regional anesthetic technique for postoperative analgesia in healthy patients after shoulder surgery. However, the major disadvantage of the interscalene block is the risk of ipsilateral phrenic nerve paralysis, with an incidence as high as 100% [2], depending on the volume, concentration, and location of local anesthetic administered. Consequently, hemidiaphragmatic paralysis depresses respiratory function, specifically decreasing forced vital capacity, forced expiratory volume in 1 second, and peak expiratory flow rates, which may be detrimental to patients with poor pulmonary reserve [3].

Given the increasing number of patients with preexisting pulmonary conditions undergoing shoulder surgery, current research is directed at diaphragm-sparing nerve block techniques. An example of these techniques is combining an infraclavicular brachial plexus block and a suprascapular nerve block [4, 5]. To date, there is limited literature regarding the analgesic efficacy of this combined technique. We report the successful application of a combined ultrasound-guided infraclavicular brachial plexus block and suprascapular nerve block in a patient with moderate-to-severe chronic obstructive lung disease undergoing total shoulder arthroplasty. The patient provided written consent to review and report this case.

2. Case Report

A 67-year-old man (American Society of Anesthesiologists physical status class IV; height, 170 cm; weight, 84.3 kg) was seen for a right reverse total shoulder arthroplasty. He had multiple comorbid conditions, including a history of a traumatic brain injury resulting in residual right-sided hemiparesis complicated by limb spasticity and neck contractures (making him wheelchair bound), poor functional status, and significant pulmonary disease. His pulmonary history included moderate-to-severe chronic obstructive pulmonary disease secondary to a 50-pack-year smoking history (Global Initiative for Obstructive Lung Disease Class C; forced vital capacity, 59%; forced expiratory volume in 1 second, 55%; diffusing capacity of the lungs for carbon monoxide, 53%), severe thoracic kyphosis resulting in restrictive lung disease, bronchiectasis complicated by impaired mucociliary clearance with mucus pooling notable on imaging studies, neuromuscular weakness in the setting of traumatic brain injury leading to poor respiratory effort, and obstructive sleep apnea necessitating continuous positive airway pressure therapy. The patient's baseline pain in his right shoulder was 9 out of 10 on a numeric pain rating scale (NRS), which he treated with scheduled acetaminophen and tramadol 75 mg per day.

Given the risk of hemidiaphragmatic paralysis after interscalene block, as well as the technical difficulty of performing nerve blocks above the clavicle because of the patient's neck contracture, the anesthesia team opted to perform a combined ultrasound-guided infraclavicular and suprascapular nerve block in the preoperative period. After appropriate monitoring and sedation, the ultrasound-guided infraclavicular block was performed via paracoracoid approach by visualizing the neurovascular bundle in a parasagittal plane just medial and inferior to the coracoid process. A 21-gauge, 100-mm insulated needle was advanced in-plane in a cephalad-to-caudad trajectory under direct visualization, with the needle tip positioned cephaloposteriorly to the axillary artery. A single injection of 15 mL of 0.5% bupivacaine with 1 : 200,000 epinephrine and 25 mcg of dexmedetomidine was administered, evaluating for a U-shaped spread, defined as local anesthetic distribution in a cephalad, posterior, and caudad position to the axillary artery, as described by Dingemans et al. [6].

An ultrasound-guided suprascapular nerve block, described by Harmon and Hearty [7], was performed by advancing the needle beneath the transverse scapular ligament into the suprascapular notch within the vicinity of the suprascapular nerve. A single injection of 10 mL of 0.5% bupivacaine with 1 : 200,000 epinephrine and 25 mcg of dexmedetomidine was administered.

The patient underwent the procedure supported, uneventfully, with general anesthesia and received a total of 100 mcg fentanyl, 10 mg ketamine, and 4 mg dexamethasone, all intravenously. During wound closure, the surgeon injected the incision site with 0.25% ropivacaine. The patient was successfully extubated and transported to the postanesthesia care unit, where he reported an NRS score of 0 and received no additional pain medication. He required minimal oxygen (2-L nasal cannula) and had an appropriate motor and sensory blockade in the expected infraclavicular distribution from the ipsilateral deltoid muscle to his fingers.

On the inpatient surgical unit, the postoperative pain regimen consisted of scheduled acetaminophen 1,000 mg every 6 hours and tramadol 25 mg every 6 hours as needed for breakthrough pain. In the first 20 hours postoperatively, the patient's NRS score remained 0, he did not receive any opioids, his pulmonary function was back to baseline with no additional oxygen requirement, and he continued to display motor blockade and sensory numbness of his right upper extremity, although he slowly regained motor function in his fingers. At 24 hours postoperatively, the patient's NRS score remained 0, he received 25 mg of oral tramadol for left arm spasticity pain, and his motor and sensory blockade resolved. At 27 hours postoperatively, the patient began to experience discomfort in his right shoulder, NRS score of 4, at which point he resumed his daily 75-mg tramadol pain regimen.

No adverse respiratory events or complications occurred throughout the patient's hospitalization. Although patients undergoing total shoulder arthroplasty at our institution are typically discharged on postoperative day 1, the patient was awaiting skilled nursing facility placement and was therefore discharged on postoperative day 2.

3. Discussion

The majority of the glenohumeral joint is innervated by the suprascapular nerve (C5-C6; originates from upper trunk of brachial plexus) and the axillary nerve (C5-C6; originates from posterior cord of brachial plexus). Furthermore, the shoulder joint and adjacent soft tissues receive minor contributions from the subscapular nerve (C5-C6; originates from posterior cord of brachial plexus), lateral pectoral nerve (C5-C6; originates from lateral cord of brachial plexus), and musculocutaneous nerve (C5-C7; originates from lateral cord of brachial plexus) [8]. The cutaneous innervation of the shoulder is supplied by the superficial cervical plexus (C1–C4).

An interscalene block performed at the level of the roots (C5–C7) or trunks (specifically upper trunk) of the brachial plexus, in combination with a superficial cervical plexus block, essentially allows for a complete analgesic technique to the shoulder joint. The phrenic nerve (C3–C5) and brachial plexus lie deep to the prevertebral fascia, thus local anesthetic administration after a brachial plexus block can result in medication "spilling" over onto the phrenic nerve. Kessler et al. [9] showed that the phrenic nerve and C5 nerve root are within 2 mm of each other at the level of the cricoid cartilage (also referred to C6 level). The distance between the phrenic nerve and brachial plexus increases approximately 3 mm for every centimeter caudal to the cricoid cartilage. Therefore, the risk of hemidiaphragmatic paralysis would be notably reduced, if not eliminated, if the local anesthetic injection were focused on the terminal nerves and associated articular branches of the brachial plexus, a distance considerably away from the phrenic nerve. Conversely, performing distal nerve blocks to minimize phrenic nerve blockade, such as the combined suprascapular and axillary nerve block approach, results in an incomplete analgesic technique. This would lead to suboptimal pain control due to the remaining unblocked minor neural contributors to the shoulder capsule (i.e., subscapular nerve, lateral pectoral nerve, musculocutaneous nerve, and superficial cervical plexus) [10]. Selective targeting of the posterior and lateral cords of the brachial plexus, in combination with suprascapular and superficial cervical plexus block, would provide improved postoperative analgesia by covering a greater part of the innervation to the shoulder joint. Tran et al. [4] stated that the combined infraclavicular plus suprascapular nerve block for shoulder surgery has been overlooked and forgotten. Our own literature search yielded only 1 case report from 2003 that described a combined infraclavicular plus suprascapular nerve block with nerve stimulator and high local anesthetic volumes to achieve surgical anesthesia in a patient with obstructive airway disease undergoing humeral head surgery [5].

Several considerations regarding the infraclavicular nerve block should be highlighted. First, there remains a potential concern for phrenic nerve paralysis after an infraclavicular nerve block. Petrar et al. [11] reported a 3% incidence of complete paralysis and a 13% incidence of complete or partial paralysis after a paracoracoid infraclavicular block entailing 30 mL of 0.5% ropivacaine injection for upper extremity surgery. This study used a large volume of local anesthetic to achieve surgical anesthesia before upper extremity surgery. It is important to distinguish local anesthetic volume and concentration necessary for surgical anesthesia versus postoperative analgesia. Classically, higher doses of local anesthetic (i.e., volume and concentration) are required to achieve surgical anesthesia, with consideration of providing complete anesthesia to the surgical site, along with enhanced sensory and motor block onset times. In comparison, peripheral nerve blocks intended solely for postoperative analgesia typically require lower local anesthetic doses. Furthermore, ultrasound guidance allows for a more targeted local anesthetic injection (i.e., to neural structures responsible for postsurgical pain) with a decrease in local anesthetic volume. In our case, the local anesthetic was injected in a cephaloposterior position to target mainly the posterior and lateral cords that provide innervation to the shoulder joint. In addition, we used a perineural dexmedetomidine/local anesthetic combination to potentially decrease the total dose of local anesthetic administered, while prolonging analgesia [12]. Further studies are necessary to elucidate the minimum effective volume to prevent hemidiaphragmatic paralysis while providing postoperative analgesia (as opposed to surgical anesthesia) for the infraclavicular block.

Second, the location of the infraclavicular brachial plexus block is important. The cords of the brachial plexus are labeled based on their position to the axillary artery. The infraclavicular block is commonly performed in the lateral infraclavicular fossa (also known as the *paracoracoid approach*). However, the cords in the lateral infraclavicular fossa can appear deep on ultrasonography, are difficult to visualize, and display variable anatomic positions around the axillary artery [13].

Fortunately, a single-injection technique of local anesthetic posterior to the axillary artery results in blockade of all 3 cords, even if the cords are not visualized [6, 13]. One of the challenges of a paracoracoid infraclavicular block is needle visualization, which becomes more difficult with increasing depth and extreme needle angulation. Abduction of the arm to 90° has been shown to decrease the distance from skin to the brachial plexus via ultrasound guidance [14]; however, performing abduction maneuvers would be extremely difficult in patients with severe shoulder and/or rotator cuff pathologic processes. Another approach to the infraclavicular block is the costoclavicular technique, which blocks the brachial plexus at the mid infraclavicular fossa, located under the midpoint of the clavicle. At this location, the cords of the brachial plexus are easier to visualize, the depth of the brachial plexus is superficial compared with the

paracoracoid approach, and the 3 cords are reliably located lateral to the axillary artery in a compact space [15]. Given the satisfactory ultrasound imaging of the brachial plexus and the possible benefit of a more distal location from the phrenic nerve, we used the paracoracoid approach for this case. We cannot recommend one approach to the infraclavicular block over another, and further investigations are essential to determine the utility of either technique for postoperative pain control after shoulder surgery while minimizing phrenic nerve blockade.

In conclusion, knowledge of the anatomical innervation to the shoulder joint is critical in tailoring postoperative pain management and analgesic outcome expectations after shoulder surgery. The combined low-volume, ultrasound-guided, infraclavicular plus suprascapular nerve block effectively targets most of the neural innervations to the shoulder joint, thereby providing satisfactory postoperative analgesia, as demonstrated in this case report for a total shoulder arthroplasty. Future investigations should be directed at comparing the postoperative analgesic efficacy for total shoulder arthroplasty between ultrasound-guided interscalene blocks and the combination of infraclavicular plus suprascapular nerve blocks.

Abbreviations

NRS: Numeric pain rating scale.

Additional Points

Implication Statement. Phrenic nerve paralysis is a common adverse event after an interscalene brachial plexus block; it results in respiratory compromise, particularly in patients with pulmonary disease. Combined infraclavicular and suprascapular nerve blocks provide adequate analgesic coverage after shoulder replacement surgery while minimizing the risk of phrenic nerve blockade.

Authors' Contributions

Jason K. Panchamia acquired case patient's consent and was involved in case patient's care and manuscript writing. David A. Olsen was involved in case patient's care and manuscript writing. Adam W. Amundson was involved in case patient's care, manuscript writing, and critical revision of manuscript. All authors approved the final manuscript.

References

[1] H. Ullah, K. Samad, and F. A. Khan, "Continuous interscalene brachial plexus block versus parenteral analgesia for postoperative pain relief after major shoulder surgery," *Cochrane Database of Systematic Reviews*, vol. 2, p. CD007080, 2014.

[2] W. F. Urmey, K. H. Talts, and N. E. Sharrock, "One hundred percent incidence of hemidiaphragmatic paresis associated with interscalene brachial plexus anesthesia as diagnosed by ultrasonography," *Anesthesia & Analgesia*, vol. 72, no. 4, pp. 498–503, 1991.

[3] W. F. Urmey and M. McDonald, "Hemidiaphragmatic paresis during interscalene brachial plexus block: effects on pulmonary function and chest wall mechanics," *Anesthesia & Analgesia*, vol. 74, no. 3, pp. 352-257, 1992.

[4] D. Q. H. Tran, M. F. Elgueta, J. Aliste, and R. J. Finlayson, "Diaphragm-sparing nerve blocks for shoulder surgery," *Regional Anesthesia and Pain Medicine*, vol. 42, no. 1, pp. 32–38, 2017.

[5] J. Martinez, X. Sala-Blanch, I. Ramos, and C. Gomar, "Combined infraclavicular plexus block with suprascapular nerve block for humeral head surgery in a patient with respiratory failure: an alternative approach," *Anesthesiology*, vol. 98, no. 3, pp. 784-785, 2003.

[6] E. Dingemans, S. R. Williams, G. Arcand et al., "Neurostimulation in ultrasound-guided infraclavicular block: a prospective randomized trial," *Anesthesia & Analgesia*, vol. 104, no. 5, pp. 1275–1280, 2007.

[7] D. Harmon and C. Hearty, "Ultrasound-guided suprascapular nerve block technique," *Pain Physician*, vol. 10, no. 6, pp. 743–746, 2007.

[8] O. C. Aszmann, A. Lee Dellon, B. T. Birely, and E. G. McFarland, "Innervation of the human shoulder joint and its implications for surgery," *Clinical Orthopaedics and Related Research*, no. 330, pp. 202–207, 1996.

[9] J. Kessler, I. Schafhalter-Zoppoth, and A. T. Gray, "An Ultrasound Study of the Phrenic Nerve in the Posterior Cervical Triangle: Implications for the Interscalene Brachial Plexus Block," *Regional Anesthesia and Pain Medicine*, vol. 33, no. 6, pp. 545–550, 2008.

[10] S. Dhir, R. V. Sondekoppam, R. Sharma, S. Ganapathy, and G. S. Athwal, "A comparison of combined suprascapular and axillary nerve blocks to interscalene nerve block for analgesia in arthroscopic shoulder surgery an equivalence study," *Regional Anesthesia and Pain Medicine*, vol. 41, no. 5, pp. 564–571, 2016.

[11] S. D. Petrar, M. E. Seltenrich, S. J. Head, and S. K. W. Schwarz, "Hemidiaphragmatic paralysis following ultrasound-guided supraclavicular versus infraclavicular brachial plexus blockade: a randomized clinical trial," *Regional Anesthesia and Pain Medicine*, vol. 40, no. 2, pp. 133–138, 2015.

[12] N. Hussain, V. P. Grzywacz, C. A. Ferreri et al., "Investigating the efficacy of dexmedetomidine as an adjuvant to local anesthesia in brachial plexus block a systematic review and meta-analysis of 18 randomized controlled trials," *Regional Anesthesia and Pain Medicine*, vol. 42, no. 2, pp. 184–196, 2017.

[13] A. R. Sauter, H.-J. Smith, A. Stubhaug, M. S. Dodgson, and O. Klaastad, "Use of magnetic resonance imaging to define the anatomical location closest to all three cords of the infraclavicular brachial plexus," *Anesthesia amp Analgesia*, vol. 103, no. 6, pp. 1574–1576, 2006.

[14] A. Ruiz, X. Sala, X. Bargalló, P. Hurtado, M. J. Arguis, and A. Carrera, "The influence of arm abduction on the anatomic relations of infraclavicular brachial plexus: an ultrasound study," *Anesthesia & Analgesia*, vol. 108, no. 1, pp. 364–366, 2009.

[15] M. K. Karmakar, X. Sala-Blanch, B. Songthamwat, and B. C. H. Tsui, "Benefits of the costoclavicular space for ultrasound-guided infraclavicular brachial plexus block: description of a costoclavicular approach," *Regional Anesthesia and Pain Medicine*, vol. 40, no. 3, pp. 287-288, 2015.

36

Pharmacological Management of Severe Neuropathic Pain in a Case of Eosinophilic Meningitis Related to Angiostrongylus cantonensis

Jennifer Busse,[1] David Gottlieb,[1] Krystal Ferreras (ID),[1]
Jennifer Bain,[2] and William Schechter (ID)[3]

[1] Anesthesiology, Morgan Stanley Children's Hospital of New York-Presbyterian at Columbia University Irving Medical Center, USA
[2] Neurology, Morgan Stanley Children's Hospital at Columbia University Irving Medical Center, USA
[3] Anesthesiology and Pediatrics, Morgan Stanley Children's Hospital at Columbia University Irving Medical Center, New York, NY, USA

Correspondence should be addressed to William Schechter; ws5@cumc.columbia.edu

Academic Editor: Chun-Sung Sung

Angiostrongylus cantonensis, the rat lungworm, is the most common infectious cause of eosinophilic meningitis and can be fatal. The parasite can be found throughout Southeast Asia and Pacific Islands and the global distribution is expanding. We present the case of a fourteen-year-old female who had previously traveled to Hawaii and developed severe neuropathic pain related to A. cantonensis infection refractory to gabapentin and pregabalin monotherapy, who was eventually managed with an ultralow dose ketamine infusion, methadone, and serotonin-norepinephrine reuptake inhibitor.

1. Introduction

Neuropathic pain related to Angiostrongylus cantonensis (A. cantonensis) has not been well described but may be severe, debilitating, and difficult to treat. A. cantonensis, the rat lungworm, can be found throughout Southeast Asia and the Pacific Islands, but its prevalence has been spreading globally and cases have been identified originating in the southwestern United States [1, 2]. Infection is caused by eating raw or uncooked foods containing the infective stage larvae of A. cantonensis. A. cantonensis is the most common cause of eosinophilic meningitis (EM) [1–4]. Symptomatology is not consistent among those infected, so initial diagnosis can be challenging and effective treatment of pain symptoms is difficult. The most commonly described symptoms include severe, persistent headaches caused by increased intracranial pressure and leptomeningeal inflammation [5], paresthesias [1, 4], and cranial nerve palsies [6]. Lesions associated with A. cantonensis have been reported in both cerebral hemispheres and the cerebellum with spinal nerve root involvement being the most likely primary cause of the sensory disturbance; therefore the origin of the pain is likely central and peripheral in nature [7].

Improvement in symptoms is generally seen within 3 to 6 weeks after diagnosis and they are rarely persistent after this time [1, 3]. In unusual refractory cases, patients may develop severe permanent neurological deficits [3, 6]. For mild cases, analgesics such as acetaminophen or nonsteroidal anti-inflammatory agents suffice; however, steroids are often recommended for severe refractory symptoms. Primary anthelmintic therapy is controversial because the helminth's life-cycle is limited in humans and treatment may accelerate a robust and detrimental immune response [3, 5–10].

We present a case of A. cantonensis infection in a 14-year-old female during a trip to Hawaii who developed severe ascending neuropathic pain initially involving both distal lower extremities and the mid abdominal region. It was refractory to mild analgesics, steroids, and commonly recommended doses of gabapentin and pregabalin.

1.1. Consent for Publication. The authors reviewed the case report with the patient and her parents. The patient gave verbal assent and the parents provided verbal permission for the authors to publish this report.

2. Case Description

A fourteen-year-old 48.9 kilogram (kg) female with a history of intermittent, infrequent migraines presented to our institution's emergency department with bilateral distal leg pain, severe mechanical allodynia, and truncal rash which began two weeks previously while in Hawaii after ingestion of uncooked spinach. Initial symptoms consisted of full body itching, initially without a rash, rhinorrhea, congestion, or cough. A maculopapular rash evolved to cover her entire truncal region and thighs. She then developed intense bilateral distal lower extremity pain in a stocking-like distribution from feet to knee, which became exquisitely painful to light touch and ambulation. She described the pain as "sharp" and "shooting". She then developed spontaneous tingling and numbness in both feet and hands, as well as tremors in all four extremities. She complained of burning pain across her abdomen at dermatome T10. Pain was rated at 10/10 and constant. She additionally complained of headache, diplopia, lightheadedness, and urinary retention. Before she was admitted to the hospital her pain was managed with acetaminophen, ibuprofen, and gabapentin. After the trial of gabapentin failed to reduce pain it was discontinued and pregabalin was started while still an outpatient.

A brain MRI, with and without contrast, was normal but the total spine MRI showed slight increased signal in the right dorsal cord especially at the level of T_{11}-T_{12}. A lumbar puncture revealed an opening pressure of 46 and closing pressure of 15 cm H_2O, a protein of 82, and glucose of 54 mg/dL with leukocytosis of 390 cells/μL and 17% eosinophils. Cerebrospinal fluid (CSF) serology was sent. The complete blood count (CBC) was normal except for an elevated white blood cell count of 11.46. X 10^3 cells/μL. A diagnosis of eosinophilic meningitis was made. Prednisone, 20 milligrams (mg), every eight hours was started, as were around-the-clock acetaminophen, ketorolac, and topical 5% lidocaine patches. Additionally, hydroxyzine 12.5 mg was given, as needed, for pruritus to good effect. The hydroxyzine and clonazepam given for sleep were discontinued because of excessive sedation.

Despite the above interventions, the pain remained refractory and so the following day ketamine was started at 0.02 milligrams (mg) per kilogram (kg) per hour, which was increased over five hours to 0.05 mg per kg per hour. Duloxetine, 20 mg, was administered at bedtime and methadone 2.5 mg every twelve hours was also added for continued pain that night. The following morning, the patient reported reduction in her pain to a numeric pain score of 6/10. Her leg pain resolved with the exception of the dorsum of her feet bilaterally; however, the burning pain persisted at approximately the T10 dermatome. Pregabalin continued to be slowly titrated upward to its maximum dose of 100 mg every eight hours. She did have one report of a vivid dream, but no hallucinations, tachycardia, hypertension, or signs of serotonergic or noradrenergic syndrome were present. On day 5 of admission, albendazole was started as per the

recommendations of the Hawaii Department of Health. She had no additional side effects to the analgesic medications and her mental status remained normal. Diplopia, headache, and urinary retention resolved within four days of hospitalization. Ketamine was weaned and the patient was discharged with duloxetine, methadone, pregabalin, and prednisone with plans to be tapered by Pediatric Neurology as an outpatient. Of note, within two weeks of discharge, pregabalin and methadone weaning was initiated with recrudescence of pain despite continued administration of prednisone. The weaning was then restarted the following week at a slower rate and was better tolerated. CSF serologies confirmed diagnosis of A. cantonensis infection.

3. Discussion

This case report reflects that of a teenager infected with A. cantonensis with subsequent eosinophilic meningitis causing severe headache and neuropathic pain, which is likely both central and peripheral in origin. Neuropathic pain is known to be poorly responsive to opioids [11], as well as acetaminophen and nonsteroidal anti-inflammatory, but may often be effectively treated with anticonvulsants, such as the gabapentin and pregabalin, with minimal risk. In this case, these usual medications were not effective for the patient's pain control; however the addition of ketamine was effective.

The mainstay of most treatments for neuropathic pain includes utilization of gabapentin and pregabalin, which decrease cellular excitability through hyperpolarization [12, 13]. Other pharmacologic approaches to pain management include utilizing the antidepressant class such as amitriptyline and nortriptyline or the newer amine reuptake inhibitors such as the SNRI duloxetine, which exert their effects through a multiplicity of mechanisms of action [14, 15] including descending inhibition via the nucleus tractus solitarius [16]. Methadone [17], lidocaine infusions [18, 19], and a variety of other anticonvulsants have also been shown to be efficacious in some patients with severe neuropathic pain syndromes.

Ketamine has also been reported to be effective in the treatment of acute neuropathic pain [20]. Its putative role as an analgesic is as an N-methyl-D-aspartate (NMDA) receptor antagonist to inhibit wind-up by inducing synthesis and release of nitric oxide as well as indirectly modulating mu opioid receptor signaling and myriad other mechanisms [21, 22]. Doses of 0.2mg/kg/h to 0.5mg/kg/h of IV ketamine given for short periods have been shown to be safe in pediatric patients [23]. Because of her complex neurological presentation, we used extreme caution in our dosing of ketamine and were surprised to see a rapid effect on pain at doses many times lower than that reported in the literature.

Neuropathic pain related to A. cantonensis can be severe, persistent, and difficult to treat. Neither ketamine, methadone, pregabalin nor duloxetine has ever been reported as treatment for acute neuropathic pain in eosinophilic meningitis. In this case, ketamine, methadone, and duloxetine were used as adjuvants to pregabalin, providing a clinically observable and rapid improvement in pain scores resulting in the ability of the patient to return to functionality. While prednisone and the lumbar puncture may have had an effect on her urinary retention and headache, there was no clear clinical observation that they were beneficial for her neuropathic pain.

The ketamine infusion was selected over other pharmacologic pain treatment modalities including lidocaine infusion because the safety profile was deemed better despite the historical admonition against its use in patients with increased intracranial pressure [24]. Contemporary literature on ketamine's effect on intracranial pressure is mixed and it is not clear whether this is a dose-related phenomenon, especially when given by infusion, since it has not been studied in patients receiving low dose infusions of ketamine for pain [25]. Medications such as pregabalin, duloxetine, and methadone require titration and several half-lives to take effect and so it was thought that they would not provide the immediate relief of this patient's severe pain that ketamine might provide even though the latter exerts some analgesic effect via NMDA antagonism. To minimize the need for additional titration of ketamine and prepare for outpatient treatment, methadone and duloxetine were also simultaneously initiated. Opioids such as methadone may also increase intracranial pressure by depressing ventilation, increasing $PaCO_2$, and contributing to cerebral vasodilation. Therefore, a reduced dose of 0.1 mg/kg/day divided every twelve hours was chosen as adjuvant therapy. The reduction in ICP following lumbar puncture also provided a margin of safety during initiation of both ketamine and methadone.

Once pain was under control and in preparation for discharge, ketamine was stopped and methadone, pregabalin, and duloxetine were continued with plans of weaning as an outpatient. It is of note that her pain recrudesced as pregabalin, methadone, and steroids were weaned as an outpatient but improved when she returned to original doses. She has since tolerated the steroid weaning with methadone, pregabalin, and duloxetine continuing to manage her pain.

This report presents a difficult-to-manage case of neuropathic pain, likely of central and peripheral origin. Ultimately, the patient was clinically most responsive to ketamine. Certainly of concern is administration of ketamine to patients with increased intracranial pressure. Because of this, more study is required on the effects of subanesthetic dosing of ketamine in patients at risk of increased intracranial pressure. Ketamine appears to be an excellent adjuvant that works quickly for acute neuropathic pain in patients with eosinophilic meningitis but requires caution and administration only by those trained in its use. Duloxetine and carefully dosed methadone also appeared to be of significant benefit in this patient when immediate pain relief was required in the setting of pregabalin titration.

References

[1] V. L. Re III and S. J. Gluckman, "Eosinophilic meningitis," *American Journal of Medicine*, vol. 114, no. 3, pp. 217–223, 2003.

[2] P. Eamsobhana, "Eosinophilic meningitis caused by Angiostrongylus cantonensis–a neglected disease with escalating importance," *Tropical Biomedicine*, vol. 31, no. 4, pp. 569–578, 2014.

[3] G. S. Murphy and S. Johnson, "Clinical aspects of eosinophilic meningitis and meningoencephalitis caused by Angiostrongylus cantonensis, the rat lungworm," *Hawaii Journal of Medicine and Public Health*, vol. 72, 2, no. 6, pp. 35–40, 2013.

[4] T. J. Slom, M. M. Cortese, S. I. Gerber et al., "An outbreak of eosinophilic meningitis caused by Angiostrongylus cantonensis in travelers returning from the Caribbean," *The New England Journal of Medicine*, vol. 346, no. 9, pp. 668–675, 2002.

[5] V. Chotmongkol, K. Sawanyawisuth, and Y. Thavornpitak, "Corticosteroid treatment of eosinophilic meningitis," *Clinical Infectious Diseases*, vol. 31, no. 3, pp. 660–662, 2000.

[6] W. Alto, "Human infections with Angiostrongylus cantonensis," *Pac Health Dialog*, vol. 8, no. 1, pp. 176–182, 2001.

[7] P. D. Clouston, A. J. Corbett, D. S. Pryor, and R. Garrick, "Eosinophilic meningitis: Cause of a chronic pain syndrome," *Journal of Neurology, Neurosurgery & Psychiatry*, vol. 53, no. 9, pp. 778–781, 1990.

[8] L. Rosen, G. Loison, J. Laigret, and G. D. Wallace, "Studies on eosinophilic meningitis. 3. Epidemiologic and clinical observations on pacific Islands and the possible etiologic role of Angiostrongylus cantonensis," *American Journal of Epidemiology*, vol. 85, no. 1, pp. 17–44, 1967.

[9] Q.-P. Wang, D.-H. Lai, X.-Q. Zhu, X.-G. Chen, and Z.-R. Lun, "Human angiostrongyliasis," *The Lancet Infectious Diseases*, vol. 8, no. 10, pp. 621–630, 2008.

[10] L. Ramirez-Avila, S. Slome, F. L. Schuster et al., "Eosinophilic meningitis due to Angiostrongylus and Gnathostoma species," *Clinical Infectious Diseases*, vol. 48, no. 3, pp. 322–327, 2009.

[11] S. Arner and B. A. Meyerson, "Lack of analgesic effect of opioids on neuropathic and idiopathic forms of pain," *Pain*, vol. 33, no. 1, pp. 11–23, 1988.

[12] J. Hendrich, A. T. Van Minh, F. Heblich et al., "Pharmacological disruption of calcium channel trafficking by the alpha 2 delta ligand gabapentin," *Proceedings of the National Academy of Sciences*, vol. 105, no. 9, pp. 3628–3633, 2008.

[13] C. P. Taylor, N. S. Gee, T.-Z. Su et al., "A summary of mechanistic hypotheses of gabapentin pharmacology," *Epilepsy Research*, vol. 29, no. 3, pp. 233–249, 1998.

[14] D. Fornasari, "Pharmacotherapy for Neuropathic Pain: A Review," *Pain and Therapy*, vol. 6, no. S1, pp. 25–33, 2017.

[15] Y. Deng, L. Luo, Y. Hu, K. Fang, and J. Liu, "Clinical practice guidelines for the management of neuropathic pain: a systematic review," *BMC Anesthesiology*, vol. 16, no. 1, 2015.

[16] C. Bridgestock and C. P. Rae, "Anatomy, physiology and pharmacology of pain," *Anaesthesia and Intensive Care Medicine*, vol. 14, no. 11, pp. 480–483, 2013.

[17] I. W. Tremont-Lukats, V. Challapalli, E. D. McNicol, J. Lau, and D. B. Carr, "Systemic administration of local anesthetics to relieve neuropathic pain: a systematic review and meta-analysis," *Anesthesia & Analgesia*, vol. 101, no. 6, pp. 1738–1749, 2005.

[18] R. H. Dworkin, A. B. O'Connor, M. Backonja et al., "Pharmacologic management of neuropathic pain: evidence-based recommendations," *Pain*, vol. 132, no. 3, pp. 237–251, 2007.

[19] I. W. Tremont-Lukats, P. R. Hutson, and M.-M. Backonja, "A randomized, double-masked, placebo-controlled pilot trial of extended IV lidocaine infusion for relief of ongoing neuropathic

pain," *The Clinical Journal of Pain*, vol. 22, no. 3, pp. 266–271, 2006.

[20] J. L. Zeballos, P. Lirk, and J. P. Rathmell, "Low-dose ketamine for acute pain medication management: A Timely Nudge toward Multimodal Analgesia," *Regional Anesthesia and Pain Medicine*, vol. 43, no. 5, pp. 453–455, 2018.

[21] M. Backonja, G. Arndt, K. A. Gombar, B. Check, and M. Zimmermann, "Response of chronic neuropathic pain syndromes to ketamine: a preliminary study," *PAIN*, vol. 56, no. 1, pp. 51–57, 1994.

[22] M. B. Max, M. G. Byas-Smith, R. H. Gracely, and G. J. Bennett, "Intravenous infusion of the NMDA antagonist, ketamine, in chronic posttraumatic pain with allodynia: A double-blind comparison to alfentanil and placebo," *Clinical Neuropharmacology*, vol. 18, no. 4, pp. 360–368, 1995.

[23] A. L. Bredlau, R. Thakur, D. N. Korones, and R. H. Dworkin, "Ketamine for pain in adults and children with cancer: a systematic review and synthesis of the literature," *Pain Medicine*, vol. 14, no. 10, pp. 1505–1517, 2013.

[24] J. Evans, M. Rosen, R. D. Weeks, and C. Wise, "Ketamine in neurosurgical procedures," *The Lancet*, vol. 1, no. 7688, pp. 40-41, 1971.

[25] N. Kramer, D. Lebowitz, M. Walsh, and L. Ganti, "Rapid Sequence Intubation in Traumatic Brain-injured Adults," *Cureus*, vol. 10, no. 4, Article ID e2530, 2018.

37

A Minimal-Invasive Metabolic Test Detects Malignant Hyperthermia Susceptibility in a Patient after Sevoflurane-Induced Metabolic Crisis

Frank Schuster, Stephan Johannsen, and Norbert Roewer

Department of Anesthesia and Critical Care, University of Wuerzburg, Oberduerrbacher Street 6, 97080 Wuerzburg, Germany

Correspondence should be addressed to Frank Schuster; schuster_f@klinik.uni-wuerzburg.de

Academic Editors: A. Han, H. Shankar, and C.-S. Sung

Malignant hyperthermia is a rare but life-threatening complication of general anesthesia in predisposed patients usually triggered by potent inhalation anesthetics and/or the depolarizing muscle relaxant succinylcholine. The authors present a case of delayed sevoflurane-induced malignant hyperthermia in a 21-year-old male patient that was sufficiently treated by discontinuation of trigger agent application and dantrolene infusion. After surviving an MH episode diagnostic procedures are indicated to increase patient safety. In the presented case, the use of a novel minimal-invasive metabolic test with intramuscular injection of halothane and caffeine successfully confirmed MH susceptibility and hence might be an alternative for invasive in vitro contracture testing in selected cases.

1. Introduction

Malignant hyperthermia (MH) is a rare but potentially lethal pharmacological induced disease of skeletal muscle. Exposure to triggering agents such as volatile anesthetics and/or the depolarizing muscle relaxant succinylcholine may induce a hypermetabolic muscular syndrome characterized by hypoxemia, hypercapnia, tachycardia, muscular rigidity, acidosis, hyperkalemia, and hyperthermia, due to an uncontrolled sarcoplasmic calcium release via functionally altered ryanodine receptors subtype 1 or dihydropyridine receptors [1]. Currently, the in vitro contracture test (IVCT) requiring an open muscle biopsy is the only reliable procedure to diagnose MH susceptibility in affected patients. However, due to its invasive characteristics this test is associated with severe risks to the patients, for example, wound infections, postoperative bleeding, or persistent dysesthesia. Important progress was made within the last years by screening for causative MH mutations, which allows a genetic diagnosis in 30% to 50% of MH families [2]. Unfortunately, a negative genetic result does not sufficiently exclude MH susceptibility and hence must be confirmed by IVCT [3]. Recently, a minimal-invasive metabolic test was proposed to analyze muscular alterations in MH patients under in vivo conditions. The local monitoring of interstitial lactate concentrations after pharmacological stimulation induced by MH trigger agents allowed a differentiation between MH susceptible (MHS) and MH nonsusceptible (MHN) patients [4].

In the presented case report, we used this minimal-invasive test to screen for MH susceptibility in a patient who developed clinical sings of MH during general anesthesia with sevoflurane while undergoing an elective shoulder arthroscopy.

2. Case Presentation

2.1. Intra- and Postoperative Course. With approval of the local ethics committee (application number: 263/11, ethics committee of the University of Wuerzburg), we report the case of a 21-year-old male patient weighting 100 kg, who was scheduled for elective shoulder arthroscopy. Neither the patient nor his family had any history of neuromuscular disease or MH. According to the medical records, the patient underwent two uneventful anesthesias using halothane combined with oxygen (O_2) and nitrous oxide (N_2O) for cleft lip revision at the age of 5 months and at the age of 4 years, respectively. The preoperative laboratory examinations were within normal values. Initial heart rate (95 bpm), blood pressure (145/80 mmHg), and peripheral oxygen saturation (96%) were unremarkable. Anesthesia was induced by intravenous application of 0.1 mg/kg piritramid, an initial bolus of 2.5 mg/kg propofol followed by an additional application of 1.5 mg/kg propofol, and 1.5 mg/kg succinylcholine. To secure patient's airways, a size 8,0 mm cuffed endotracheal tube was inserted after direct laryngoscopy. Afterwards, anesthesia was maintained by sevoflurane 1.5 vol% supplemented by O_2/N_2O and application of 0.05 mg/kg piritramid if needed. During the initial period of surgery, hemodynamic and metabolic parameters were within normal limits with end-tidal carbon dioxide values between 38 and 39 mmHg. Suddenly, after 290 min a slightly increase of heart rate from 60 bpm to 80 bpm and a rise in systolic blood pressure from 120 mmHg to 135 mmHg were noticed. Furthermore, end-tidal carbon dioxide concentration rapidly increased from 39 mmHg to 85 mmHg within 5 min after the onset of sinus tachycardia. Simultaneously, oxygen saturation decreased from 98% to 93%. Unfortunately, there was no monitoring of body temperature, but the attending anesthesiologist observed and documented warming of head and chest during this episode. After MH was suspected, the anesthesiologist immediately stopped sevoflurane and hyperventilated the patient with 100% oxygen (25 L/min). In addition, 240 mg dantrolene was applied twice and anesthesia was continued intravenously by infusion of 5 mg/kg/h propofol and repeated fentanyl applications. After these interventions, hemodynamic and metabolic parameters were stabilized within 10 min. The surgical procedure was stopped, and the patient was transferred to the intensive care unit (ICU) in stable conditions.

Laboratory analyses performed after admission to the ICU detected a significant rhabdomyolysis with creatine kinase levels about 20.000 U/L and a hyperkalemia (6.4 mmol/L). Further laboratory data were unremarkable. Interestingly, blood gas analysis drawn one hour after the MH suspected event did not show signs of metabolic or respiratory acidosis. Four hours after the admission, the patient was extubated without neurological deficits.

3. Diagnostic Findings

Due to the suspected MH event, the patient was informed about the possible risk of MH susceptibility and a diagnostic workup was recommended. Hence, after written and oral informed consent of the patient, we decided to perform the recently developed minimal-invasive metabolic test three days after the suspected MH episode. In brief, after regional anesthesia of the skin, two microdialysis probes with a semipermeable membrane for measurement of interstitial metabolites were inserted into the lateral vastus muscle and perfused with 1 μL/min Ringer's solution. 15 min after equilibration either a single bolus of 200 μL halothane 4 vol% dissolved in soy bean oil or 200 μL caffeine 80 mM was injected into the muscular tissue. Dialysate samples were collected after 15-minute intervals, and lactate concentration was measured spectrophotometrically. If lactate values

exceeded a threshold of 2.8 mM after halothane or 1.6 mM after caffeine, which had been defined by a previous set of tests, MH susceptibility was assumed [4]. Prior to halothane or caffeine application, the baseline lactate levels did not significantly differ between both microdialysis probes (0.4 mM versus 0.8 mM). After halothane injection the lactate values significantly increased to a maximum of 3.7 mM. Similarly, caffeine induced a significant increase of lactate to 3.1 mM (Table 1).

Even though MH susceptibility had been confirmed by this metabolic test, the patient decided to undergo further diagnostic testing due to personal reasons. Due to the MH suspected course of the described case and to avoid invasive IVCT, we determined to screen the hotspots of the ryanodine receptor subtype 1 gene for MH related alterations. Unfortunately, genetic analysis did not detect MH associated mutations. Hence, twelve weeks after the MH suspected event an open muscle biopsy and IVCT according to published guidelines of the European MH Group were performed at our lab [3]. In few words, 2.5 g muscle tissue was excised of the left vastus lateral muscle after femoral nerve block. Single muscle bundles were mounted in a tissue bath and exposed to incremental concentrations of caffeine (0.5; 1; 1.5; 2; 3; 4; and 32 mM) or halothane (0.11; 0.22; 0.44; and 0.66 mM) at 3 min intervals. Since significant contractures ≥ 2 mN occurred at the defined threshold concentrations of caffeine 2 mM and halothane 0.44 mM, the MH-susceptibility of the patient was confirmed (Table 2).

4. Discussion

Malignant hyperthermia is a rare but life-threatening complication of general anesthesia usually triggered by volatile anesthetics and/or succinylcholine in susceptible patients. While genetic frequency of MH predisposition is stated to be 1 : 2.000, the prevalence of MH-episodes varies regionally between 1 : 10.000 and 1 : 220.000 [5].

Nowadays, due to continuous progress in anesthesia, it seems that the incidence of fulminant MH crisis decreases. Since the potent MH trigger halothane is no longer used in clinical routine in industrialized countries, the presently utilized inhalation anesthetics appear to delay the onset of MH or lead to abortive MH reactions with alleviated symptoms. For instance, Hopkins and colleagues reported that the onset of MH was significantly faster after halothane exposure (median: 20 min, range: 5–45 min) compared to sevoflurane (median: 60 min, range: 10–210 min) [6]. Hence, the intraoperative course in the presented case with development of MH signs 290 min after induction of general anesthesia seems consistent with these findings. However, in some cases application of sevoflurane induces MH symptoms within few minutes [7].

In addition, anesthesiologists must be aware that previous uneventful anesthesia does not exclude MH susceptibility [8]. On average, susceptible patients undergo three uneventful anesthesias until the first MH episode occurs [5]. In this context, it is not surprising that the presented patient reported two unremarkable anesthesias in the past. The underlying

TABLE 1: Local lactate increase following interstitial application of 200 μL caffeine 80 mM and 200 μL halothane 4 vol%.

Time	0 min	15 min	30 min	45 min	60 min	75 min
Caffeine 80 mM	0.4 mM	0.6 mM	0.7 mM	2.7 mM	3.1 mM	2.7 mM
Halothane 4 vol%	0.8 mM	0.7 mM	0.9 mM	2.1 mM	3.7 mM	2.8 mM

0 min: baseline lactate levels; 15 min: time point of caffeine or halothane injection.

TABLE 2: In vitro contracture test results. A contracture $\geq$ 2 mN at the defined threshold concentrations of caffeine 2 mM and halothane 0.44 mM confirmed MH susceptibility.

Caffeine	Predrug	0,5 mM	1 mM	1,5 mM	2 mM	3 mM	4 mM	32 mM
Test 1	14.0 mN	13.5 mN	15.6 mN	19.6 mN	25.6 mN	29.1 mN	29.1 mN	144 mN
Test 2	12.7 mN	12.2 mN	13.0 mN	17.8 mN	24.7 mN	35.7 mN	32.2 mN	209 mN
Halothane	Predrug	0,11 mM	0,22 mM	0,44 mM	0,66 mM			
Test 1	11.6 mN	23.0 mN	35.1 mN	32.1 mN	26.5 mN			
Test 2	19.1 mN	20.9 mN	28.1 mN	29.5 mN	26.8 mN			

pathomechanism why some patients develop MH during the first exposition to triggering agents while others do not still remains unclear. A possible explanation might be the presence of an individual compensation mechanism at a cellular level lowering myoplasmic calcium concentrations in these patients.

Based on these observations, attending anesthesiologists must keep in mind that MH may occur at any time during general anesthesia and prior unremarkable anesthesias, are not a prove for the absence of MH susceptibility.

In case of a suspected MH, application of trigger agents must be discontinued immediately and causal therapy by dantrolene infusion should be initiated to avoid serious harm to the patient [9]. The mode of action of dantrolene is based on inhibition of the sarcoplasmic calcium release during an MH episode without increasing sarcoplasmic calcium reuptake [10]. The return of metabolic parameters to normal values reflects the therapeutic success of MH treatment, comparable to the absent of metabolic or respiratory acidosis in the presented case.

Due to the possible risk in case of future anesthesia, patients should be referred to a MH-center to initiate further diagnostics after surviving a suspected MH event. In the reported case, the authors decided to apply a novel minimal-invasive metabolic test with intramuscular halothane and caffeine injection to screen for MH susceptibility. Based on the metabolic alterations in the course of an MH episode, measurement of interstitial lactate concentration was assumed as a suitable method to detect MH in affected patients. The measured increase of local lactate concentrations following halothane and caffeine application clearly indicated the diagnosis "MHS" in our patient. In contrast to the IVCT, the metabolic test is less invasive; since the induced metabolic reactions are limited to an area < 10 mm around the inserted microdialysis probes and due to the expected dilutional effects of the administered drugs in the tissue, serious systemic, or local adverse effects are unlikely [11]. Furthermore, previous histological examination of rat muscular tissue after application of caffeine 80 mM revealed only unspecific morphological changes [12].

Although MH susceptibility was proven by the metabolic test, the patient decided to undergo further diagnostic testing. Due to the clinical course of the reported MH reaction and in contrast to the diagnostic guidelines of the European MH Group, we decided to perform genetic screening at first. Unfortunately, no mutation of the ryanodine receptor subtype 1 could be detected in the patient. Hence, IVCT was carried out eight weeks after the suspicious event, since the absence of a mutation does not reliably exclude MH [13].

In summary, the authors present a case of a delayed sevoflurane-induced MH in a 21-year-old male patient, who was sufficiently treated by dantrolene and discontinuation of trigger agent application. After surviving an MH episode diagnostic procedures are indicted to increase patient safety. In the presented case, the use of a novel minimal-invasive metabolic test with intramuscular application of MH triggering agents such as halothane and caffeine successfully proved MH susceptibility and hence might avoid invasive in vitro contracture testing in selected cases.

Acknowledgments

The publication of this investigation was funded by the German Research Foundation (DFG) and the University of Wuerzburg in the funding programme Open Access Publishing.

References

[1] F. Schuster and C. R. Müller-Reible, "Malignant hyperthermia diagnostics, treatment and anaesthetic management," *Anasthesiologie Intensivmedizin Notfallmedizin Schmerztherapie*, vol. 44, no. 11-12, pp. 758–763, 2009 (German).

[2] T. Girard, S. Treves, E. Voronkov, M. Siegemund, and A. Urwyler, "Molecular genetic testing for malignant hyperthermia susceptibility," *Anesthesiology*, vol. 100, no. 5, pp. 1076–1080, 2004.

[3] F. R. Ellis, P. J. Halsall, and H. Ording, "A protocol for the investigation of malignant hyperpyrexia (MH) susceptibility. The European malignant hyperpyrexia group," *British Journal of Anaesthesia*, vol. 56, no. 11, pp. 1267–1269, 1984.

[4] F. Schuster, T. Metterlein, S. Negele et al., "An in-vivo metabolic test for detecting malignant hyperthermia susceptibility in humans: a pilot study," *Anesthesia and Analgesia*, vol. 107, no. 3, pp. 909–914, 2008.

[5] O. Bandschapp and T. Girard, "Malignant hyperthermia," *Swiss Medical Weekly*, vol. 142, no. 7, Article ID w13652, 2012.

[6] P. M. Hopkins, "Malignant hyperthermia: pharmacology of triggering," *British Journal of Anaesthesia*, vol. 107, no. 1, pp. 48–56, 2011.

[7] Y. S. Lee, W. Y. Kim, S. H. Lee et al., "A case of malignant hyperthermia during anesthesia induction with sevoflurane," *Korean Journal of Anesthesiology*, vol. 59, pp. S6–S8, 2010.

[8] H. Adam, U. Gottschaldt, N. C. Pausch, H. Rüffert, and K. M. Sipli, "Fulminant MH crisis during the ninth general anaesthesia," *Anästhesiologie, Intensivmedizin, Notfallmedizin und Schmerztherapie*, vol. 42, no. 10, pp. 692–699, 2007 (German).

[9] K. P. E. Glahn, F. R. Ellis, P. J. Halsall et al., "Recognizing and managing a malignant hyperthermia crisis. Guidelines from the European Malignant Hyperthermia Group," *British Journal of Anaesthesia*, vol. 105, no. 4, pp. 417–420, 2010.

[10] T. Krause, M. U. Gerbershagen, M. Fiege, R. Weißhorn, and F. Wappler, "Dantrolene—a review of its pharmacology, therapeutic use and new developments," *Anaesthesia*, vol. 59, no. 4, pp. 364–373, 2004.

[11] F. Schuster, H. Schöll, M. Hager, R. Müller, N. Roewer, and M. Anetseder, "The dose-response relationship and regional distribution of lactate after intramuscular injection of halothane and caffeine in malignant hyperthermia-susceptible pigs," *Anesthesia and Analgesia*, vol. 102, no. 2, pp. 468–472, 2006.

[12] F. Schuster, P. Tas, R. Müller, N. Roewer, and M. Anetseder, "Pharmacologic modulation of skeletal muscle metabolism: a microdialysis study," *Basic and Clinical Pharmacology and Toxicology*, vol. 98, no. 4, pp. 372–376, 2006.

[13] A. Urwyler, T. Deufel, T. McCarthy, and S. West, "Guidelines for molecular genetic detection of susceptibility to malignant hyperthermia," *British Journal of Anaesthesia*, vol. 86, no. 2, pp. 283–287, 2001.

38

Mobitz Type II Atrioventricular Block Followed by Remifentanil in a Patient with Severe Aortic Stenosis

Mehryar Taghavi Gilani and Majid Razavi

Anesthesia Department, Imam-Reza Hospital, School of Medicine, Mashhad University of Medical Sciences, Mashhad, Iran

Correspondence should be addressed to Majid Razavi; razavim@mums.ac.ir

Academic Editors: U. Buyukkocak, M. R. Chakravarthy, and J. Malek

Opioids have been considered for their hemodynamic stability. Remifentanil is an opioid analgesic with rapid metabolism and fast primary effect and recovery. In this paper, a very rare effect of using remifentanil along with propofol was presented. An 84-year-old male patient with severe aortic stenosis underwent general anesthesia. In order to induce anesthesia and maintain it, fentanyl, pancuronium, and propofol, along with a combination of propofol and remifentanil, were used, respectively. At beginning of remifentanil infusion, bradycardia and then Mobitz type II conduction block with a hemodynamic disorder occurred for the patient. The decreased blood pressure responded to injection of atropine and ephedrine; however, dysrhythmia only improved after cessation of remifentanil. Therefore remifentanil should be used with caution in aortic stenosis.

1. Introduction

Remifentanil is a congener of fentanyl family of narcotics which is separable from others for the ester structure. Complications of this drug are like those of other opioids and include bradycardia, itching, nausea, vomiting, and muscular rigidity [1]. Aortic stenosis is the most common valvular disorder of heart which is seen in cardiac rheumatic disease and old ages and is divided to slight, moderate, and severe types based on valvular diameter and transvalvular pressure gradient. Anesthesia in these patients could be accompanied by decreased cardiac output, and cardiopulmonary resuscitation is hardly done at this situation.

In this study, a serious complication of remifentanil was considered during management of anesthesia in a patient with severe aortic stenosis.

2. Case Description

The patient was an 84-year-old man, weighting 72 kg, who was hospitalized for open prostate surgery. In records, the patient was only complaining from exertional dyspnea, had no obvious cardiopulmonary problems, and did not mention using any specific drugs. In the conducted examination,

pulmonary auscultation had no problems. Examination of abdomen and organs was normal, and only IV/VI systolic murmur and a thrill were heard in the aortic area. In order to evaluate the patient before the operation, blood tests, electrocardiogram, and echocardiogram were requested. The only positive point in the lab tests was prothrombin time (PT) = 15.6 sec. In the electrocardiogram (ECG), heart rate was 65 beats per minute, and the rhythm was regular; however, left axis deviation and left ventricle hypertrophy were observed. In echo, ejection fraction was 57%, severe hypertrophy of left ventricle, calcified and narrow aortic valve were reported; also, 52 mm Hg was reported for transvalvular aortic gradient; but, no functional and wall motion disorder was seen for left ventricle.

Vital signs of the patient before the induction were blood pressure of 150/90 mm Hg and heart rate of 60 beats per minute. For anesthetic induction with caution and low dose, 100 μg of fentanyl, 4 mg of pancuronium, and 80 mg of propofol were used. After tracheal intubation, in order to maintain anesthesia, a combination of propofol and remifentanil (200 mg + 500 μg) along with 50% oxygen and N_2O was used. The rate of infusion was 0.2 μg/kg/min for remifentanil. After induction and beginning the infusion of remifentanil and propofol, the patient suffered from decreased heart rate

(35–40 beats per minute) and decreased blood pressure (80/50 mm Hg); after a few moments, he experienced Mobitz II atrioventricular block (Figure 1). To increase heart rate and sinus control, first, 0.5 mg atropine and then 10 mg ephedrine were injected; however, atrioventricular block was not modified (heart rate of about 40 beats per minute) despite increased blood pressure to 110/75 mm Hg. Then, infusion of remifentanil was stopped and propofol with rate of 50 μg/kg/min was used alone. After about 2-3 min, atrioventricular block and bradyarrhythmia were overcome (Figure 2), and the patient's blood pressure was raised to 130/90 mm Hg. The patient had no hemodynamic problem during the operation, and recovery and was completely under control. He had a little restlessness during the recovery and improved after some minutes. Then, he was transferred to the ward in total awareness with blood pressure of 130/80 and heart rate of 62 beats per minute.

3. Discussion

Remifentanil is a narcotic from the fentanyl's family, which has a rapid primary effect and has a short half life (about 3 min) even after long-term usage; therefore, it is a good choice in total intravenous anesthesia (TIVA) and pain relief in ICU [2]. Due to hemodynamic stability, remifentanil is used in many cardiac diseases such as eisenmenger [3], coarctation of aorta [4], and severe aortic stenosis [5, 6], cardiomyopathies [7]. In the elderly, the pharmacokinetic and pharmacodynamic of remifentanil differ, and there is increased sensitivity of brain to remifentanil. Also, potency of the drug is twice, and it is required to decrease primary dosage of the drug. Central distribution volume and also clearance decrease, and the amount of infusion should be decreased to 1/3 [8, 9]. However, in some cases, this drug could decrease cardiovascular function, and the patient may suffer from bradycardia and hypotension. Sometimes, severe variations are observed in heart rate which has been reported as a result of predominance of parasympathetic over sympathetic tone and is seen in the patients with junctional rhythms and even temporary sinusoidal arrest, which rapidly improves by injection of anticholinergic drug (atropine) [10, 11]. In Fattorini et al.'s study, as a consequence of stimulating sinus node with increased heart rate to less than 140 beats per minute, Wenckebach atrioventricular block was observed in 7 out of 40 patients, which indicated specific increase in refractory period of the atrioventricular node [10].

Aortic stenosis is one of the most common valvular disorders among the elderly. This disorder occurs in children as a result of bicuspid valve and rheumatic diseases, and, in the elderly, it happens mostly because of degenerative disorders, calcification, and fibrous aortic valve. Aortic stenosis is divided to three: slight, moderate, and severe grades according to the difference in transvalvular gradient (left ventricle and aorta). In the severe and fatal type, gradient difference is more than 50 mm Hg and diameter of aortic valve is less than 0.7 cm^2 in this case [6].

In patients with severe aortic stenosis, performing anesthesia has many risks, and, even performing CPR and using defibrillator have a low degree of success. In these patients,

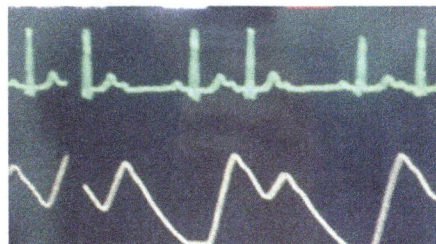

FIGURE 1: After remifentanil infusion.

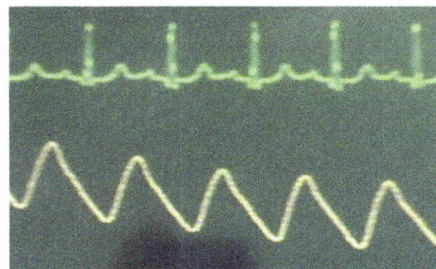

FIGURE 2: After remifentanil cessation.

due to hypertrophy of left ventricle, the amount of intravascular liquid should be maintained at a desirable and upper normal level; therefore, sometimes, central venous pressure and pulmonary artery pressure are monitored. Increased heart rate could cause ischemia of heart muscle as a result of the decrease in the circulation of coronary blood along with increase in oxygen demand; also, bradycardia causes decrease in cardiac output. Systemic vascular resistance should be also maintained at normal level in order to maintain cardiac output. Increased resistance with increased gradient prevents aortic flow, and decreased resistance of vessels also causes decreased peripheral perfusion and ischemia problems. Decreased blood pressure should be immediately modified by alpha agonists like phenylephrine and metaraminol. Atrial contraction in normal people includes 15–20% of cardiac output; but, in people with severe aortic stenosis, about 40% of cardiac output is caused by atrial contraction, and any nonsinusoidal rhythm decreases cardiac output.

In the surgeries on patients with severe aortic stenosis, regional anesthesia [12] and also general anesthesia could be used; but, regional anesthesia causes sympathectomy and can decrease peripheral vascular resistance. Moreover, bradycardia which follows anesthesia can decrease cardiac output. Thus, in this patient who had 52 mm Hg differences in gradient pressure, general anesthesia was performed. For hemodynamic stability, an opioid base using infusion of remifentanil was used. Since opioids are not adequately anesthetic by themselves, low dosage of propofol was used for induction, and also remifentanil was applied for infusion. In order to prevent decreased heart rate, pancuronium was used. In this patient, severe decrease of heart rate was accompanied by Mobitz cardiac block type II, and this variation in heart rate and rhythm caused hemodynamic disorder which did not respond to injection of atropine and ephedrine; only stopping remifentanil caused improvement.

There have been a limited number of reports on creation of complete heart block following concurrent consumption of propofol, remifentanil, vecuronium, and sevoflurane [13, 14], but, no case of Mobitz cardiac block type II has been observed. Also, in most of the studies, using anticholinergic before remifentanil or after the rhythm disorder improves or prevents that signs; however, in this patient, using atropine and also indirect sympathomimetic compound of ephedrine did not solve the rhythm disorder. In the study by Mizuno et al. on a 17-year-old patient, an intermittent bundle branch block followed by bradycardia was reported in the consumption of sevoflurane and remifentanil, which responded to atropine [15]. In Nishio et al.'s study, a 66-year-old patient with sick sinus syndrome, propofol was used along with sevoflurane and remifentanil, which did not intensify the disorder in the patient [16]. In Fujii et al.'s investigation (2011), effect of remifentanil on sinus node and atrial conduction was studied among 60 children, in both of them conduction pathway was inhibited, and no disorder was observed in atrioventricular conduction [17], but, in this paper, the patient suffered from atrioventricular conduction disorder and Mobitz type II block followed by bradycardia.

4. Final Conclusion

In patients with severe aortic stenosis, remifentanil can be used for hemodynamic stabilization, but, remifentanil along with propofol could cause conduction disorder and conduction block and should be used with caution in aortic stenosis. In this patient, dysrhythmia and atrioventricular block did not respond to atropine and ephedrine treatment, and only remifentanil cessation solved the problem.

Authors' Contribution

M. T. Gilani contributed to paper preparation and approved the final paper. M. T. Gilani attests to the integrity of the original data and the analysis reported in this paper.

References

[1] T. D. Egan, "The clinical pharmacology of remifentanil: a brief review," *Journal of Anesthesia*, vol. 12, no. 4, pp. 195–204, 1998.

[2] C. L. Westmoreland, J. F. Hoke, P. S. Sebel, C. C. Hug Jr., and K. T. Muir, "Pharmacokinetics of remifentanil (GI87084B) and its major metabolite (GI90291) in patients undergoing elective inpatient surgery," *Anesthesiology*, vol. 79, no. 5, pp. 893–903, 1993.

[3] A. Duman, G. Sarkilar, M. Dayioglu, M. Özden, and N. Görmüs, "Use of remifentanil in a patient with eisenmenger syndrome requiring urgent cesarean section," *Middle East Journal of Anesthesiology*, vol. 20, no. 4, pp. 577–580, 2010.

[4] R. Sinha and R. Garg, "Anesthetic management for laparoscopy surgery in a patient with residual coarctation of aorta and mild aortic stenosis," *Journal of Anaesthesiology, Clinical Pharmacology*, vol. 27, no. 3, pp. 412–413, 2011.

[5] T. T. Lao, M. Sermer, L. MaGee, D. Farine, and J. M. Colman, "Congenital aortic stenosis and pregnancy—a reappraisal," *American Journal of Obstetrics and Gynecology*, vol. 169, no. 3, pp. 540–545, 1993.

[6] A. M. Ioscovich, E. Goldszmidt, A. V. Fadeev, S. Grisaru-Granovsky, and S. H. Halpern, "Peripartum anesthetic management of patients with aortic valve stenosis: a retrospective study and literature review," *International Journal of Obstetric Anesthesia*, vol. 18, no. 4, pp. 379–386, 2009.

[7] C. F. Minto, T. W. Schnider, and S. L. Shafer, "Pharmacokinetics and pharmacodynamics of remifentanil II. Model application," *Anesthesiology*, vol. 86, no. 1, pp. 24–33, 1997.

[8] C. F. Minto, T. W. Schnider, T. D. Egan et al., "Influence of age and gender on the pharmacokinetics and pharmacodynamics of remifentanil I. Model development," *Anesthesiology*, vol. 86, no. 1, pp. 10–23, 1997.

[9] C. P. McCarroll, L. D. Paxton, P. Elliott, and D. B. Wilson, "Use of remifentanil in a patient with peripartum cardiomyopathy requiring Caesarean section," *British Journal of Anaesthesia*, vol. 86, no. 1, pp. 135–138, 2001.

[10] F. Fattorini, R. Romano, A. Ciccaglioni et al., "Effects of remifentanil on human heart electrical system: a transesophageal pacing electrophysiological study," *Minerva Anestesiologica*, vol. 69, no. 9, pp. 673–679, 2003.

[11] K. Maruyama, Y. Nishikawa, H. Nakagawa, J. Ariyama, A. Kitamura, and M. Hayashida, "Can intravenous atropine prevent bradycardia and hypotension during induction of total intravenous anesthesia with propofol and remifentanil," *Journal of Anesthesia*, vol. 24, no. 2, pp. 293–296, 2010.

[12] J. C. Hemming and S. T. Thomas, "Management of patients with valvular heart disease," in *International Pracice of Anesthesia*, C. Prys-Roberts and B. R. Thmas Brown, Eds., pp. 3–6, Butterworth Heinemann, Oxford, UK, 1996.

[13] K. Tanaka, Y. Adachi, S. Suzuki, K. Nishiwaki, and N. Matsuda, "ECG changes after the induction of general anesthesia with remifentanil: a report of three cases," *Masui*, vol. 61, no. 10, pp. 1128–1132, 2012.

[14] E. Hamaguchi, H. Kawano, S. Kawahito, H. Kitahata, and S. Oshita, "Torsade de pointes associated with severe bradycardia after induction of general anesthesia," *Masui*, vol. 60, no. 9, pp. 1097–1100, 2011.

[15] J. Mizuno, S. Kato, K. Ino, T. Yoshimura, S. Yunokawa, and S. Morita, "Intermittent bradycardia-dependent bundle branch block during sevoflurane and remifentanil anesthesia," *Masui*, vol. 58, no. 8, pp. 976–979, 2009.

[16] Y. Nishio, K. Hara, G. Obara, and T. Sata, "General anesthesia with remifentanil for a patient having sinoatrial block and constrictive pulmonary disorder," *Masui*, vol. 57, no. 8, pp. 1002–1004, 2008.

[17] K. Fujii, H. Iranami, Y. Nakamura, and Y. Hatano, "High-dose remifentanil suppresses sinoatrial conduction and sinus node automaticity in pediatric patients under propofol-based anesthesia," *Anesthesia and Analgesia*, vol. 112, no. 5, pp. 1169–1173, 2011.

39

Epidural Anesthesia Complicated by Subdural Hygromas and a Subdural Hematoma

Christine Vien,[1] Paul Marovic,[2] and Brendan Ingram[1]

[1]*Monash Health, 246 Clayton Road, Clayton, Melbourne, VIC 3168, Australia*
[2]*Alfred Health, 55 Commercial Road, Melbourne, VIC 3004, Australia*

Correspondence should be addressed to Christine Vien; ckt.vien@gmail.com

Academic Editor: Ehab Farag

Inadvertent dural puncture during epidural anesthesia leads to intracranial hypotension, which if left unnoticed can cause life-threatening subdural hematomas or cerebellar tonsillar herniation. The highly variable presentation of intracranial hypotension hinders timely diagnosis and treatment. We present the case of a young laboring adult female, who developed subdural hygromas and a subdural hematoma following unintentional dural puncture during initiation of epidural anesthesia.

1. Introduction

Inadvertent dural puncture during epidural anaesthesia leads to intracranial hypotension, which if left unnoticed can cause life-threatening complications such as subdural hematomas and cerebellar tonsillar herniation [1, 2]. The highly variable presentation of intracranial hypotension hinders timely diagnosis and treatment.

2. Case Presentation

A twenty-seven-year-old otherwise healthy nulliparous patient requested epidural anesthesia for pain relief during spontaneous labor.

Following informed consent and using an aseptic technique, an 18 g Tuohy needle was inserted into the L3-4 epidural space, guided by a loss of resistance to normal saline. Unfortunately, the thecal sac was breached and the needle was immediately withdrawn. A second attempt, through the L2-L3 interspinous space, resulted in the successful placement of an epidural catheter and this was confirmed with a test dose of 10 mL of 0.2% ropivacaine. Further analgesia was provided via patient controlled epidural analgesia (PCEA) using 5 mL of 0.125% bupivacaine with a lockout of 15 minutes, as per the institution's protocol. There was no evidence of a high block. Six hours after the initiation of epidural analgesia, the patient required instrumental delivery with Kielland's rotational forceps.

The patient developed a mild, intermittent, nonpostural headache on day one following delivery but was able to continue caring for her newborn child. Her neurological examination and vital signs were normal. The symptoms were not indicative of a Postdural Puncture Headache (PDPH) and she was treated with intravenous hydration and oral analgesia.

On day two, the patient's headache became persistent and postural, and she developed nausea and vomiting. This was attributed to PDPH and she was informed of the potential treatments including autologous blood patching. She declined the blood patch and wished to continue with conservative management of paracetamol, ibuprofen, metoclopramide, and ondansetron with reasonable control. On day three, the Medical Emergency Team urgently attended the patient's bedside due to the onset of bradycardia (heart rate of forty beats per minute) in the setting of severe headache and vomiting. The patient was promptly investigated with Computed Tomography (CT).

Brain CT demonstrated bilateral cerebral convexity subdural hygromas and a small right frontal subdural hematoma (Figure 1), while a head CT venogram was unremarkable. The patient also underwent a brain MRI, which demonstrated

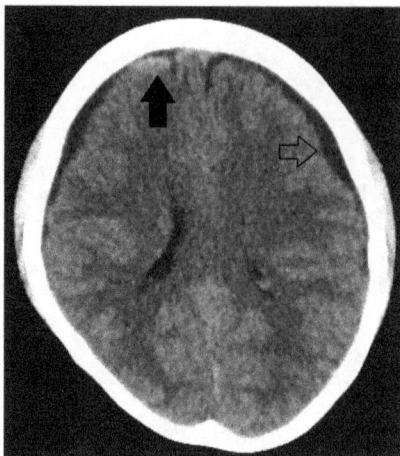

FIGURE 1: Nonintravenous contrast enhanced brain CT demonstrates bilateral CSF-density subdural hygromas (left subdural hygroma labelled with an open arrow) and a hyperdense acute right frontal subdural hematoma (solid arrow).

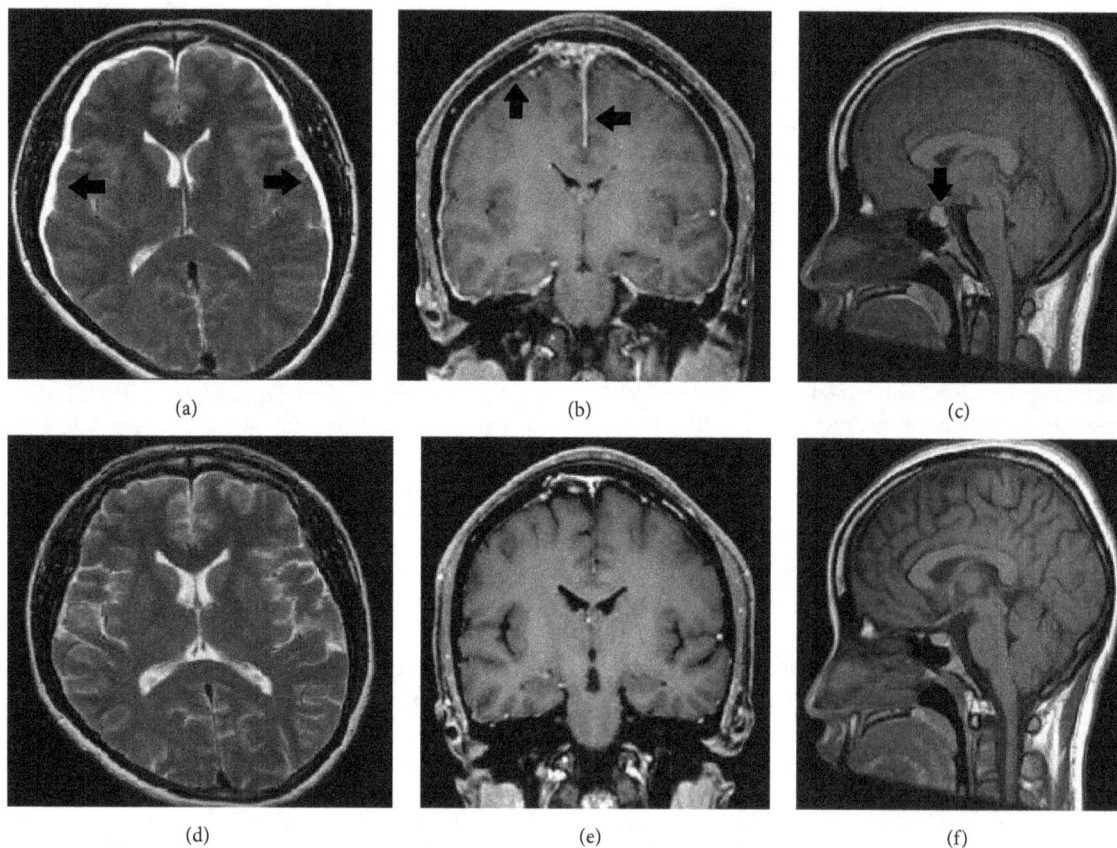

(a)

(b)

(c)

(d)

(e)

(f)

FIGURE 2: (a) Axial T2 weighted sequence demonstrates bilateral CSF-intensity subdural hygromas (arrows). (b) Coronal T1 weighted gadolinium enhanced sequence demonstrates pachymeningeal thickening and enhancement (arrows). (c) Sagittal T1 weighted sequence demonstrates pituitary gland enlargement. (d)–(f) Posttreatment MRI examination demonstrates complete radiological resolution.

further classical signs of intracranial hypotension, namely, slit-like lateral ventricles, an enlarged pituitary gland, and aseptic pachymeningitis (Figure 2) [3].

On day four, an epidural blood patch was performed without complication using 25 mL of autologous blood, resulting in rapid relief of the patient's headache.

A follow-up brain MRI was performed one month later, which demonstrated complete resolution of the subdural hygromas (Figure 2). The patient was symptom-free.

3. Discussion

Postpartum headache is extremely common, reportedly occurring in up to 80% of patients [4]. The commonest causes are tension headache and migraine, which in combination are twenty times more common than PDPH, let alone the rarer complications of subdural hygromas and hematomas [5].

Subdural hygromas are composed of xanthochromic fluid and result from intracranial hypotension [6]. The prevailing theory is that cerebrospinal fluid (CSF) leaks into the epidural space via the dural defect leading to compensatory vasodilatation of the pachymeningeal blood vessels (Monro-Kellie doctrine), which subsequently become leaky [3, 7–10]. Some investigators have proposed that arachnoid granulation rupture may be a contributing factor [10]. Subdural hygromas occur in 10–69% of patients with intracranial hypotension and can occur as early as five hours or as late as five months after dural puncture [11–14].

If a dural tear is left untreated, continued spinal CSF leakage can lead to caudal sagging of the intracranial contents (occurring after $\geq$250 mL of CSF is lost) [15]. Traction-related tearing of subdural veins is the likely mechanism by which hygromas are complicated by hematomas, which may be unilateral or bilateral [14]. The risk of subdural hygroma and hematoma formation increases proportionally with the degree of intracranial hypotension and the number of dural punctures, as well as with coexistent cerebral atrophy, cerebral aneurysm, vascular malformation, pregnancy, dehydration, and use of anticoagulants.

The true incidence of subdural hematoma following dural puncture remains elusive as most patients are managed without imaging investigation. Studies have reported that, of the patients who develop subdural hygromas, 47% go on to develop subdural hematomas [16–18].

The cardinal feature of intracranial hypotension is an orthostatic headache, which is of variable quality, typically most severe within the first twenty-four hours and usually resolving within ten days [19, 20]. Altered conscious state, meningism, nausea, vomiting, dizziness, cranial nerve palsies, visual disturbance, photophobia, and rarely seizures have also been described [21]. Bradycardia has also been described and is thought to occur due to rostral migration of the brain with subsequent compression of the hypothalamus. Mass effect on the hypothalamus can cause alterations in autonomic outflow [22, 23].

If the headache persists, loses its postural nature, returns following initial resolution, or is associated with haemodynamic changes, neuroradiological investigation is advocated to assess sequelae of intracranial hypotension as a delay in diagnosis can be catastrophic [14]. Studies have demonstrated that dural puncture complicated by subdural hematoma carries a mortality rate of a value between 17 and 29% [14, 24].

Subdural fluid collections (hematomas or hygromas) can be managed safely with conservative methods, such as bed rest, hydration, and caffeine. If the patient is still symptomatic despite these measures, an epidural blood patch (EBP) should be performed [17]. Craniotomy or burr hole evacuation is rarely required even if the subdural fluid collection is large and exerts significant mass effect; however they may take up to three months to resolve [13, 25].

Anaesthetists need to be cognisant of the possibility of subdural hematomas in the setting of PDPH, especially in parturients experiencing persistent headache with neurological or haemodynamic disturbance. Early radiological investigation is encouraged, as a delay in diagnosis can be fatal.

Competing Interests

The authors declare no competing interests.

References

[1] A. Francia, P. Parisi, A. M. Vitale, and V. Esposito, "Life-threatening intracranial hypotension after diagnosti lumbar puncture," *Neurological Sciences*, vol. 22, no. 5, pp. 385–389, 2001.

[2] I. K. Hart, I. Bone, and D. M. Hadley, "Development of neurological problems after lumbar puncture," *British Medical Journal (Clinical Research Edition)*, vol. 296, no. 6614, pp. 51–52, 1988.

[3] S. C. Pannullo, J. B. Reich, G. Krol, M. D. F. Deck, and J. B. Posner, "MRI changes in intracranial hypotension," *Neurology*, vol. 43, no. 5, pp. 919–926, 1993.

[4] L. Scharff, D. A. Marcus, and D. C. Turk, "Headache during pregnancy and in the postpartum: a prospective study," *Headache*, vol. 37, no. 4, pp. 203–210, 1997.

[5] E. Goldszmidt, R. Kern, A. Chaput, and A. Macarthur, "The incidence and etiology of postpartum headaches: a prospective cohort study," *Canadian Journal of Anesthesia*, vol. 52, no. 9, pp. 971–977, 2005.

[6] K. S. Lee, W. K. Bae, Y. T. Park, and I. G. Yun, "The pathogenesis and fate of traumatic subdural hygroma," *British Journal of Neurosurgery*, vol. 8, no. 5, pp. 551–558, 1994.

[7] R. Bakshi, L. L. Mechtler, S. Kamran et al., "MRI findings in lumbar puncture headache syndrome: abnormal dural-meningeal and dural venous sinus enhancement," *Clinical Imaging*, vol. 23, no. 2, pp. 73–76, 1999.

[8] R. E. Gordon, F. G. Moser, B. D. Pressman, and W. Young, "Resolution of pachymeningeal enhancement following dural puncture and blood patch," *Neuroradiology*, vol. 37, no. 7, pp. 557–558, 1995.

[9] A. Sabharwal and G. M. Stocks, "Postpartum headache: diagnosis and management," *Continuing Education in Anaesthesia, Critical Care and Pain*, vol. 11, no. 5, pp. 181–185, 2011.

[10] S. Miyazaki, H. Fukushima, K. Kamata, and S. Ishii, "Chronic subdural hematoma after lumbar-subarachnoid analgesia for a cesarean section," *Surgical Neurology*, vol. 19, no. 5, pp. 459–460, 1983.

[11] R. J. de Noronha, B. Sharrack, M. Hadjivassiliou, and C. A. J. Romanowski, "Subdural haematoma: a potentially serious consequence of spontaneous intracranial hypotension," *Journal of Neurology Neurosurgery and Psychiatry*, vol. 74, no. 6, pp. 752–755, 2003.

[12] T.-H. Lai, J.-L. Fuh, J.-F. Lirng, P.-H. Tsai, and S.-J. Wang, "Subdural haematoma in patients with spontaneous intracranial hypotension," *Cephalalgia*, vol. 27, no. 2, pp. 133–138, 2007.

[13] W. I. Schievink, M. M. Maya, F. G. Moser, and J. Tourje, "Spectrum of subdural fluid collections in spontaneous intracranial hypotension," *Journal of Neurosurgery*, vol. 103, no. 4, pp. 608–613, 2005.

[14] P. E. Vos, W. A. de Boer, J. A. L. Wurzer, and J. van Gijn, "Subdural hematoma after lumbar puncture: two case reports and review of the literature," *Clinical Neurology and Neurosurgery*, vol. 93, no. 2, pp. 127–132, 1991.

[15] G. B. Yildirim, S. Colakoglu, T. Y. Atakan, and H. Büyükkirli, "Intracranial subdural hematoma after spinal anesthesia," *International Journal of Obstetric Anesthesia*, vol. 14, no. 2, pp. 159–162, 2005.

[16] I. Aysel, N. Sertoz, and M. Uyar, "A case report of a cranial subdural hematoma due to a rare complication of spinal anesthesia," *The Internet Journal of Anesthesiology*, vol. 29, no. 1, 2010.

[17] H. K. Wang, P. Liliang, C. Liang, K. Lu, K. Hung, and H. Chen, "Delayed subdural hematoma after epidural blood patching in a patient with spontaneous intracranial hypotension—case report," *Neurologia Medico-Chirurgica*, vol. 50, no. 6, pp. 479–481, 2010.

[18] D. B. Scott and B. M. Hibbard, "Serious non-fatal complications associated with extradural block in obstetric practice," *British Journal of Anaesthesia*, vol. 64, no. 5, pp. 537–541, 1990.

[19] C. L. Stella, C. D. Jodicke, H. Y. How, U. F. Harkness, and B. M. Sibai, "Postpartum headache: is your work-up complete?" *American Journal of Obstetrics and Gynecology*, vol. 196, no. 4, pp. 318.e1–318.e7, 2007.

[20] D. Bezov, R. B. Lipton, and S. Ashina, "Post-dural puncture headache: part I diagnosis, epidemiology, etiology, and pathophysiology," *Headache*, vol. 50, no. 7, pp. 1144–1152, 2010.

[21] C. E. Beck, N. W. Rizk, L. T. Kiger, D. Spencer, L. Hill, and J. R. Adler, "Intracranial hypotension presenting with severe encephalopathy," *Journal of Neurosurgery*, vol. 89, no. 3, pp. 470–473, 1998.

[22] J. D. Wasnick, C. A. Lien, L. A. Rubin, and R. A. R. Fraser, "Unexplained bradycardia during craniotomy closure: the role of intracranial hypotension," *Anesthesia & Analgesia*, vol. 76, no. 2, pp. 432–433, 1993.

[23] M. C. Rogers, J. A. Abildskov, and J. B. Preston, "Neurogenic ECG changes in critically ill patients: an experimental model," *Critical Care Medicine*, vol. 1, no. 4, pp. 192–196, 1973.

[24] P. Newrick and D. Read, "Subdural haematoma as a complication of spinal anaesthetic," *British Medical Journal*, vol. 285, no. 6338, pp. 341–342, 1982.

[25] W. I. Schievink, M. M. Maya, B. K. Pikul, and C. Louy, "Spontaneous spinal cerebrospinal fluid leaks as the cause of subdural hematomas in elderly patients on anticoagulation: report of 3 cases," *Journal of Neurosurgery*, vol. 112, no. 2, pp. 295–299, 2010.

40

Unintended Avulsion of Hypertrophic Adenoids in Posterior Nasopharynx: A Case Report of a Rare Complication Caused by Nasotracheal Intubation

Hao-Hu Chen,[1] Li-Chuan Chen,[1] Yu-Hui Hsieh,[1] Mao-Kai Chen,[1] Chung-Ho Chen,[2] and Kuang-I Cheng[1,3]

[1] Department of Anesthesiology, Kaohsiung Medical University Hospital, Kaohsiung 807, Taiwan
[2] Department of Oral and Maxillofacial Surgery, College of Dental Medicine, Kaohsiung Medical University, Kaohsiung 807, Taiwan
[3] Faculty of Medicine, Department of Anesthesiology, College of Medicine, Kaohsiung Medical University, Kaohsiung 807, Taiwan

Correspondence should be addressed to Kuang-I Cheng; kuaich@gmail.com

Academic Editor: Pavel Michalek

The enlarged adenoid serves as a mechanical obstacle on the nasopharynx to intricate nasotracheal intubation. No matter what video or direct laryngoscopic techniques are applied, nasotracheal tube navigation from the nasal valve area through the nasal cavity to the nasopharynx is always blind; trauma is not uncommon. Here we report a case of unintended avulsed adenoids that plugged the tube tip while the nasotracheal tube blindly navigated through the nasopharyngeal space. After failing to insert a bent tip of gum elastic bougie passing through the nasopharynx, an alternative method of NTI was performed by mounting the nasotracheal tube on a fiberoptic bronchoscope. The nasotracheal tube was successfully railroaded along the insertion tube of the fiberscope to the trachea.

1. Introduction

The adenoids (pharyngeal tonsils) are lymphoid tissue in the upper posterior aspect of the nasopharynx, designed to process infections in the nose and throat. Though the cause of adenoid hyperplasia is not really understood, many facts such as repeated infections [1], chronic inflammation [2], allergic rhinitis [2, 3], and heavy cigarette smoking [4] all trigger its hypertrophy. The enlarged adenoid serves as a mechanical obstacle on the nasopharynx to intricate nasotracheal intubation. Nasotracheal intubation (NTI) is needed for elective oromaxillofacial surgery. No matter what video or direct laryngoscopic techniques for NTI are used, nasotracheal tube insertion from the nasal valve through the nasal cavity to the nasopharynx is always blind; trauma is not uncommon. Herein, we report a case of unintended avulsed adenoids that plugged the tube tip while the nasotracheal tube was blindly navigated through the nasopharyngeal space. After failure to insert a bent tip of gum elastic bougie passing through the nasopharynx, an alternative method of NTI was performed by mounting the nasotracheal tube on a fiberoptic bronchoscope. The nasotracheal tube was successfully railroaded along the insertion tube of the fiberscope to the trachea.

2. Case Report

A 40-year-old man, with American Society of Anesthesiologists physical status II, height 167 cm, weight 63.5 kg, was scheduled for wide excision of oral tissue leukoplakia on the right buccal mucosa and tongue. He had a white patch over the right buccal area for 3 years and his right tongue ulcer had appeared for one year. His history included hypertension and diabetes mellitus with regular treatment, allergic rhinitis, and a heavy cigarette smoker (2 packs per day). His radiologic and laboratory test findings were not abnormal except for slightly elevated C-reaction protein.

(a)

(b)

(c)

(d)

(e)

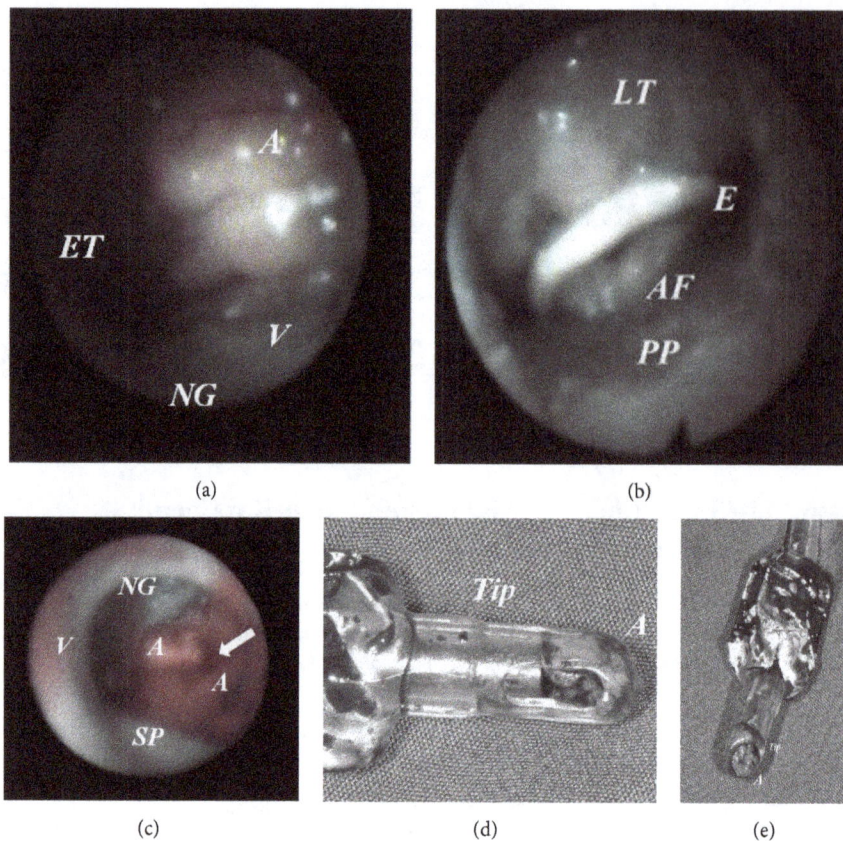

FIGURE 1: Hypertrophic adenoid avulsed by a nasotracheal tube. Hypertrophic adenoid viewing by a fiberscope (a). Hypertrophic lingual tonsil (b). Avulsed hypertrophic adenoid; a groove appear on the adenoid (c). Tip of the nasotracheal tube was filled with adenoid tissue but side hole was not occluded (d and e). A: adenoid hypertrophy; AF: arytenoid folds; E: epiglottis; ET: eustachian tube; LT: lingual tonsil; NG: nasogastric tube; PP: posterior pharyngeal wall; SP: soft palate; V: vomer.

An otolaryngologist examined his nasal cavities and selected his left nostril for nasotracheal intubation before he was taken to the operating room (OR). In OR, fentanyl (1 μg/kg) and midazolam (0.03 mg/kg) were administered intravenously for sedation. An anesthesiologist examined his left nasal airway patency with a fiberscope. Turbinates were swollen, narrowing the nasal pathway, and nasopharynx with grade II adenoid hypertrophy [5] and oropharynx with lingual hyperplasia were found (Figures 1(a) and 1(b)). Four cotton-tipped applicators dipped with 6% cocaine were properly placed for at least five minutes for vasoconstriction and to blunt the branches of the trigeminal nerve under standard monitoring, including electrocardiogram, pulse oximetry, and noninvasive blood pressure measurement.

After that, intravenous induction agents including fentanyl 2 μg/kg, thiopental 5 mg/kg, and propofol 1 mg/kg were intravenously administered. Mask ventilation was easily performed uneventfully. Nasotracheal intubation was facilitated with 0.6 mg/kg of rocuronium; the nasotracheal tube (RAE Nasal, Mallinckrodt Medical Athlone, Ireland of 7.0 inner diameter) was thermosoftened and lubricated with 2% lidocaine gel coating its tip and cuff.

The nasotracheal tube was inserted with bevel of the tube facing medially, and the tube passed through the nasal pathway along the space between the inferior turbinate and the floor of the nose. Mild resistance was encountered during tube insertion through the nasal pathway and on the nasopharyngeal space. However, a mass was filled with inlet of the tube as the tip of the nasotracheal tube was on the oropharynx, (Figure 1(d)). The plugged tube was withdrawn. Then, viewing from a fiberscope, a groove appeared on the hypertrophic adenoid (Figure 1(c)) and a bleeding point on the lower margin of the adenoid but not on the middle or inferior turbinate was found. After failure to insert a bent tip of gum elastic bougie passing through the nasopharynx from the selected nostril, we chose an alternative method of NTI by mounting the nasotracheal tube on a fiberoptic bronchoscope (outer diameter: 4 mm, working length: 600 mm, Olympus LF-2, Tokyo, Japan). The tip of the fiberscope was carefully passed through the nasal cavity and nasopharynx to the trachea. The nasotracheal tube was railroaded along the shaft of the fiberscope to the trachea. Surgical procedures were uneventful. The damaged retropharyngeal tissues did not bleed actively after operation as viewed by a fiberscope. Pathology of the specimen submitted tissue fragment of

0.5 × 0.2 × 0.1 showed eroded respiratory mucosa with exuberant lymphoid stroma. The patient recovered smoothly without obvious nasal pain, sore throat, or hoarseness.

3. Discussion

Nasal damage following NTI most frequently involves mucosa overlying the inferior turbinate and adjacent septum [6]. The most significant site of nasal obstruction is also at the nasal valve area or the anterior part of the inferior turbinate in the case of turbinate hypertrophy [7]. However, hypertrophic adenoid injuries during insertion of the nasotracheal tube through the nasopharyngeal space are an important but often neglected issue during conventional NTI. The hypertrophic adenoid is mainly composed of lymphoid tissues with a mound of cobblestone features. While the nasotracheal tube is blindly passing through the nasopharynx in a sharp curve, the posterior nasopharyngeal wall may impact its advancement. Hypertrophic adenoids are fragile and easily bleed during NTI.

In a case presentation, the unusual complication of avulsed adenoid might occur. The possible nasopharyngeal tissue damage during NTI includes retropharyngeal dissection [8], laceration [9], bleeding [8, 9], and tissues avulsion [10]. The nasotracheal tube advancing under a forward force avulsed hypertrophy adenoid not only induced tissue bleeding but also occluded the tube. Ng and Yew [10] reported that the avulsed adenoid that occluded the tube was not found till the critical point of nasotracheal tube into trachea, but ventilation could not occur. For early detection of hypertrophic adenoid not merely via fiberoptic bronchoscope or flexible nasopharyngoscopy, a noninvasive method with a lateral X-ray of the neck remains a reliable and valid diagnostic test [11].

Although avulsion of hypertrophic adenoid is an unusual complication, a routine assessment for patients with high risk is needed. In normal subjects without nasal obstruction, the prevalence incidence of hypertrophic adenoid is 55.1% and with nasal obstruction is 63.6% [12]. A history of allergic rhinitis [2] or being a heavy cigarette smoker [4] should alert the anesthetist to encounter potentially enlarged adenoids. Hypertrophic adenoids are often underestimated and ignored for those patients undergoing NTI. However, avulsion of hypertrophic adenoid is usually based on using improper pressure or forced advancement of the nasotracheal tube against opposing resistance on the nasopharynx. A groove on the hypertrophic adenoid, a bleeding point beneath it, and a lymphoid tissue filled with the tube tip can readily demonstrate the injured adenoid being cut by the nasotracheal tube.

In this case, after hypertrophic adenoid was avulsed, a blindly inserted gum elastic bougie failed because we were not able to navigate the soft bend with a fixed angle tip without resistance through the nasopharynx. The main reason is that the fixed tip of bougie did not match the curvature of the nasopharynx. Ng and Yew [10] also met the situation of adenoid occlusion from the nasotracheal tube, and orotracheal intubation was determined finally. However,

a flexible fiberscope assisted by bleeding suction successfully went through the nasopharyngeal space in our case.

4. Conclusion

High-risk patients with allergic rhinitis and heavy smoking history should be assessed for abnormally enlarged lymphoid tissues to prevent unintentional avulsion hypertrophic adenoid during NTI. Hypertrophic adenoid injury should not be overlooked during NTI. However, under injured hypertrophic adenoid with bleeding, a flexible fiberoptic bronchoscope combined with a catheter bleeding suction is recommended for NTI.

Acknowledgment

This case report and accompanying images are published with the written informed consent of the patient.

References

[1] J. M. Bernstein, E. Hasse, F. Scannapieco et al., "Bacterial interference of penicillin-sensitive and -resistant Streptococcus pneumoniae by Streptococcus oralis in an adenoid organ culture: implications for the treatment of recurrent upper respiratory tract infections in children and adults," *Annals of Otology, Rhinology and Laryngology*, vol. 115, no. 5, pp. 350–356, 2006.

[2] N. Yildirim, M. Şahan, and Y. Karslioğlu, "Adenoid hypertrophy in adults: clinical and morphological characteristics," *Journal of International Medical Research*, vol. 36, no. 1, pp. 157–162, 2008.

[3] S.-W. Huang and C. Giannoni, "The risk of adenoid hypertrophy in children with allergic rhinitis," *Annals of Allergy, Asthma and Immunology*, vol. 87, no. 4, pp. 350–355, 2001.

[4] Y. Finkelstein, Z. Malik, J. Kopolovic, J. Bernheim, M. Djaldetti, and D. Ophir, "Characterization of smoking-induced nasopharyngeal lymphoid hyperplasia," *Laryngoscope*, vol. 107, no. 12, pp. 1635–1642, 1997.

[5] S. R. Parikh, M. Coronel, J. J. Lee, and S. M. Brown, "Validation of a new grading system for endoscopic examination of adenoid hypertrophy," *Otolaryngology—Head and Neck Surgery*, vol. 135, no. 5, pp. 684–687, 2006.

[6] J. E. O'Connell, D. S. Stevenson, and M. A. Stokes, "Pathological changes associated with short-term nasal intubation," *Anaesthesia*, vol. 51, no. 4, pp. 347–350, 1996.

[7] O. Hilberg, "Objective measurement of nasal airway dimensions using acoustic rhinometry: methodological and clinical aspects," *Allergy*, vol. 57, no. 70, pp. 5–39, 2002.

[8] M. J. Krebs and T. Sakai, "Retropharyngeal dissection during nasotracheal intubation: a rare complication and its management," *Journal of Clinical Anesthesia*, vol. 20, no. 3, pp. 218–221, 2008.

[9] J. E. Tintinalli and J. Claffey, "Complications of nasotracheal intubation," *Annals of Emergency Medicine*, vol. 10, no. 3, pp. 142–144, 1981.

[10] S. Y. Ng and W. S. Yew, "Nasotracheal tube occlusion from adenoid trauma," *Anaesthesia and Intensive Care*, vol. 34, no. 6, pp. 829–830, 2006.

[11] K. Lertsburapa, J. W. Schroeder, and C. Sullivan, "Assessment of adenoid size: a comparison of lateral radiographic measurements, radiologist assessment, and nasal endoscopy," *International Journal of Pediatric Otorhinolaryngology*, vol. 74, no. 11, pp. 1281–1285, 2010.

[12] A.-L. Hamdan, O. Sabra, and U. Hadi, "Prevalence of adenoid hypertrophy in adults with nasal obstruction," *Otolaryngology—Head and Neck Surgery*, vol. 37, no. 4, pp. 469–473, 2008.

41

Subarachnoid Fluid Lactate and Paraplegia after Descending Aorta Aneurysmectomy: Two Compared Case Reports

Enrico Giustiniano, Silvia Eleonora Malossini, Francesco Pellegrino, and Franco Cancellieri

Department of Anesthesia and Intensive Care Unit, Humanitas Clinical and Research Center, Via Manzoni 56, 20089 Rozzano, Italy

Correspondence should be addressed to Enrico Giustiniano; enrico.giustiniano@gmail.com

Academic Editors: D. Lee and E. A. Vandermeersch

We report a comparison of two cases regarding subjects who underwent thoracoabdominal aorta aneurysmectomy. During the procedure we monitored cerebrospinal fluid lactate concentration. One patient experienced postoperative paraplegia and his cerebrospinal fluid lactate concentration was much higher than that in the other case, whose postoperative outcome was uneventful. Consequently we consider that monitoring the lactate concentration in cerebrospinal fluid during thoracic aorta surgical procedures may be a helpful tool to predict the ischemic spine-cord injury allowing for trying to recover it precociously.

1. Introduction

During descending aorta surgical repair, spinal cord deficit due to ischemia is a dreadful complication that comes with paraparesis/paraplegia in 6–40% of patients [1, 2].

In this setting, lactate releasing is the epiphenomenon of cellular suffering due to insufficient oxygen delivery. When spinal cord experiences an ischemic event, lactate production occurs as neurons switch on anaerobic metabolism. As literature reports, when blood brain barrier (BBB) is intact, subarachnoid lactate level depends on local production, then it is due to neuronal hypoxic suffering [3]. To prevent spinal cord injury cerebrospinal fluid (CSF) drainage, aimed to reduce intrathecal pressure to provide a better blood perfusion, is a technique now accepted by anesthesiologists and cardiovascular surgeons, although its effectiveness is controversial [4, 5].

During descending aorta surgery, we usually monitor the lactate trend in CSF, as this type of operation exposes the patient to the risk of spinal ischemia due to aortic clamping proximally to Adamkiewicz artery.

Normal spinal fluid lactate concentration ranges from 0.6 to 3.1 mmol/L. Its level is age related and it can rise when spinal ischemic event occurs, also depending on the lasting of the low flow state [6, 7].

In our hospital, descending aorta surgical repair is performed without cardiopulmonary by-pass. Our experience on this kind of operation arises from a series of 8–10 cases per year.

Out of 8 cases observed in the last year, we report two comparable cases of thoracic aorta repair with different neurological outcome that could have been predicted by intraoperative trend of lactate in subarachnoid fluid.

2. Case Report 1

A 61-year-old male patient (ASA 3; BMI 26.0 kg/mq body surface area) underwent general anesthesia for thoracic aorta aneurysmectomy. Preoperative blood test did not show any significant alteration but high level of serum creatinine (4.0 mg/dL) due to chronic renal failure (CRF) not needing of renal replacement therapy (RRT); electrocardiogram showed atrial flutter with 2 : 1–3 : 1 conduction (heart rate 55–65 bpm) as a consequence of a previous myocardial infarction surgically treated with coronaric-artery by-pass graft (CABG) three years before. Preoperative echocardiogram showed a good global kinesis (ejection fraction 65%; left ventricle end-diastolic volume 113 mL). Aneurysm maximum diameter was 7.5 cm.

Surgical approach consisted of thoraco-phreno-laparo-tomic incision, and before left emithorax opening, one lung ventilation (OLV) started and tidal volume (TV) was set to 6 mL/kg. After 90 minutes from the beginning; surgeon clamped aorta 3 cm below the isthmus. The clamping phase lasted 60 minutes.

During the operation i.v. administration of Nitrate (0.5 mcg/kg/min) was needed to assure safe values of blood pressure, particularly during clamping phase, and "to protect" coronary circulation.

Before aortic clamping, patient received N-acetyl-cysteine 2.4 g i.v. bolus, Methyl-Prednisolone 2 g i.v. bolus, and Mannitol 18% 100 ml, aiming to protect kidney and as free-radicals scavenging.

Global intraoperative fluid administration was 7200 mL including 10 units of red blood cells and 7 units of fresh frozen plasma; bleeding resulted in about 5000 mL and 2700 mL was readministered by a red cells storage device. Subarachnoid fluid withdrawal was 75 mL.

Postoperatively, he was admitted to ICU, awakened, and successfully extubated on the day after. Unfortunately he experienced paraplegia, although intrathecal pressure was ≤10 mmHg. CSF lactate concentration raised during operation and returned to normal level (3.2 mmol/L) within 12 hours, postoperatively. Magnetic resonance exam of spinal cord excluded local bleeding.

He was dismissed to ward after 6 days and left hospital 24 days after the operation.

3. Case Report 2

A 72-years-old male patient (ASA 3; BMI 23.1 kg/mq body surface area) underwent general anesthesia for thoracic aorta aneurysmectomy. Preoperative blood test did not show any significant alteration but Kaliemia 5.1 mmol/L and serum creatinine 1.29 mg/dL; electrocardiogram showed a sinus rhythm (68 bpm); echocardiogram reported a good global kinesis (ejection fraction 60%; left ventricle end-diastolic volume 78 ml). Eight years before, he experienced a myocardial infarction treated with percutaneous angioplasty and stenting. Aneurism maximum diameter was 6.7 cm.

Nitrate was not administered even during clamping phase; conversely, hemodynamics needed to be supported by Dopamine administration (8–10 mcg/kg/min).

Surgical approach consisted of thoraco-phreno-laparo-tomic incision, and before left emithorax opening, OLV started and TV lowered at 6 mL/kg.

After 100 minutes from the beginning, surgeon clamped aorta 5 cm below the isthmus. The clamping phase lasted 105 minutes.

Before aortic clamping patient received N-acetyl-cysteine 2 g i.v. bolus, Methyl-Prednisolone 2 g i.v. bolus, and Mannitol 18% 100 ml, aiming to protect kidney and as free-radicals scavenging.

Global intraoperative fluid administration was 8500 mL including 4 units of red blood cells and 4 units of fresh frozen plasma; bleeding resulted in about 2000 mL and 625 mL was

TABLE 1: Intraoperative data.

	Case report 1	Case report 2
Preclamping		
HR (bpm)	62	73
SpO$_2$ (%)	98	100
MAP (mmHg)	80	80
CI (L/min/mq BSA)	2.4	2.7
SVV (%)	9	4
pH	7.33	7.35
pCO$_2$ (mmHg)	40	38
p/F ratio	230	250
EtCO$_2$ (mmHg)	25	29
Subarachnoid fluid withdrawal (mL)	40	60
P_{Lq}/spinal perfusion pressure (mmHg)	20/60	20/60
Diuresis (mL)	300	500
Serum lactate (mmol/L)	2.2	1.7
Subarachnoid lactate (mmol/L)	1.2	1.6
During clamping		
HR (bpm)	80	62
SpO$_2$ (%)	99	99
MAP (mmHg)	90	60
CI (L/min/mq BSA)	4.1	3.8
SVV (%)	4	5
pH	7.31	7.35
pCO$_2$ (mmHg)	39	41
p/F ratio	165	154
EtCO$_2$ (mmHg)	26	30
Subarachnoid fluid withdrawal (mL)	70	95
P_{Lq}/spinal perfusion pressure (mmHg)	15/75	13/47
Diuresis (mL)	400	620
Serum lactate (mmol/L)	8.9	5.2
Subarachnoid lactate (mmol/L)	2.5	1.2
After unclamping		
HR (bpm)	83	86
SpO$_2$ (%)	97	98
MAP (mmHg)	70	80
CI (L/min/mq BSA)	3.0	2.4
SVV (%)	7	14
pH	7.29	7.32
pCO$_2$ (mmHg)	46	41
p/F ratio	208	240
EtCO$_2$ (mmHg)	31	27
Subarachnoid fluid withdrawal (mL)	80	100
P_{Lq}/spinal perfusion pressure (mmHg)	7/63	18/62
Diuresis (mL)	450	700
Serum lactate (mmol/L)	10.5	8.3
Subarachnoid lactate (mmol/L)	6.3	2.0

HR: heart rate; MAP: mean arterial pressure; BSA: body surface area; SVV: stroke volume variation; p/F: pO$_2$/FiO$_2$ ratio.

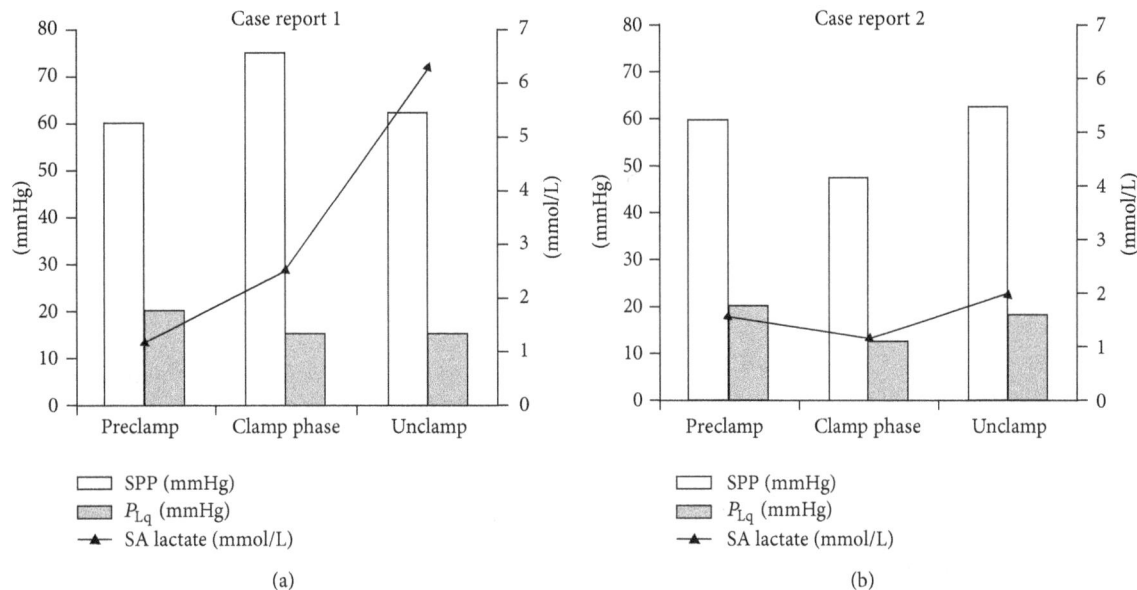

FIGURE 1: Subarachnoid pressure and Lactate. SPP = Spinal perfusion pressure (MAP-P_{Lq}); P_{Lq} = intrathecal pressure; SA Lactate = lactate level in subarachnoid fluid.

readministered by a red cells storage device. Subarachnoid fluid withdrawal was 100 mL.

Postoperatively, he was admitted to ICU, awakened, and successfully extubated on the day after. Patient did not experience any neurological postoperative complication and was dismissed to ward after 2 days and left hospital 15 days after the operation.

3.1. Common Features. In both of the two cases, aortic aneurysm involved the supradiaphragmatic tract of the vessel.

General anesthesia was induced with Fentanyl 1 mcg/kg i.v. + Propofol 2 mg/kg i.v. after preanesthesia administration of Morphine 5 mg + Atropine 0.5 mg i.m. Orotracheal intubation (double-lumen tube n.39) was performed after myorelaxation with cis-Atracurium 10 mg i.v. bolus and further administration of 0.15 mg/kg every 30 minutes. Anesthesia continued with administration of a gas mixture of air and oxygen (FiO_2 0.5-0.6, according to blood gas-analysis (BGA) results) and Sevoflurane 1-2%. Mechanical ventilation setting was tidal volume (TV) 5–8 mL/kg according to one-lung ventilation (OLV) or bilateral lung ventilation (BLV) phase; respiratory rate was 12 apm and it was modified to assure normal pCO_2; positive end-expiratory pressure (PEEP) was 5–7 cmH$_2$O.

Intraoperative monitoring included electrocardiogram (D2 and V5) and ST line analysis, heart rate (HR), not-invasive blood pressure (NIBP) and invasive blood pressure (IBP) after right radial artery line insertion connected with FloTrac/Vigileo sensor (Edwards Lifesciences, Irvine, USA) for Cardiac Output (CO; Cardiac Index, CI) monitoring, peripheral oxygen saturation (SpO_2), central venous pressure (CVP), end-tidal carbon dioxide ($EtCO_2$), and diuresis. A subarachnoid catheter was inserted (Lumbar Drainage Catheter 46 cm, Codman and Shurtleff, Inc., Raynham, MA, USA) at lumbar level L3-L4 and connected to standard multichannel patient monitoring system to measure intrathecal pressure (P_{Lq}) and withdraw CSF to lower it when necessary. Transesophageal echocardiogram (TEE) was used to value cardiac performance, particularly during the clamping period. BGA was tested after surgical incision, after OLV starting, every 15 minutes during aortic clamping, after unclamping, and after BLV restoring (Table 1).

Postoperative analgesia started before the end of operation with i.v. infusion of a saline solution containing Morphine 30 mg/50 ml (2.1 mL/h). After the operation, the patient was sedated with Propofol 100 mg/h and admitted to ICU as planned to continue postoperative care and monitoring.

4. Discussion

Here are two case samples that we report to point out that liquor lactate level could be predictive of postoperative spinal cord damage due to ischemic event occurred during clamping phase of thoracic aorta surgical repair.

Preoperatively, the two cases were very similar. They differed by the neurological outcome. The second patient did not experienced any complication, although he needed pharmacological hemodynamic support to provide an adequate blood flow. The former came out of operation with paraplegia. It happened although we lowered subarachnoid pressure significantly to assure a good spinal blood perfusion pressure (Figure 1).

What may the cause be? Anatomical differences of vascular bed regarding Adamkiewicz artery origin, inadequate spinal perfusion pressure despite being in normal range, insufficient cerebrospinal fluid drainage could be some possible reasons of spinal suffering. Furthermore, another possible reason may be the different level at which aorta was clamped below the isthmus, although it consisted of only 2 cm. Anyway, whatever the cause, we expected a postoperative injured spinal cord in case 1 because, after the aortic clamping, subarachnoid lactate level rose progressively to a warning concentration.

As literature reports, when aorta is clamped subarachnoid pressure raises, probably due to a sympathetically mediated vasoconstriction that increases the tone of spinal veins with consequent venous engorgement [4]. Because of this issue, CSF withdrawal according to cerebrospinal fluid pressure is performed aiming to prevent spinal suffering from intrathecal hypertension.

Spinal cord low flow state can be detected by subarachnoid level of lactate production as it does not cross throughout blood brain barrier when it is not injured and then lactate blood-CSF mixing does not occur. It is a warning sign of neuronal anaerobic metabolism due to low flow state and its raising occurs earlier than other markers such as S-100 protein, [8].

The literature reports that CSF lactate level and other biochemical markers could raise without any postoperative neurological impairment [9]. We consider it may be only a possibility, not the rule. Since our habit is to monitor CSF lactate concentration, it was just the one case of postoperative paraplegia with significant intraoperative high level of subarachnoid fluid lactate concentration (>3 mmol/L).

Consequently, may CSF lactate level predict postoperative neurological outcome of spinal cord after descending aorta surgical repair? Several studies showed contrasting results and we are persuaded that a wide prospective trial should be performed aiming to answer the question.

In any case, CSF lactate concentration raising after descending aorta clamping should be a warning sign to make anesthesiologist do his best to prevent spinal cord ischemia/reperfusion injury even when all other parameters say that all is going well. Conversely, we consider that, whatever he does, it could be insufficient and postsurgical spinal damage is unavoidable.

References

[1] C. S. Cinà, A. Laganà, G. Bruin et al., "Thoracoabdominal aortic aneurysm repair: a prospective cohort study of 121 cases," *Annals of Vascular Surgery*, vol. 16, no. 5, pp. 631–638, 2002.

[2] E. Weigang, M. Hartert, M. P. Siegenthaler et al., "Perioperative management to improve neurologic outcome in thoracic or thoracoabdominal aortic stent-grafting," *Annals of Thoracic Surgery*, vol. 82, no. 5, pp. 1679–1687, 2006.

[3] A. H. M. Bashar, K. Suzuki, T. Kazui et al., "Changes in cerebrospinal fluid and blood lactate concentrations after stent-graft implantation at critical aortic segment: A preliminary study," *Interactive Cardiovascular and Thoracic Surgery*, vol. 7, no. 2, pp. 262–266, 2008.

[4] B. Drenger, S. D. Parker, S. M. Frank, and C. Beattie, "Changes in cerebrospinal fluid pressure and lactate concentrations during thoracoabdominal aortic aneurysm surgery," *Anesthesiology*, vol. 86, no. 1, pp. 41–47, 1997.

[5] C. S. Cinà, L. Abouzahr, G. O. Arena, A. Laganà, P. J. Devereaux, and F. Farrokhyar, "Cerebrospinal fluid drainage to prevent paraplegia during thoracic and thoracoabdominal aortic aneurysm surgery: a systematic review and meta-analysis," *Journal of Vascular Surgery*, vol. 40, no. 1, pp. 36–44, 2004.

[6] I. Holbrook, R. Beetham, A. Cruickshank et al., "National audit of cerebrospinal fluid testing," *Annals of Clinical Biochemistry*, vol. 44, no. 5, pp. 443–448, 2007.

[7] W. G. Leen, M. A. Willemsen, R. A. Wevers, and M. M. Verbeek, "Cerebrospinal fluid glucose and lactate: age-specific reference values and implication for clinical practice," *PloS ONE*, vol. 7, no. 8, Article ID e42745, 2012.

[8] N. Khaladj, O. E. Teebken, C. Hagl et al., "The role of cerebrospinal fluid S_{100} and lactate to predict clinically evident spinal cord ischaemia in thoraco-abdominal aortic surgery," *European Journal of Vascular and Endovascular Surgery*, vol. 36, no. 1, pp. 11–19, 2008.

[9] R. E. Anderson, A. Winnerkvist, L.-O. Hansson et al., "Biochemical markers of cerebrospinal ischemia after repair of aneurysms of the descending and thoracoabdominal aorta," *Journal of Cardiothoracic and Vascular Anesthesia*, vol. 17, no. 5, pp. 598–603, 2003.

42

Anesthetic Management of a Surgical Patient with Chronic Renal Tubular Acidosis Complicated by Subclinical Hypothyroidism

Hiroe Yoshioka, Haruyuki Yamazaki, Rie Yasumura, Kosuke Wada, and Yoshiro Kobayashi

Department of Anesthesiology, National Hospital Organization Tokyo Medical Center, 2-5-1 Higashigaoka, Meguro-ku, Tokyo 152-8902, Japan

Correspondence should be addressed to Hiroe Yoshioka; hiroe_y_0614@hotmail.co.jp

Academic Editor: Renato Santiago Gomez

A 53-year-old man with chronic renal tubular acidosis and subclinical hypothyroidism underwent lower leg amputation surgery under general anesthesia. Perioperative acid-base management in such patients poses many difficulties because both pathophysiologies have the potential to complicate the interpretation of capnometry and arterial blood gas analysis data; inappropriate correction of chronic metabolic acidosis may lead to postoperative respiratory deterioration. We discuss the management of perioperative acidosis in order to achieve successful weaning from mechanical ventilation and promise a complete recovery from anesthesia.

1. Introduction

Metabolic acidosis is categorized clinically as high or normal anion gap based on the presence or absence of unmeasured anions in serum. Renal tubular acidosis (RTA) is characterized by normal anion-gap metabolic acidosis, originating from excessive urinary loss of bicarbonate or defective urinary acidification [1]. Therefore, unlike high anion-gap acidoses (e.g., lactic acidosis or ketoacidosis), RTA must be treated with administration of sodium bicarbonate. However, perioperative acid-base management in such cases poses many difficulties because the total carbon dioxide (CO_2) content in blood as well as actual blood pH must be fully taken into consideration for successful weaning from mechanical ventilation. In addition, thyroid function is associated with basal metabolic rate and CO_2 production; thus, subclinical hypothyroidism presents specific challenges for anesthesiologists.

This case highlights the perioperative acid-base management of a patient who has suffered from untreated chronic RTA complicated by subclinical hypothyroidism while undergoing lower leg amputation surgery under general anesthesia. We report this case because the anesthetic management of similar cases has rarely been reported; in addition, there has been no prior report detailing the management of perioperative acidosis, which is the focal point of this case.

2. Case Presentation

A 53-year-old man (height: 167 cm; weight: 48 kg) who presented difficulty in walking due to severe pain in his lower leg was brought to our hospital by an ambulance. The patient had a prior history of chronic kidney disease, arteriosclerosis obliterans, and insulin-dependent diabetes mellitus. Physical and laboratory examination revealed ulcerative formations in the left lower leg and severe metabolic acidosis (Table 1). An intravenous subsequently oral administration of sodium bicarbonate resulted in marked improvement of the acidosis. Upon detailed examination, polyarteritis nodosa was strongly suspected as the etiology of the refractory ulcer in the lower leg; simultaneously, RTA type 4 was diagnosed based on a prior history of hyperkalemia and diabetes, accompanying a low serum aldosterone level.

For suspected pathophysiology, a 10 mg daily oral dose of prednisolone had been administered for about 2 months but his ulcerative lesions deteriorated; therefore, the patient was

TABLE 1: Perioperative blood gas analysis.

	On admission	Preoperative	Immediately after intubation	Postoperative
pH	7.031	7.345	7.286	7.345
$PaCO_2$ (mmHg)	13.6	27.7	34.4	37.1
HCO_3^- (mmol/L)	3.5	14.8	16.0	19.8
BE (mmol/L)	−25.3	−10.0	−9.7	−5.4
AnGap (mmol/L)	18.1	3.6	4.8	2.7
Lactate (mg/dL)	15.4	17.4	—	—

AnGap: anion gap; BE: base excess; HCO_3^-: bicarbonate; $PaCO_2$: arterial carbon dioxide partial pressure.

TABLE 2: Preoperative laboratory test values.

	Test value (normal range)
HGB (g/dL)	7.1 (13.5–17.0)
PLT ($\times 10^9$/L)	59 (150–350)
BUN (mg/dL)	32.7 (8.0–22.0)
Cre (mg/dL)	2.6 (0.6–1.1)
TP (g/dL)	4.6 (6.3–8.2)
Alb (g/dL)	2.1 (3.5–5.2)
Na (Mmol/L)	128 (138–146)
K (Mmol/L)	5.3 (3.6–4.9)
Cl (Mmol/L)	106 (99–109)
PRA (ng/mL/h)	0.3 (0.2–2.7)
PAC (pg/mL)	13 (36–240)
TSH (U/dL)	6.17 (0.3–4.5)
T3 (pg/mL)	1.2 (2.0–4.5)
T4 (ng/dL)	1.1 (0.7–1.8)

Alb: albumin; BUN: blood urea nitrogen; Cl: chloride; Cre: creatinine; HGB: hemoglobin; K: potassium; Na: sodium; PAC: plasma aldosterone concentration; PRA: plasma renin activity; TP: total protein; TSH: thyroid-stimulating hormone; T3: triiodothyronine; T4: thyroxine.

scheduled for lower leg amputation surgery about 3 months after admission.

Preoperative laboratory tests (Table 2) revealed impaired renal function and hyperkalemia, while those findings were compatible with RTA type 4. With regard to endocrine function, we suspected subclinical hypothyroidism due to reduced plasma triiodothyronine (T3) levels and elevated thyroid-stimulating hormone (TSH). Blood gas analysis showed severe metabolic acidosis accompanied by normal anion gap corrected for albumin and compensatory respiratory alkalosis (Table 1), because the oral sodium bicarbonate therapy had been discontinued 2 months before the surgery. Despite severe metabolic acidosis, the history and physical examination did not indicate any obvious evidence of hyperventilation. The patient had a body temperature of 36.4°C, blood pressure of 121/73 mmHg, a heart rate of 89 beats per minute (bpm), a respiratory rate of 10 breaths per minute, and an oxygen saturation level of 98% (room air); chest radiography and electrocardiogram examinations revealed no abnormalities.

General anesthesia was scheduled instead of regional anesthesia because of low platelet count. Oral prednisolone (10 mg/day) was continued until the day of the surgery.

Preoperative values of blood pressure, heart rate, respiratory rate, and body temperature were almost within normal ranges: 142/91 mmHg, 84 bpm, 10 breaths per minute, and 35.8°C, respectively. Endotracheal intubation under general anesthesia was provided with intravenous induction of 50 μg fentanyl, 70 mg propofol, and 40 mg rocuronium; and anesthesia was maintained by 1.2–1.8% sevoflurane with intermittent intravenous administration of fentanyl. The total amount of fentanyl was 250 μg during operation. The end tidal CO_2 ($ETCO_2$) level of the patient was 22 mmHg immediately after intubation; then his minute volume was set at 3 L/min. However, the blood gas analysis revealed that the arterial carbon dioxide partial pressure ($PaCO_2$) of the patient was within the normal range (Table 1). The frequency of ventilation was subsequently adjusted to and maintained at a rate of 3–3.5 L/min, in order to ensure that the $PaCO_2$ remained within the normal range. During this time, $ETCO_2$ levels were 22–29 mmHg.

The total time of surgery was 1 h and 48 min; 1250 mL of crystalloid solution (normal saline and hypotonic solution which contains no potassium), 280 mL of red blood cell transfusion, and 100 mL of 8.4% sodium bicarbonate were administered during the surgery. The total blood loss and urine volume were determined to be 170 mL and 150 mL, respectively. Although the patient continued to exhibit mild signs of metabolic acidosis upon completion of surgery (Table 1), this did not appear to impact his circulatory condition. A chest radiograph taken upon completion of surgery revealed a small amount of bilateral pleural effusion. The patient was given a muscle relaxant antagonist (200 mg of sugammadex) after awakening and was extubated after a spontaneous breathing trial. There was no appreciable event during the surgery, except a red blood cell transfusion. No subsequent problems related to hyperventilation or apnea were observed, and the patient was sent back to his room without incident.

3. Discussion

RTA is classified into three types based on pathophysiology. Among them, RTA type 4 is characterized by distal tubular aldosterone resistance or aldosterone deficiency, resulting in hyperkalemia and onset of metabolic acidosis [1]. RTA type 4 is usually asymptomatic with only mild acidosis but can be occasionally accompanied by life-threatening electrolyte disturbances and severe decrease in bicarbonate concentration. In addition, its clinical course tends to be prolonged and thus complicated as with this case. Therefore, rather than actual blood pH, time-dependent changes in contained CO_2 in the whole body should be taken into consideration for successful weaning from mechanical ventilation when perioperative corrective treatment is performed.

Literature reviews of anesthetic management of patients with severe acute metabolic acidosis have focused on the maintenance of adequate blood pressure and tissue perfusion. However, in chronic cases, anesthesiologists should give attention to intraoperative acid-base status in order to ensure adequate spontaneous breathing immediately after surgery.

In general, respiratory drive is stimulated by low pH, particularly in patients with chronic metabolic acidosis. Therefore, any arterial pH, which is higher than preoperative value, can be associated with a higher risk for postoperative hypoventilation to various degrees, even if normal acid-base balance without hypercapnia has been achieved at the time of weaning from mechanical ventilation. Rapid or excessive correction of chronic metabolic acidosis during surgery leads to either life-threatening hypoventilation or sudden onset of apnea [2].

With regard to correction of acidosis, there is no conclusive evidence to support bicarbonate administration to surgical patients with chronic metabolic acidosis. In contrast, patients of RTA type 4 need administration of bicarbonate at a daily rate of 1.5–2 mmol/kg [1]; nevertheless, the dose and rate of perioperative bicarbonate administration remain controversial in particular cases.

In general, severe metabolic acidosis with arterial pH < 7.2 is associated with higher mortality in critically ill patients [3]; therefore, we adjusted the ventilator settings and bicarbonate administration to maintain arterial pH at a value simultaneously less than the preoperative value and higher than 7.2 along with normocapnia.

On the other hand, the clinical picture of this case was remarkable in the light of perioperative $PaCO_2$ level when compared to that of most patients with severe metabolic acidosis.

Firstly, although the preoperative $PaCO_2$ of the patient was extremely low (27.7 mmHg), which seems to be respiratory overcompensation, no obvious signs of deep breathing or hyperventilation were observed. Secondly, despite the adjustment of the minute volume in order to bring the $PaCO_2$ level within the normal range, low minute volume was required for this patient. For comparison, the minute volume and the $PaCO_2$ level were assessed in other surgical patients without metabolic acid-base disorders (Table 3). The minute volume and the $PaCO_2$ level exhibited by the patient in this case were lower than the group average. Based on these observations, we speculated that any underlying pathophysiologies might lead to a decrease in $PaCO_2$ without an increase in alveolar ventilation.

Specifically, the body equilibrium of RTA patients is known to shift to the left as follows: $H^+ + HCO_3^- \rightleftarrows H_2CO_3 \rightleftarrows H_2O + CO_2$; as such, if the bicarbonate level is not replenished, the internal CO_2 level will be depleted, resulting in a decline in $PaCO_2$.

As another speculation, subclinical hypothyroidism may possibly lead to decreased CO_2 production in the body

TABLE 3: Minute volume and $PaCO_2$ levels of 29 male patients (aged 48–90) subjected to nonlaparoscopic surgery.

	Mean (SD)
Age (years)	74.0 (11.2)
Height (cm)	165.0 (5.2)
Weight (kg)	48.7 (2.2)
Minute volume (L/min)	4.8 (1.0)
$PaCO_2$ (mmHg)	39.1 (5.0)

$PaCO_2$: arterial carbon dioxide partial pressure.

because decreased thyroid function is associated with diminished basal metabolic rate, thus resulting in reduced tissue CO_2 production [4]; similarly, subclinical hypothyroidism is reported to induce a decrease in resting energy expenditure [5].

Definitely, subclinical hypothyroidism and RTA type 4 have the potential to complicate the reading and interpretation of capnometry and $PaCO_2$ measurements.

In order to avoid postoperative respiratory deterioration in patients with chronic metabolic acidosis, anesthesiologists should give basic consideration to the previously documented pitfalls: type of anesthesia, dose of opioids used in combination, methods of postoperative pain management, and body temperature of the patient. Besides, perioperative acid-base management on the basis of the abovementioned goal of pH and $PaCO_2$ will probably determine success of weaning from mechanical ventilation and promise a complete recovery from anesthesia in patients with RTA complicated by subclinical hypothyroidism. Given that hemodynamic stability has already been achieved in patients suffering from long-term preoperative exposure to RTA with low serum bicarbonate concentration, the main anesthetic concerns should include the dose and rate of bicarbonate administration tailored according to the patient's usual acid-base balance and preoperative respiratory status: $PaCO_2$ levels, the minute volume, and the presence of signs of deep breathing or hyperventilation.

Ethical Approval

Written informed consent from the patient was not obtained because of the patient's death. The authors received permission from the Institutional Review Board of National Hospital Organization Tokyo Medical Center to publish this case report.

Competing Interests

The authors declare that there is no conflict of interests regarding the publication of this paper.

References

[1] J. R. Soriano, "Renal tubular acidosis: the clinical entity," *Journal of the American Society of Nephrology*, vol. 13, no. 8, pp. 2160–2170, 2002.

[2] D. Chan, S. Thong, and O. Ng, "Postoperative apnoea in an adult patient after rapid correction of metabolic acidosis," *OA Case Reports*, vol. 3, no. 2, article 16, 2014.

[3] B. Jung, T. Rimmele, C. Le Goff et al., "Severe metabolic or mixed acidemia on intensive care unit admission: incidence, prognosis and administration of buffer therapy. A prospective, multiple-center study," *Critical Care*, vol. 15, no. 5, article R238, 2011.

[4] H. T. Lee and M. Levine, "Acute respiratory alkalosis associated with low minute ventilation in a patient with severe hypothyroidism," *Canadian Journal of Anaesthesia*, vol. 46, no. 2, pp. 185–189, 1999.

[5] M. Tagliaferri, M. E. Berselli, G. Calò et al., "Subclinical hypothyroidism in obese patients: relation to resting energy expenditure, serum leptin, body composition, and lipid profile," *Obesity Research*, vol. 9, no. 3, pp. 196–201, 2001.

43

Anesthetic Management of a Patient with Sustained Severe Metabolic Alkalosis and Electrolyte Abnormalities Caused by Ingestion of Baking Soda

Jose Soliz, Jeffrey Lim, and Gang Zheng

Department of Anesthesiology and Perioperative Medicine, MD Anderson Cancer Center, Houston, TX 77030, USA

Correspondence should be addressed to Jose Soliz; jsoliz@mdanderson.org

Academic Editor: Kuang I. Cheng

The use of alternative medicine is prevalent worldwide. However, its effect on intraoperative anesthetic care is underreported. We report the anesthetic management of a patient who underwent an extensive head and neck cancer surgery and presented with a severe intraoperative metabolic alkalosis from the long term ingestion of baking soda and other herbal remedies.

1. Introduction

Little is known about the impact of alternative medicine on perioperative anesthetic care. We present a case of a patient who was under the long term management of a naturalistic doctor for a history of colon cancer. His prescribed treatment remedy constituted of a combination of herbs and alkaline fluid. This history was not elicited preoperatively. His intraoperative arterial blood gas test revealed unexpected profound metabolic alkalosis and multiple electrolytes abnormalities. This case presented some unique challenges in intraoperative hemodynamic and electrolyte management.

2. Case Report

A 63-year-old 75 kg male with a history of sinonasal melanoma presented for an endoscopic ethmoidectomy, sphenoidectomy, maxillectomy, palatectomy, and bilateral neck dissection. His past medical history included a 12-year history of colon cancer, which had been managed with a "nature remedy" in Mexico. His remedy included 4Life Transfer Factor Plus, Choice Fifty, Orasal, Boluoke, Grano Derma, Resveratrol Plus, and vitamins C, E, and D. He denied any other medical or surgical issues in the past. His laboratory report 14 days prior to surgery revealed potassium 3.2 mEq/L, chloride 94 mEq/L, and bicarbonate 31 mEq/L. All other electrolyte, renal, and liver function labs were within normal

range. On preoperative anesthesia assessment, his vital signs were within normal limits, and his physical exam was normal with the exception of a large mass on the right side of his face.

He was brought to operating room with 2 mg of midazolam premedication. Upon arrival at the operating room he became difficult to arouse. General anesthesia was induced with 150 mg of propofol, 20 mcg of sufentanil, and 70 mg of rocuronium and was maintained with air, oxygen, and 0.6-0.7 MAC of desflurane plus 0.1 mcg/kg/hr of sufentanil infusion. After 1.5 hours of surgery, the patient received one liter of plasmalyte with minimal blood loss. A baseline arterial blood gas reported severe metabolic alkalosis and multiple electrolytes derangements (Table 1 at 0919). A blood chemistry test confirmed the accuracy of blood gas report. Therefore, 1 gram of calcium chloride, 2 grams of magnesium sulfate, 40 mEq of potassium chloride in 800 mL of normal saline (an institutional policy for peripheral IV potassium), and 100 mg of hydrocortisone were given. The ventilator settings were adjusted to target the $ETCO_2$ of 40 mmHg. After about 2.5 hours into the surgery, his blood pressure decreased from 110s/70s mmHg to 80s/60s mmHg. Meantime, he had a total fluid balance of 4,000 mL of plasmalyte, 700 mL of blood loss, and 175 mL of urine output. After several boluses of vasopressin and phenylephrine, a 4-unit/hr vasopressin infusion was added to his treatment. His BP remained low in 80s/60s mmHg, for which he frequently required boluses of phenylephrine and ephedrine. His EKG showed regular

TABLE 1: Intraoperative laboratory values.

	Time					
	0919	0954	1115	1226	1435	1738
pH	7.65	7.53	7.48	7.49	7.51	7.44
CO_2	35	44	47	44	41	46
O_2	198	193	183	205	202	266
HCO_3	39	37	35	34	33	31
Base excess	17	13	10	9	9	6
Sodium	123	124	127	126	127	129
Potassium	2.6	2.5	3.3	3.4	2.9	3.2
Glucose	157	208	230	258	271	225
Calcium (ionized)	0.89	1.16	1.18	1.03	0.98	1.11
Lactate	1.3	1.8	1.9	2.3	3.1	3.5
Hematocrit	42	38	31	26	34	31

sinus rhythm with rate of low 80s bpm. The total anesthetic duration was 12 hours. At the end of surgery, he received a total of 7600 mL of plasmalyte, 1100 mL of colloid, and 797 mL of packed blood cells, with 1000 mL of estimated blood loss and 595 mL of urine output. In addition, he also received second dose of 1 gram of calcium at the 7th hour and 40 mEq potassium at the 9th hour of surgery. Table 1 illustrates his intraoperative arterial blood gas results at different time points. He was extubated at the end of surgery in the operating room.

Postoperatively, he developed hallucinations described as "constantly dreaming and difficulty to close eyes." The hallucination disappeared on postoperative day 3 without intervention. His K, Na, and CL remained low until postoperative day 6. His postoperative EKG showed a normal sinus rhythm with a rate of 70s bpm. No other issues were identified in his postoperative course. The patient was discharged to home on postoperative day 7.

On postoperative followup, we learned that, for the past 12 years, the patient used herbal medications and also drank an "alkaline liquid": a mixture of 1 liter of pH 7.8–8 water, typically with bottled water, key lime juice, and a quarter of tablespoon baking soda. The endpoint of the remedy was to achieve urine pH of 7.58–8. He stopped all the herbs 5 days prior to surgery per his doctor's advice but kept his "alkaline liquid" until the night before surgery. He never experienced muscular cramping, weakness, or alter mental status in the past.

3. Discussion

Baking soda (sodium bicarbonate) has been widely used by people for reasons ranging from increasing excise tolerance to treating acid reflux disease and other medical conditions. Severe cardiac dysrhythmia and death after ingestion of sodium bicarbonate have been reported [1–4]. Ingestion of baking soda results in multiple issues including metabolic and electrolytes derangement. Details on pathophysiological influences of metabolic alkalosis and electrolytes abnormalities are beyond the scope of a case report.

Generally, treating severe metabolic and electrolyte abnormalities during anesthesia is based on patient's baseline

condition and clinical symptoms. In our case, the lack of knowledge of etiology and baseline values led to difficulty in determining the endpoint of electrolyte correction. Our goal for this case was to partially restore potassium to a range of 3–3.5 mEq/L in light of his previous potassium 3.2 mEq/L to minimize the risk of intraoperative cardiac dysrhythmia. Without knowing his baseline sodium value we decided to use plasmalyte rather than hypertonic saline to avoid the risk of acute sodium overcorrection from his baseline level. This case presented a couple of unique issues. First, the patient developed refractory hypotension despite fluid replacement with the volume that seemed adequate in other similar cases. This might reflect the combined effects of hypovolemia and direct vasodilation from bicarbonate. Kaplan et al. found in their study that bicarbonate is a direct peripheral vasodilator. Under general anesthesia with halothane it caused profound hypotension in health volunteers [5]. Another study showed that even mild metabolic alkalosis induced by bicarbonate resulted in symptomatic hypotension during renal dialysis and required a larger volume infusion than in non-alkalotic patients [6]. Attenuated response to vasopressors was also observed in this case. Despite multivasopressor therapy in addition to fluid replacement, we were not able to achieve sustained blood pressure close to his baseline level. This might have reflected that, under a state of severe alkalosis, the response to vasoactive agents is blunted. Indeed, combined effects of left shift hemoglobin dissociation curve with tissue hypoxia caused by alkalosis, a low perfusion status, and multielectrolyte derangement had put the patient in a high risk of an ischemic event.

Secondly, we observed that the patient presented with a decreased response to stimuli. As described above, with a low anesthetic level, without extra adjustment of anesthetics the patient did not show HR and BP changes in response to multiple skin incisions and head repositions. We suspect that the decrease in anesthetic demand was secondary to a decrease in central nervous system (CNS) response to stimuli secondary to the CSF alkalosis. Sustained metabolic alkalosis with significant multiple electrolyte derangements under general anesthesia is a rare clinical scenario. Little is known about the potential complications and drug pharmacodynamics and pharmacokinetics under this situation.

It is a very common and misleading opinion that alternative medicines are benign and safe, as these remedies have been used worldwide. Lack of regulation and standardization of alternative medicine has made clinical evaluation of patients and their remedies challenging. More importantly, not knowing the impacts of alternative medicine to perioperative patient care will significantly undermine the perioperative risk stratification. Hence, developing an interview protocol and actively seeking history of alternative remedies rather than "patient to tell" during preoperative interview should be as important as the retrieval of any other medical and surgical information.

References

[1] L. J. Fitzgibbons and E. R. Snoey, "Severe metabolic alkalosis due to baking soda ingestion: case reports of two patients with unsuspected antacid overdose," *Journal of Emergency Medicine*, vol. 17, no. 1, pp. 57–61, 1999.

[2] M. H. Nichols, S. Wason, J. G. Del Rey, and M. Benfield, "Baking soda: a potentially fatal home remedy," *Pediatric Emergency Care*, vol. 11, no. 2, pp. 109–111, 1995.

[3] M. Price, P. Moss, and S. Rance, "Effects of sodium bicarbonate ingestion on prolonged intermittent exercise," *Medicine and Science in Sports and Exercise*, vol. 35, no. 8, pp. 1303–1308, 2003.

[4] I. B. Gawarammana, J. Coburn, S. Greene, P. I. Dargan, and A. L. Jones, "Severe hypokalaemic metabolic alkalosis following ingestion of gaviscon," *Clinical Toxicology*, vol. 45, no. 2, pp. 176–178, 2007.

[5] J. A. Kaplan, G. L. Bush, J. H. Lecky, A. J. Ominsky, and H. Wollman, "Sodium bicarbonate and systemic hemodynamics in volunteers anesthetized with halothane," *Anesthesiology*, vol. 42, no. 5, pp. 550–558, 1975.

[6] L. Gabutti, N. Ferrari, G. Giudici, G. Mombelli, and C. Marone, "Unexpected haemodynamic instability associated with standard bicarbonate haemodialysis," *Nephrology Dialysis Transplantation*, vol. 18, no. 11, pp. 2369–2376, 2003.

44

Glucose Management during Insulinoma Resection Using Real-Time Subcutaneous Continuous Glucose Monitoring

Yuki Sugiyama ⓘ,[1] Chiaki Kiuchi,[1] Maiko Suzuki,[1] Yuki Maruyama,[1] Ryo Wakabayashi,[1] Yasunari Ohno,[2] Shugo Takahata,[2] Takumi Shibazaki,[3] and Mikito Kawamata[1]

[1]*Department of Anesthesiology and Resuscitology, Shinshu University School of Medicine, Japan*
[2]*Division of Pediatric Surgery, Department of Surgery, Shinshu University School of Medicine, Japan*
[3]*Department of Pediatrics, Shinshu University School of Medicine, Japan*

Correspondence should be addressed to Yuki Sugiyama; ysugiyama@shinshu-u.ac.jp

Academic Editor: Renato Santiago Gomez

Insulinoma is a rare neuroendocrine tumor that causes hypoglycemia due to unregulated insulin secretion. Blood glucose management during insulinoma resection is therefore challenging. We present a case in which real-time subcutaneous continuous glucose monitoring (SCGM) in combination with intermittent blood glucose measurement was used for glycemic control during surgery for insulinoma resection. The SCGM system showed the trends and peak of interstitial glucose in response to glucose loading and the change of interstitial glucose before and after insulinoma resection. These data were helpful for adjusting the glucose infusion; therefore, we think that an SCGM system as a supportive device for glucose monitoring may be useful for glucose management during surgery.

1. Introduction

Insulinoma is a rare neuroendocrine tumor that causes hypoglycemia, and surgical resection is indicated for all localized tumors [1]. Ten percent of insulinomas occur as a part of multiple endocrine neoplasia type 1 (MEN-1), in which insulinoma occurs at a relatively young age [2]. It is challenging for anesthesiologists to control blood glucose (BG) during surgery for insulinoma resection [3]. A subcutaneous continuous glucose monitoring (SCGM) system, which allows real-time monitoring of interstitial glucose (IG), has been developed and is used in diabetic patients [4]. We present a case of insulinoma in which an SCGM system provided the change of IG and played a role as a supportive device for glucose management during insulinoma resection.

Written informed consent was obtained from the patient's parents for publication of this case report.

2. Case Presentation

A 12-year-old girl (height, 144 cm; weight, 40 kg) was presented to the hospital with an episode of seizure with impaired consciousness. Her BG at that time was 60 mg/dL (normal value of casual BG: 70–200 mg/dL). Glucose was administered and she recovered consciousness. She had no significant comorbidities prior to hospital admission. From her family history and further investigation, she was diagnosed as having insulinoma and hyperparathyroidism in MEN-1. Arterial phase images of computed tomography showed a vascularity-rich tumor of 20 mm in diameter located in the head of the pancreas. The feeding artery of the tumor was not clearly demonstrated by angiography and selective arterial calcium injection. We considered that extended surgical procedures such as pancreatoduodenectomy might be required depending on intraoperative findings; therefore, open abdominal surgery rather than laparoscopic surgery was scheduled. Her intact parathyroid hormone level was 66.0 pg/ml (normal value: 10–65 pg/mL) and her adjusted serum calcium level was 10.3 mg/dL (normal value: 8.7–9.9 mg/dL), although parathyroid ultrasound examination revealed no parathyroid tumor. Other tumors complicated with MEN-1 were not detected. The results of other preoperative examinations were unremarkable. On the

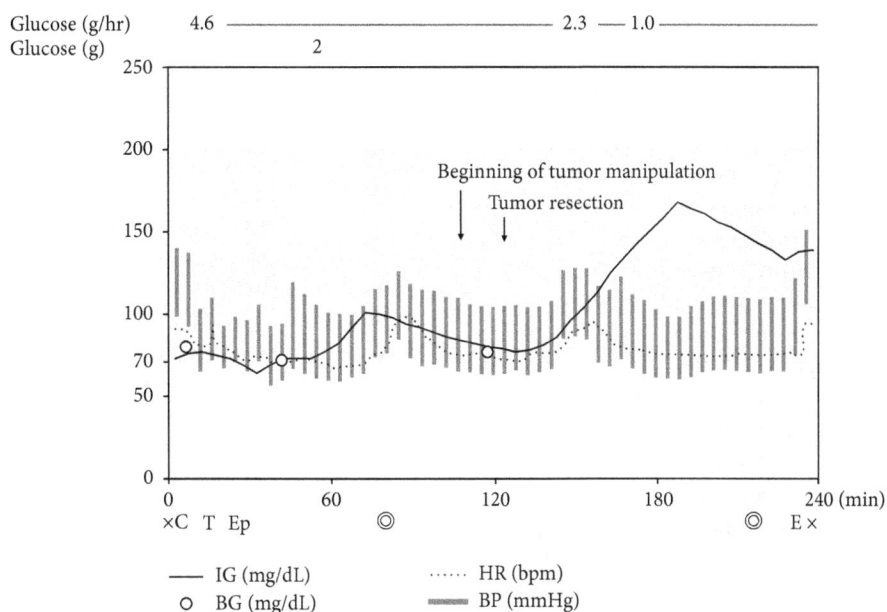

FIGURE 1: Changes of interstitial glucose level measured by the subcutaneous continuous glucose monitoring system (IG) (black line), blood glucose level (BG) (white circle), and hemodynamics during general anesthesia for resection of insulinoma. The light grey zone indicates the normal value of casual BG (70–200 mg/dL). The dotted line indicates heart rate (HR) and the grey bar indicates blood pressure (BP). C indicates calibration of the subcutaneous continuous glucose monitoring system; T: tracheal intubation; Ep: epidural catheterization; E: extubation; ◎: start or end of the operation; ×: start or end of anesthesia.

day before surgery, an Enlite™ sensor of MiniMed™ 620G (Medtronic Diabetes, Northridge, CA, USA) SCGM system was inserted into her upper arm. Although MiniMed 620G was combined with an insulin pump, we did not use the pump. The SCGM system was calibrated as recommended by the manufacturer with capillary BG measured by OneTouch® UltraVue™ Blood Glucose Meter (Johnson & Johnson, New Brunswick, NJ, USA).

No premedication was given and she walked into the operating room. Capillary BG was 80 mg/dL and the SCGM system was calibrated. Continuous glucose infusion was started at 4.6 g/hr, and general anesthesia was induced with 80 mg of propofol, 50 mcg of fentanyl, and 0.02 mcg/kg/min of remifentanil. Muscle relaxation was obtained by administration of 30 mg of rocuronium, and the trachea was intubated. After induction of general anesthesia, an epidural catheter was inserted at the eighth and ninth thoracic interspace. Anesthesia was maintained with 1.7% sevoflurane, 0.01–0.02 mcg/kg/min of remifentanil, and intermittent thoracic epidural administration of 0.25% levobupivacaine (3 ml). An arterial catheter was inserted, and arterial BG measured by an ABL800 Flex Blood Gas Analyzer (Radiometer, Brea, CA, USA) was 71 mg/dL, which was compatible with IG of 73 mg/dL. An additional 2 g of glucose was given intravenously before the start of surgery, and IG increased from 77 mg/dL to 101 mg/dL at 20 minutes (Figure 1). After that, IG mildly decreased and returned to almost the same level after 1 hour. The surgeon informed us that the tumor would be removed by enucleation shortly. Just before tumor resection, arterial BG was 76 mg/dL and IG was 80 mg/dL. At

20 minutes after tumor resection, IG showed a rapid increase. We therefore decreased the continuous glucose infusion rate to the usual dose of 1 g/hr, and IG gradually decreased and was stabilized at about 140 mg/dL. During surgery, blood pressure was between 90/50 and 120/70 mmHg, and heart rate was between 60 and 90 bpm. She was extubated in the operating room and transferred to the general surgery ward. The operation time was 2 h and 24 min, and the anesthesia time was 3 h and 53 min. Postoperative pain was controlled well by continuous epidural analgesia (12 mcg of fentanyl and 0.2% levobupivacaine at 4 ml/hr) and administration of 600 mg of acetaminophen (every 6 hr). Her postoperative course was uneventful and she was discharged on POD 10.

3. Discussion

An SCGM system has been used to monitor glucose level and has improved long-term glycemic control in diabetic patients [5]. The MiniMed 620G SCGM system is composed of a small sensor (6 g) and a transmission device (130 g), which can record real-time data from its wireless sensor. The SCGM sensor, which has a small electrode inserted into subcutaneous tissue, can measure IG by the glucose oxidase method.

In this case, we used the MiniMed 620G SCGM system as a supportive device for continuous monitoring of IG trends in combination with intermittent BG measurements. Fortunately, the operation was completed within 2.5 hr and resection of the insulinoma per se was completed within 30 min. During surgery, we performed 3 measurements of

BG and those measurements showed close correlation with IG measurements (Figure 1). A single injection of glucose was administered before the surgery because the patient's BG remained relatively low despite continuous glucose infusion. IG gradually increased in response to the single glucose injection and the delay of IG to BG in our case was found to be about 20 min from this response (Figure 1). Based on this finding, we could estimate the change in BG by the real-time change in IG. A gradual decrease and increase in IG were also seen before and after resection of the insulinoma, respectively (Figure 1). Since the SCGM system provided trends and peak of IG change, which are difficult to know by only BG measurement, SCGM could be considered as being complementary to intermittent BG measurement.

The SCGM system can provide such useful information for glucose management; however, attention should be paid to the fact that the SCGM system has not been completely established as a substitutable device for BG measurement in the perioperative period because dissociation between BG and IG sometimes occurs [6–9]. For this reason, BG measurement is recommended before administration of insulin and/or glucose, and we avoided the use of automatic control by the insulin pump of the SCGM system. The dissociation is considered to be caused by some factors including the delay of IG to BG as shown in our case. The delay of IG to BG in diabetic patients has been reported to range from 4 to 10 minutes in the abdomen [10] and to be 12 minutes in both the abdomen and arm [11]. Other possible factors related to sensor performance are the site of sensor insertion, physiological changes including impaired peripheral perfusion induced by hypotension and/or use of vasopressors [6, 7], and calibration. The site for sensor insertion recommended by the manufacturer is a site where subcutaneous fat is thick, such as the upper arm, belly, upper hip, and thigh. Involvement of peripheral perfusion in sensor performance was indicated in some studies [6, 7]; however, another study demonstrated that the accuracy of SCGM was not influenced by the change of peripheral perfusion [12]. The timing and interval of calibration are also important factors to accurately use the SCGM system, and it has been shown that enhanced calibrations improved sensor accuracy [13]. Since such many factors have the potential to change the sensor accuracy, additional calibrations are recommended when the physiological situation drastically changes or surgery is prolonged and extended.

The usefulness of continuous glucose monitoring during insulinoma resection using an artificial endocrine pancreas has been reported [14]. Although an artificial endocrine pancreas can strictly control BG by automatically measuring BG and administering both glucose and insulin, it requires a large and complicated machine (36 kg) with additional venous catheterization. On the other hand, the SCGM system is small, less invasive, and easy to use. SCGM might be more acceptable to anesthesiologists and patients in clinical use.

In conclusion, we showed the utility of the use of a combination of SCGM and intermittent BG measurement for glucose management during insulinoma resection.

References

[1] T. Okabayashi, Y. Shima, T. Sumiyoshi et al., "Diagnosis and management of insulinoma," *World Journal of Gastroenterology*, vol. 19, no. 6, pp. 829–837, 2013.

[2] A. Abu-Zaid, L. A. Alghuneim, M. T. Metawee et al., "Sporadic insulinoma in a 10-year-old boy: A case report and literature review," *Journal of the Pancreas*, vol. 15, no. 1, pp. 53–57, 2014.

[3] J. Goswami, P. Somkuwar, and Y. Naik, "Insulinoma and anaesthetic implications," *Indian Journal of Anaesthesia*, vol. 56, no. 2, pp. 117–122, 2012.

[4] D. Rodbard, "Continuous glucose monitoring: A review of recent studies demonstrating improved glycemic outcomes," *Diabetes Technology & Therapeutics*, vol. 19, pp. S25–S37, 2017.

[5] W. V. Tamborlane, R. W. Beck, B. W. Bode et al., "Continuous glucose monitoring and intensive treatment of type 1 diabetes," *The New England Journal of Medicine*, vol. 359, no. 14, pp. 1464–1476, 2008.

[6] R. van Hooijdonk, J. H. Leopold, T. Winters et al., "Point accuracy and reliability of an interstitial continuous glucose-monitoring device in critically ill patients: a prospective study," *Critical Care*, vol. 19, no. 1, article no. 34, 2015.

[7] F. Schierenbeck, A. Franco-Cereceda, and J. Liska, "Accuracy of 2 Different Continuous Glucose Monitoring Systems in Patients Undergoing Cardiac Surgery," *Journal of Diabetes Science and Technology*, vol. 11, no. 1, pp. 108–116, 2017.

[8] I.-K. Song, J.-H. Lee, J.-E. Kang, Y.-H. Park, H.-S. Kim, and J.-T. Kim, "Continuous glucose monitoring system in the operating room and intensive care unit: any difference according to measurement sites?" *Journal of Clinical Monitoring and Computing*, vol. 31, no. 1, pp. 187–194, 2017.

[9] M. Munekage, T. Yatabe, M. Sakaguchi et al., "Comparison of subcutaneous and intravenous continuous glucose monitoring accuracy in an operating room and an intensive care unit," *The International Journal of Artificial Organs*, vol. 19, no. 2, pp. 159–166, 2016.

[10] M. S. Boyne, D. M. Silver, J. Kaplan, and C. D. Saudek, "Timing of Changes in Interstitial and Venous Blood Glucose Measured with a Continuous Subcutaneous Glucose Sensor," *Diabetes*, vol. 52, no. 11, pp. 2790–2794, 2003.

[11] B. P. Kovatchev, D. Shields, and M. Breton, "Graphical and numerical evaluation of continuous glucose sensing time lag," *Diabetes Technology & Therapeutics*, vol. 11, no. 3, pp. 139–143, 2009.

[12] S. E. Siegelaar, T. Barwari, J. Hermanides, P. H. J. Van Der Voort, J. B. L. Hoekstra, and J. H. Devries, "Microcirculation and its relation to continuous subcutaneous glucose sensor accuracy in cardiac surgery patients in the intensive care unit," *The Journal of Thoracic and Cardiovascular Surgery*, vol. 146, no. 5, pp. 1283–1289, 2013.

[13] L. Leelarathna, S. W. English, H. Thabit et al., "Accuracy of subcutaneous continuous glucose monitoring in critically ill adults: Improved sensor performance with enhanced calibrations," *Diabetes Technology & Therapeutics*, vol. 16, no. 2, pp. 97–101, 2014.

[14] K. Hirose, S. Kawahito, N. Mita et al., "Usefulness of artificial endocrine pancreas during resection of insulinoma," *Journal of Medical Investigation*, vol. 61, no. 3-4, pp. 421–425, 2014.

45

A Case Report of Suspected Malignant Hyperthermia: How Will the Diagnosis Affect a Patient's Insurability?

Brian M. Osman (ID),[1] **Isabela C. Saba,**[2] **and William A. Watson**[3]

[1]University of Miami, Miller School of Medicine, Department of Anesthesiology, 1400 NW 12th Avenue, Suite 3075, Miami, FL 33136, USA

[2]University of Miami, Miller School of Medicine, Department of Anesthesiology, 1801 NW 9th Avenue, 5th Floor, Miami, FL 33136, USA

[3]University of Miami, Miller School of Medicine, Department of Anesthesiology, 1611 NW 12th Avenue, Suite C-300, Miami, FL 33136, USA

Correspondence should be addressed to Brian M. Osman; bosman@med.miami.edu

Academic Editor: Abdullah Kaki

The purpose of this case report is to increase awareness that a diagnosis of malignant hyperthermia may have long-lasting or permanent effects on a patient's insurance eligibility or premiums despite legislation providing varying levels of protection from preexisting conditions or genetic discrimination. We present a case of severe rigors, unexplained severe metabolic acidosis, and severe hyperthermia in a patient after general anesthesia for extensive head and neck surgery. The patient was treated for malignant hyperthermia and demonstrated a significant clinical improvement with the administration of dantrolene. Even with an "almost certain" diagnosis of malignant hyperthermia by clinical presentation, genetic testing was negative and the gold-standard caffeine-halothane contracture test has yet to be performed. Laboratory results, clinical grading scales, and genetic testing support a diagnosis of malignant hyperthermia but the gold standard is a live muscle biopsy and caffeine-halothane contracture test. A clinical diagnosis of MH or a positive caffeine-halothane contracture test could result in exclusion from genetic discrimination legislature due to the fact that diagnosis can be confirmed without genetic testing. The fate of the Affordable Care Act may also affect how insurance companies scrutinize this disease. Improving accuracy of MH diagnosis in hospital discharge records will be crucial.

1. Introduction

Malignant hyperthermia (MH) is a disease of pharmacogenetics which presents with an abnormal increase in the body's basal metabolic rate, usually after exposure to specific triggering agents such as volatile anesthetic gasses, depolarizing muscle relaxants, and rarely stressors such as heat and vigorous exercise [1]. The Malignant Hyperthermia Association of the United States (MHAUS) estimates that MH affects roughly 1 in 100,000 adult surgeries and 1 in 30,000 pediatric cases [2]. The gold standard for diagnosing MH involves a caffeine-halothane contracture test (CHCT) on a live muscle biopsy sample, but certain clinical diagnostic criteria, laboratory results, and genetic tests may also provide evidence of the diagnosis [3]. MH is difficult and often time-consuming to diagnose but, in the face of a developing crisis,

clinicians cannot wait on genetic testing or a CHCT to guide dantrolene treatment. We present a challenging case of a patient whom we treated as if she were experiencing an acute MH crisis after suddenly presenting with severe postoperative rigors, extreme hyperpyrexia, and an unexplained severe metabolic acidosis. While the confirmation of the diagnosis is still pending, the patient's medical record mentions a high suspicion of MH susceptibility and subsequent treatment with dantrolene. The inability to rapidly confirm a diagnosis or even perform the gold-standard biopsy test in a single hospital admission can result in suspected or inaccurately diagnosed cases ending up as a preexisting condition in a patient's permanent medical record [4]. Denial of insurance coverage, exorbitant premiums, and discrimination based on preexisting conditions has garnered enough attention to result in various legislative protections, but the risk of repeal of current policies and implementation of new healthcare campaigns may have profound effects on the affordability or eligibility of insurance for patients who carry the diagnosis of MH.

2. Case Presentation

Informed consent was obtained from the patient as well as authorization to use or disclose protected health information. A 48-year-old ASA III female with infiltrative squamous cell carcinoma in the floor of the mouth presented for an extensive composite resection, free flap reconstruction, neck dissection, and tracheostomy. She had a medical history significant for hypertension, anemia, and 55 pack-years of cigarette smoking. Surgical history included minor procedures and was negative for any anesthetic complications, and there was no reported personal or family history of problems with anesthesia or intolerance to exercise or heat. The patient had no known drug allergies and was taking 20 mg of lisinopril daily, 120 mg of verapamil daily, 5mg of oxycodone as needed for pain, transdermal 50 mcg/hr fentanyl patch, and multivitamins. The anesthetic plan included general anesthesia and a postinduction radial arterial line. Intravenous induction was performed with 100 mcg of fentanyl, 80 mg of lidocaine, 150 mg of propofol, and 30 mg of rocuronium and the patient was intubated with a 7.0 mm endotracheal tube. Anesthesia was maintained with 2% Sevoflurane gas and IV fentanyl for the remainder of the 13-hour surgery. Two units of appropriately typed and crossed packed red blood cells were administered during the case to correct anemia. The arterial blood gases drawn before the conclusion of the case were within acceptable limits (Table 1). The patient emerged from anesthesia without incident, followed commands, denied pain or feeling cold, and was breathing spontaneously through the new tracheostomy. At 22:30 hours, report was given to the Intensivist and vital signs were reported to be stable with a heart rate of 110 beats per minute, blood pressure of 135/75 mmHg, respiratory rate of 22 breaths per minute, oxygen saturation of 100%, and a temperature of 96.4 F. At 23:00 hours, the anesthesia team was called by the ICU to reevaluate the patient for the sudden onset of severe rigors and an acute rise in temperature to 102.5 F, which had occurred over the course of 15 minutes (indicating an increase of 2 degrees F every 5 minutes). An arterial-blood gas taken less than 10 minutes after the onset of symptoms demonstrated a new onset metabolic acidosis and extreme base deficit (Table 2). We observed severe generalized rigors, hyperthermia, tachycardia, and a respiratory rate of 50 breaths per minute. Ruling out the differential diagnoses of uncontrolled pain, sepsis, hypoglycemia, seizure disorder, thyroid storm, neuroleptic malignant syndrome, transfusion reaction, or medication withdrawal, we suspected a diagnosis of MH and called the MHAUS 24-hour MH Hotline. Ice packs were applied to cool the patient and we ordered the appropriate labs to support the MH diagnosis and rule out other conditions (Tables 2 and 3). Within approximately 20 minutes after the initial onset of symptoms, the MH cart was opened and dantrolene (20 mg vials reconstituted with 60 ml of sterile water) was given according to the MHAUS dosing recommendations (2.5mg/kg, followed by 1 mg/kg, and then 1 mg/kg IV every 6 hours until symptoms subside). After the second dose, within approximately 5 minutes, the patient's temperature trended down to 99 degrees F and the base excess improved (Table 2). Simultaneously, the muscle rigidity, tachycardia, and tachypnea all resolved. The patient was continuously monitored and the remaining ICU course was uneventful.

Generalized weakness and muscle soreness were reported up to 5 days afterward, but the patient fully recovered and was eventually discharged home. Genetic testing was sent to a lab for sequencing of both the RYR1 and CACNA1S genes, known to be associated with MH. After approximately one week, the results for our patient returned negative. Due to the extensive nature of the patient's surgery and financial concerns, the CHCT has yet to be performed.

3. Discussion

Malignant hyperthermia (MH) may be considered rare, but it is remarkably lethal if left untreated. Confirming a diagnosis requires harvesting a freshly biopsied muscle tissue sample to be tested at one of only four available centers in the United States. The obvious challenges to completing the caffeine-halothane contracture test can lead clinicians to treat even suspected cases of MH before having the opportunity to confirm the diagnosis. Even with a valid health insurance policy, some companies label the test as "experimental" and may limit or deny coverage altogether [2]. However, collecting a blood sample while in the ICU to send for MH susceptibility genetic testing was a viable option for our case. Mutations of the RYR1 and CACNA1S genes are associated with MH and 42 different RYR1 mutations and 2 CACNA1S mutations have been identified to date [5]. Per MHAUS, RYR1 gene sequencing is currently available at only two accredited molecular genetics laboratories in the United States [2] and substantial efforts were required on our part in order to link the laboratory at our hospital with one of these testing centers. Genetic testing for diseases is becoming more accessible, spurring medical advances, but is also increasing the interest of insurance companies to develop more accurate customer risk stratifications [6]. The outcome of these genetic tests could therefore affect the pricing or structure of insurance available to a patient found to have a genetic disease or abnormality. As this fear of genetic discrimination began to permeate society and leach into health policy and political agendas, legislation introducing some nondiscrimination provisions was included in the Health Insurance Portability and Accountability Act (HIPAA) of 1996 and the Genetic Information Nondiscrimination Act (GINA) of 2008 [7]. A handful of states in the United States also provide some additional protective provisions. The idea was to prevent health insurers or health plan adjusters from utilizing genetic information to determine a patient's coverage and premium adjustments or impose exclusions for preexisting conditions. GINA also prohibited the use of genetic information to make decisions regarding hiring, firing, promotion, or other terms

TABLE 1: Arterial-blood gases at 3 and 2 hours before end of surgery.

Date	10/10/16	10/10/16
Time	17:54 (3 hours before surgery end)	19:04 (2 hours before surgery end)
Glucose (65-99 mg/dL)[a]	151	144
pH[b] (7.35 – 7.45)	7.37	7.36
pCO2[c] (35-45 mmHg)[d]	40.7	39.2
pO2[e] (65-100 mmHg room air)[d]	173	177
BE[f] (-3- + 3 mEq/L)[g]	0	-3
HCO3[h] (22-26 mmol/L)[i]	24.3	22.6
Hb[j] (12.0-16.0 g/dL)[k]	5.5	9.5
Hct[l] (36-48 %)	17	28
O2Hb[m] (>90 %)	100	100
Potassium (3.5–5.0 mmol/L)[i]	3.8	3.7
Sodium (136-145 mmol/L)[i]	138	140

[a]mg/dL = milligrams per deciliter; [b]pH = potential of hydrogen; [c]pCO2 = partial pressure of carbon dioxide; [d]mmHg = millimeters of mercury; [e]p02 = partial pressure of oxygen; [f]BE = base excess; [g]mEq /L = milliequivalents per liter; [h]HCO3 = bicarbonate ion; [i]mmol/L = millimoles per liter; [j]Hb = hemoglobin; [k]g/dL = grams per deciliter; [l]Hct = Hematocrit; [m]O2Hb = oxygen saturation of hemoglobin.

TABLE 2: Arterial-blood gases during postoperative course.

Date	10/10/16	10/10/16	10/11/16	10/11/16	10/11/16	10/11/16	10/11/16	10/11/16	10/12/16
Time	23:07[1]	23:15	00:32[2]	02:20	03:07	09:35	15:30	21:22	04:45
pH[a] (7.35 – 7.45)	7.139	7.179	7.468	7.653	7.532	7.608	7.51	7.5	7.424
pCO2[b] (35-45 mmHg)[c]	31.6	31.4	25.8	14.4	21.7	21	26.8	28.9	36.7
pO2[d] (65-100 mmHg)[c]	221	213	157.6	123	565.7	95.5	104.7	83	67.7
BE[e] (-3 - + 3 mEq/L)[f]	-17	-15	-4.2	-3.9	-4.1	-0.4	-1.2	-0.1	-0.8
HCO3[g] (22-26 mmol/L)[h]	10.7	11.7	18.3	15.6	17.8	20.6	21	22	23.5
Hb[i] (12.0-16.0 g/dL)[j]	9.5	9.9	11	8	7.4	7.2	10.1	12.2	7.3
O2Hb[k] (>90 %)	100	100	97.9	98	98.7	97.1	97.6	95.6	92.7
Potassium (3.5-5.2 mmol/L)[h]	3.4	3.5	4.1	3.7	3.6	3.1	3.2	3.6	3.8
Sodium (135-145 mmol/L)[h]	140	142	145	141	141	142	140	140	137

[a]pH = potential of hydrogen; [b]pCO2 = partial pressure of carbon dioxide; [c]mmHg = millimeters of mercury; [d]p02 = partial pressure of oxygen; [e]BE = base excess; [f]mEq/L = milliequivalents per liter; [g]HCO3 = bicarbonate ion; [h]mmol /L = millimoles per liter; [i]Hb = hemoglobin; [j]g /dL = grams per deciliter; [k]O2Hb = oxygen saturation of hemoglobin.

[1]Time of first arterial-blood gas after anesthesia consulted for suspected MH.
[2]Time of first arterial-blood gas after treatment with dantrolene.

of employment [7]. It is important to mention that GINA may have offered many protections against genetic discrimination, but several restrictions and exceptions existed allowing for loopholes with potentially profound consequences. For example, GINA provisions did not apply to life insurance, disability, or long-term care insurance, there was no mandate to provide coverage for genetic services, GINA did not prohibit the use of genetic test information in health insurance reimbursement decisions, and once genetic information has manifested itself into an actual health condition, this condition would no longer be protected by GINA [6, 7]. More

important to the discussion of our patient with suspected MH, genetic testing is highly specific, but the sensitivity can be only about 50% [8]. Therefore, a negative test cannot rule out MH susceptibility and we relied more on the clinical signs and supportive laboratory results. A clinical diagnosis based on symptomatology or the caffeine-halothane contracture test is made without the utilization of genetic testing. Therefore, there are no provisions or protections from GINA for MH testing performed on an *in vitro* muscle biopsy. The recent Affordable Care Act (ACA) of 2010 and the GINA 2011 update enhanced consumer protections in the

TABLE 3: Postoperative supporting follow-up labs from ICU.

Date	10/11/16	10/11/16	10/11/16	10/11/16	10/11/16	10/11/16	10/11/16	10/12/16
Time	0:00	2:00	2:49	5:50	9:38	15:00	20:32	4:50
Creatine Kinase (26-192 U/L)[a]	913	1038			1022	1177		
CK-MB[b] (0-6 ng/mL)[c]	9.1	7			7		3	
Myoglobin, plasma (28-58 ng/mL)[c]			888		638	566	410	261
Troponin-T (0-0.06 ng/mL)[c]	<0.01	<0.01						
Lactic Acid, plasma (0.5-2.0 mmol/L)[d]	10			3.9				

[a]U/L = units per liter; [b]CK -MB = creatine kinase muscle/brain; [c]ng /mL = nanograms per milliliter; [d]mmol/L = millimoles per liter.

TABLE 4: Larach et al.'s clinical grading scale for malignant hyperthermia[1].

Clinical finding (maximum score)	Manifestation
Respiratory acidosis (15 points)	End-tidal CO_2 >55 mmHg, $PaCO_2$ >60 mmHg
Cardiac involvement (3 points)	Unexplained sinus tachycardia, ventricular tachycardia, or ventricular fibrillation
Metabolic acidosis (10 points)	Base deficit >8 mEq/L, pH <7.25
Muscle rigidity (15 points)	Generalized rigidity, severe masseter muscle rigidity
Muscle breakdown (15 points)	Serum creatine kinase concentration >20,000/L units, cola-colored urine, excess myoglobin in urine or serum, plasma [K+] >6 mEq/L
Temperature increase (15 points)	Rapidly increasing temperature, T >38.8° C
Other	Rapid reversal of MH signs with dantrolene (score=5 points), elevated resting serum creatine kinase concentration (score=10 points)
Family history (15 points)	Consistent with autosomal dominant inheritance

(1) From Rosenberg H, Sambuughin N, Riazi S, Dirksen R. Malignant hyperthermia susceptibility; synonym: malignant hyperpyrexia. 2003 [Updated 2013]. In: Adam MP, Ardinger HH, Pagon RA, et al., editors. GeneReviews [Internet]. University of Washington, Seattle; 1993-2018. Available from: https://www.ncbi.nlm.nih.gov/books/NBK1146/. Accessed October 13, 2018.

private health insurance market to prohibit issuers of health insurance from discriminating against patients with genetic diseases by refusing coverage or adjusting premiums because of preexisting conditions [7]. Our patient's RYRI/CACNA1S genetic test did not return with any identifiable mutations and the caffeine-halothane test is pending at the patient's discretion. Our decision to administer dantrolene was based on the guidance provided by the MHAUS 24-Hour Hotline and the utilization of the clinical grading scale developed by Larach and colleagues (Table 4), wherein a higher score implies a greater likelihood of a MH. Our patient received a raw score of 83 points, where a score of 50+ points is "almost certainly" associated with a diagnosis of MH [3, 9]. In further support of a probable diagnosis of MH, the rapid reversal of metabolic acidosis associated with dantrolene administration increased our patient's Larach scale score by 5 additional points to a total score of 88 [3, 9].

Pending confirmation, the patient's medical record mentions suspicion of MH susceptibility and treatment with dantrolene for malignant hyperthermia. This information will remain in the patient's permanent medical record and could be viewed as a preexisting condition. With the current protections put fourth by the ACA and GINA, a clinical diagnosis of MH should not put the patient at risk of being rejected by any health insurance plan, paying higher premiums, or result in refusal of payment while carrying a diagnosis of MH. However, the ACA does not cover life insurance, disability, or other types of supplemental insurance and our patient would continue to be at risk for wide variability of access or affordability. The current debates for repealing or replacing of any of the protections offered by the ACA or adopting the proposed American Health Care Act may completely change our patient's access to even basic health insurance in the future.

In conclusion, making a clinical diagnosis of MH can be problematic and confirmation of the disease is cumbersome and not usually possible on a single admission. There is no test that can be applied acutely to distinguish MH from other causes of hypermetabolism or hyperthermia [4]. The symptoms may occur at any time during the perioperative period and can be highly variable. This case is unique in that our patient developed suspicious symptoms at a very late stage of the perioperative period, given that the patient inhaled volatile anesthetic for 13 hours before any symptoms appeared. We stress the importance of considering MH even with an unusual or extremely late presentation and also pose that prompt, proactive treatment with dantrolene may significantly blunt the disease process. MHAUS recommends that all facilities where MH triggering anesthetics and depolarizing muscle relaxants are administered should stock dantrolene [10]. It is widely available, from generic formulations to more sophisticated preparations designed to reduce the number of vials needed for reconstitution of the drug. Brandom et al. demonstrated that the complications with dantrolene are rarely life-threatening but may include muscle weakness (14.6%), phlebitis (9.2%), and gastrointestinal upset (4.3%) [11]. The benefits of using dantrolene with our patient certainly outweighed the risks, resulting in a favorable outcome, but such prudent clinical decisions may have long-lasting effects. Pinyavat et al. explain that miscoding for MH, preemptively treating suspicious cases with dantrolene (as with our case), and even simply having a family member with the disease have contributed to a significant number of cases being added to Medicaid and Medicare databases, as well as individual state hospital discharge databases, listing MH as "present on admission," and have resulted in MH being identified as a preexisting condition [4]. Without confirmation via the caffeine-halothane contracture test, we will never be certain of the diagnosis with our patient. This case of suspected MH, in the arena of an uncertain health insurance market, has highlighted the importance of improving the accuracy and awareness of diagnosing someone with a serious disease capable of marring the patient's permanent health record with a preexisting condition.

References

[1] H. Rosenberg, N. Pollock, A. Schiemann, T. Bulger, and K. Stowell, "Malignant hyperthermia: a review," *Orphanet Journal of Rare Diseases*, vol. 10, no. 1, article no. 310, pp. 1–19, 2015.

[2] "MHAUS guidelines: testing for malignant hyperthermia (MH) susceptibility: how do I counsel my patients?" Malignant Hyperthermia Association of the United States, https://www.mhaus.org/testing/introduction-to-mh-testing/testing-for-malignant-hyperthermia-mh-susceptibility-how-do-i-counsel-my-patients/ ; 2018 [accessed 4 April 2018].

[3] H. Rosenberg, N. Sambuughin, S. Riazi, and R. Dirksen, *Malignant Hyperthermia Susceptibility; Synonym: Malignant Hyperpyrexia*, M. P. Adam, H. H. Ardinger, and R. A. Pagon, Eds., vol. 128, GeneReviews, University of Washington, Seattle, Washington, USA, 2003.

[4] T. Pinyavat, H. Rosenberg, B. H. Lang et al., "Accuracy of malignant hyperthermia diagnoses in hospital discharge records," *Anesthesiology*, vol. 122, no. 1, pp. 55–63, 2015.

[5] "Diagnostic MH mutations," Euoprean Malignant Hyperthermia Group, https://www.emhg.org/diagnostic-mutations , 2018 [accessed 11 April 2018].

[6] A. Nill, G. Laczniak, and P. Thistle, "The use of genetic testing information in the insurance industry: an ethical and societal analysis of public policy," *Journal of Business Ethics*, pp. 1–17, 2017.

[7] A. A. Parkman, J. Foland, B. Anderson et al., "Public Awareness of Genetic Nondiscrimination Laws in Four States and Perceived Importance of Life Insurance Protections," *Journal of Genetic Counseling*, vol. 24, no. 3, pp. 512–521, 2015.

[8] D. Schneiderbanger, S. Johannsen, N. Roewer, and F. Schuster, "Management of malignant hyperthermia: Diagnosis and treatment," *Therapeutics and Clinical Risk Management*, vol. 10, no. 1, pp. 355–362, 2014.

[9] M. G. Larach, A. R. Localio, G. C. Allen et al., "A clinical grading scale to predict malignant hyperthermia susceptibility," *Anesthesiology*, vol. 80, no. 4, pp. 771–779, 1994.

[10] "Frequently asked questions," Malignant Hyperthermia Association of the United States, https://www.mhaus.org/faqs/how-quickly-must-dantrolene-be-accessible/ ; 2011 [Accessed 15 October 2018].

[11] B. W. Brandom, M. G. Larach, M.-S. A. Chen, and M. C. Young, "Complications associated with the administration of dantrolene 1987 to 2006: A report from the North American malignant hyperthermia registry of the malignant hyperthermia association of the United States," *Anesthesia & Analgesia*, vol. 112, no. 5, pp. 1115–1123, 2011.

Early Detection and Management of Massive Intraoperative Pulmonary Embolism in a Patient Undergoing Repair of a Traumatic Acetabular Fracture

Tobechi E. Okoronkwo, XueWei Zhang, Jessica Dworet, and Matthew Wecksell ⓘD

New York Medical College-Westchester Medical Center, USA

Correspondence should be addressed to Matthew Wecksell; matthew.wecksell@wmchealth.org

Academic Editor: Ilok Lee

A 73-year-old male with history of hyperlipidemia and osteoarthritis was transferred from an outside hospital after a fall from a ladder at home. He sustained a severe right sided acetabular fracture involving the femoral head, requiring operative repair. Preoperative evaluation was unremarkable except for oxygen saturation < 95 %. After induction of anesthesia and surgical positioning, the patient went into cardiac arrest. After intraoperative cardiopulmonary resuscitation (CPR) and placement on extracorporeal membrane oxygenation (ECMO), the patient stabilized. Cardiac catheterization revealed a large left pulmonary embolism. Here, we discuss the etiology and management of intraoperative pulmonary embolism.

1. Introduction

Perioperative pulmonary emboli (PE) in trauma patients are common. The incidence of thromboembolic events in trauma patients has been estimated at up to 63% [1] and the incidence of subclinical thromboemboli is higher still. The associated mortality of PE has reportedly been greater than 50% [2]. While timely diagnosis and treatment of PE can significantly improve patient survival [3], PE can be difficult to detect prior to hemodynamic collapse. Massive pulmonary embolism is often associated with physiologic instability characterized by acute right ventricular dysfunction, hypoxemia unresponsive to conventional therapy and cardiac arrest. Treatment of patients following massive PE with persistent shock includes installation of extracorporeal membrane oxygenation (ECMO), emergent pulmonary embolectomy, and thrombolysis. There lacks an overall consensus regarding which is the gold standard treatment modality [4].

While the American Society of Anesthesiologists (ASA) standard monitors have their role in diagnosis of PE, typically by demonstrating cardiovascular collapse, monitoring modalities like transesophageal echocardiography (TEE) and pulmonary artery catheters (PACs) have greater specificity and sensitivity. TEE and PACs can aid in therapeutic management of PE, especially in the hands of experienced personnel. While diagnostically helpful, TEE and PACs are not incorporated at the beginning of a standard orthopedic operation in a patient with no significant medical history. Here, we present a case of pulmonary embolism occurring after the induction of anesthesia and positioning in a patient with an extensive right acetabulum fracture. Our goal is to evaluate the available modalities for early detection and supportive care after hemodynamic collapse. The patient's family has given written consent to publish this case report.

2. Case Presentation

The patient is a 73-year-old male who was transferred from an outside hospital for repair of a right acetabulum fracture involving the femoral head after falling approximately 8-feet from a ladder while painting his house. Past medical history was significant for hyperlipidemia and osteoarthritis. Baseline metabolic equivalents were greater than four. Aside from a cataract extraction, the patient had no other operations. He denied any allergies. Prior to presentation, the patient was on Aspirin 81 mg daily for cardiovascular disease prevention and Atorvastatin 20 mg daily for hyperlipidemia. Computed tomography (CT) without contrast showed an acute, comminuted, and displaced fracture of the right acetabulum involving both posterior and anterior acetabular walls. The right femoral head was superiorly and laterally displaced with impaction fracture to its inferior and medial aspects. There were bone fragments within the right gluteus musculature, and the high attenuation in tissue density represented blood product within. Prior to surgery, the orthopedic team made an effort to reduce the patient's right acetabulum fracture with tibial traction pin under conscious sedation with midazolam, fentanyl, and ketamine in the emergency department. During the closed reduction, the patient experienced a brief period of respiratory depression. For approximately two minutes, his oxygen saturation was 85-86%, which improved to 95% with Narcan reversal. The emergency department record also noted that the patient had premature ventricular contractions on the electrocardiogram (EKG) at this time. After the closed reduction, the orthopedic team opted to monitor the patient on continuous telemetry for 24 hours and take the patient for open reduction and internal fixation of the right acetabulum the next day. He was not on prophylactic anticoagulation for this preoperative period.

Prior to entering the operating room, the patient's vital signs were stable: blood pressure 120/64, heart rate 73 beats per minute, respiratory rate 18 per minute, oxygen saturation 95%, and temperature 98.6 Fahrenheit. Neurological exam was significant for limited right knee flexion (<30 degrees). Otherwise, overall sensation was intact and right deep tendon reflex was intact. Hemoglobin was 11.6, down from 13.4 on admission. Coagulation tests showed elevated prothrombin time at 12.8, partial thromboplastin time 26.7, and international normalized ratio 1.20. In the OR, the patient was induced with standard dosing of midazolam, fentanyl, lidocaine, propofol, and succinylcholine. Phenylephrine was given preemptively on induction to avoid hypotension. Intubation was uncomplicated. Patient had two 20g peripheral intravenous catheter in place, and a left radial arterial line was placed after intubation. Despite premedication with phenylephrine, the patient became hypotensive with systolic blood pressure (SBP) in the 80s, median arterial pressure < 65. Boluses of ephedrine and phenylephrine were given, and a phenylephrine infusion was started thirty minutes after induction. The patient initially responded appropriately to treatment (SBP > 100). Due to concern for sciatic nerve injury, intraoperative somatosensory evoked potential (SSEP) monitoring was performed, and general anesthesia was maintained with propofol at 100 mcg/kg/min and remifentanil at 0.2 mcg/kg/min, in addition to 0.5% end tidal sevoflurane.

Upon patient positioning to the right lateral decubitus position from supine, the patient's SBP acutely declined into the 50s and the patient became hypoxic with an oxygen saturation of 88%. His hypotension was no longer responsive to phenylephrine or ephedrine. Norepinephrine and epinephrine drips were started. Also, the FiO2 was increased from 50% to 100%. There was a minimal and transient response to epinephrine administration. The patient was then returned to supine position, and he arrested shortly

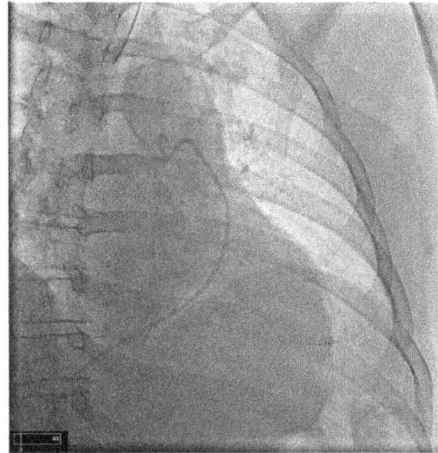

FIGURE 1: Before injection with catheter in pulmonary artery.

thereafter. Chest compressions commenced immediately upon loss of cardiac rhythm. The cardiac anesthesia team emergently responded and performed an intraoperative transesophageal echocardiography (TEE), which showed reduced left ventricular ejection fraction and reduced right ventricular systolic function. Due to unsuccessful cardiopulmonary resuscitation, the patient was placed on venoarterial ECMO via right femoral artery and vein; stable hemodynamics were achieved. A total of 8000 units of Heparin was given upon ECMO installation. At this point, the planned surgery was aborted. The patient was transported to the cardiac catheterization lab for pulmonary angiogram, cardiac catheterization, and antegrade perfusion of the right superficial femoral artery. A large thrombus in the left pulmonary artery was discovered on selective angiography (Figures 1–4). Hypothermic protocol was initiated. Heparin therapy was also continued at this point.

On hospital day 5, a CT chest with contrast showed multiple bilateral pulmonary emboli and evidence of right ventricular failure. Right heart catheterization and placement of a Swan-Ganz catheter demonstrated that the patient was found to have severe pulmonary hypertension 55/30 and elevated central venous pressure (CVP) of 18. The patient underwent bilateral pulmonary artery embolectomy, exploration of right atrium with removal of clots, discontinuation of ECMO support, and repair of right femoral artery on hospital day 9. His pulmonary artery pressure and CVP improved to 31/12 and 8, respectively. One month later, the patient was discharged to a rehabilitation facility with a plan for conservative management of his fracture.

3. Discussion

Early detection and treatment of PE are essential to improving morbidities and mortalities of patients with traumatic injuries. PE is often diagnosed clinically using the history, vital signs, and symptoms to guide in the detection of a thrombus [5]. PE is often diagnosed clinically using the history, vital signs, and symptoms to guide in the detection

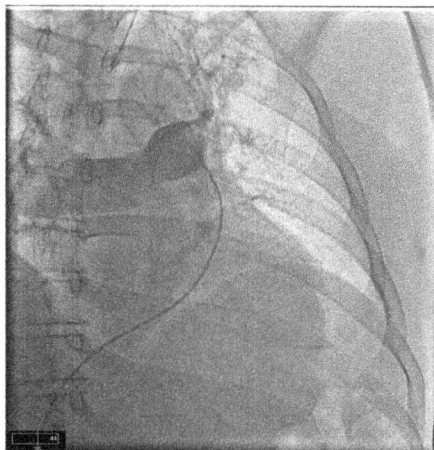

FIGURE 2: Start of injection with contrast showing mainly in the right lung with some contrast in the left upper lobe.

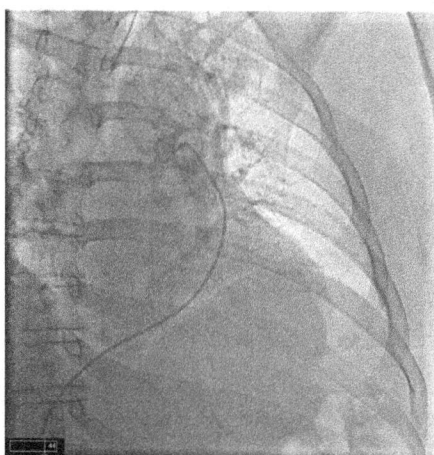

FIGURE 3: After injection with minimal perfusion of the left upper lobe and almost no perfusion of the left lower lobe.

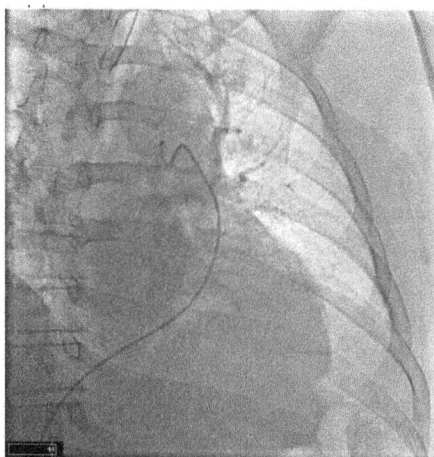

FIGURE 4: After injection without any significant perfusion of the left lung, especially in the lower lobe.

of a thrombus. When using pulse oximetry as an indicator of PE, the finding is usually a sudden and drastic drop in oxygen saturation. Retrospectively, the patient's low preoperative oxygen saturation may be secondary to the thrombus in his pulmonary artery (Figures 1–4). Indeed, the development of venous thromboembolism (VTE) likely occurred prior to surgery. He may have had small microemboli in place causing his low oxygen saturation before surgery.

As mentioned earlier, the development of venous thromboembolism (VTE) likely occurred prior to surgery. Major trauma often leads to the risk factors in Virchow's triad or hypercoagulability, endothelial injury, and venous stasis. The patient might have had microembolies derived from peripheral bone marrow cellular aggregates trapped in the lung vessels, causing his low oxygen saturation before surgery. Moreover, his injury caused direct disruption to the endothelial glycocalyx layer (EGL), which leads to release of both procoagulant and anticoagulant factors though procoagulant ones prevail [6]. This endothelial activation after trauma may be caused by vasoactive catecholamines, inflammatory mediators such as tumor necrosis factor-alpha (TN F-α), thrombin, and hypoxia [7]. This can lead both to pulmonary microemboli as well as the formation of larger deep venous emboli.

Immobility and reduced blood flow from the injury also contributed significantly to VTE development in this patient. On a microscopic level, hypoperfusion is associated with decreased level of protein C, which is an important anticoagulant because activated protein C deactivates factor Va and VIIIa [6]. Activated protein C mediated fibrinolysis is hindered as well. Trauma induced coagulopathy is a complex process, and both microembolism and classical pulmonary embolism derived from a peripheral DVT were at play in this case – leading both to preoperative mild hypoxia events, and an acute catastrophic event on positioning. The inciting event causing a venous thrombus to detach and embolize is often unknown [8], but can be associated with clot propagating maneuvers, as there have been case reports citing tourniquet placement as the initiator of clot migration [5]. Subsequent repositioning of our patient in the operating room may have caused a larger venous thrombus to become dislodged and embolize to the pulmonary arteries, leading to cardiac arrest.

Pulmonary angiogram is the gold standard for diagnosis, but it is often possible to begin the evaluation with a less invasive test. Intraoperative TEE is extremely useful for monitoring and diagnosis. One study discovered that in 19 out of 22 cardiac arrests, TEE was successful in establishing a diagnosis [9]. In addition, TEE provides a survival benefit, allowing clot visualization and initiation of specific treatment plans [2, 9]. Orthopedic and trauma patients are some of those at highest risk for thrombi, but cardiac anesthesiologists are seldom found administering these anesthetics. Although right ventricular strain is the most common finding in these cases, our patient showed a global deterioration [9]. One explanation is that the patient's extensive fracture resulted in occult bleeding which contributed to severe hemodynamic instability and cardiac arrest.

ECMO has been previously described as a treatment modality for patients with massive pulmonary embolism and resulting shock [4, 10, 11], but it is not without significant risk. Dolmatova et al. described five cases of near fatal pulmonary embolism in which ECMO was used. In these cases the overall mortality was 40%, with one death resulting from an ECMO-related complication and another death from the inability to maintain cerebral perfusion [4]. On the other hand, ECMO has been successfully implemented in patients with pulmonary embolism that remain unstable despite aggressive resuscitation. The 90-day-survival was 47% in one study where ECMO was used in 17 unstable patients with pulmonary embolism [11]. In the same study, fifteen (88%) patients suffered severe hemorrhage, but there was no influence on overall survival [11]. In a review of case reports and case series published over the past 20 years, there was an overall survival rate of 70% in patients with massive PE. When comparing thrombolysis, catheter embolectomy, and surgical embolectomy, the mortality was not affected by the treatment modality. However, patients who had ECMO instituted during cardiorespiratory arrest had a higher risk of death [5].

Trauma patients are at increased risk of VTE due to the presence of Virchow's triad of hypercoagulability, endothelial injury, and venous stasis [1]. This patient likely experienced all three. Injury to blood vessels can cause intimal damage that results in thrombosis. Prolonged bed rest and hypoperfusion cause venous stasis. A hypercoagulable state results from decreased levels of antithrombin III and suppression of thrombolysis [1]. Because of this patient's extensive fracture, his risk of VTE was particularly high. The benefits of starting anticoagulation early may outweigh the bleeding risks of doing so prior to surgery. Looking back at the course of this patient, the time from injury to repair was prolonged by interhospital transfer and initial attempt to perform closed reduction of his fracture. During this two-day period, the patient may benefit from multiple doses of anticoagulation with close monitoring for bleeding (hemoglobin and hematocrit, imaging) with the intention of holding anticoagulation just prior to the operation. However, frequently studies focus on prevention of VTE events after orthopedic surgeries, and not much has been established regarding the benefits and risks of presurgery thromboprophylaxis regimens [12–14]. Furthermore, most controlled trials compare different anticoagulant medications rather than the preoperative versus postoperative timing of the anticoagulation. In Europe, low molecular weight heparin (LMWH) is traditionally started before surgery, whereas in North America a higher dose of LMWH is usually started postoperatively due to concern for hemorrhage [15]. However, one study compared preoperative and postoperative thromboprophylaxis in patients with femoral neck fractures. They examined 25,019 patients from the Norwegian Hip Fractures Resister who underwent hemiarthroplasties for femoral neck fractures. 99% of these patients received LMWH. They found that starting anticoagulation postoperatively resulted in an increased mortality (RR 1.13) and a higher risk of reoperation (RR 1.19) compared to patients who started anticoagulation preoperatively [15]. Furthermore, there was no difference in bleeding complications. Using a lower dose of LMWH was also associated with the lower mortality and reoperation risk [15]. This study,

although not a randomized controlled trial, does support the use of a lower dose of LMWH preoperatively.

The American College of Chest Physicians (ACCP) guidelines recommends the use of low molecular weight heparin for major trauma patients as soon as it is safe to do so [1]. Trauma patients have a high incidence of VTE [16, 17]. However, patient mortality due to PE following total joint replacement was not significantly affected by the type of thromboprophylaxis regimen [14]. After elective total joint replacement in 4253 patients, the incidence of fatal PE was very low (0.07%) [15]. Overall mortality was higher in patients on potent anticoagulants than on patients receiving aspirin combined with regional anesthesia. The incidence of nonfatal PE was also higher in patients on potent anticoagulants. Thus, PE occurs despite the use of anticoagulants [16]. However, these types of elective orthopedic surgeries cannot be directly compared to trauma patients with extensive orthopedic injuries. In trauma patients, the initiation of anticoagulation is often delayed due to concerns of injury associated bleeding. In a multicenter prospective cohort study [16], VTE prophylaxis was initiated within 48 hours of injury in 25% of patients, but 25% did not receive anticoagulation for at least seven days. Early prophylaxis was associated with a 5% risk of VTE. Delay of anticoagulation beyond 4 days resulted in a threefold increase in the risk of VTE. Factors associated with the late initiation of prophylaxis included severe head injury, absence of comorbidities, and massive transfusion [16].

4. Conclusion

The current practice of withholding anticoagulation prior to surgery in trauma patients with orthopedic injuries at high risk of VTE is not indicated. The risk/benefit ratio of preoperative anticoagulation must be carefully considered and weighed against the risk of VTE. Further research is needed to clarify the use of preoperative anticoagulation in orthopedic trauma patients.

Authors' Contributions

Tobechi E. Okoronkwo wrote the case report, researched the topic, and presented the case at the 2017 cardiac anesthesia conference. Jessica Dworet helped edit the case report and contributed to the case description as the primary anesthesiologist for the case. Matthew Wecksell helped edit the case report, researched the topic, assisted in the resuscitation, and obtained consent for publication. XueWei Zhang helped edit the case report and researched the topic.

References

[1] S. Toker, D. Hak, and S. Morgan, "Deep vein thrombosis prophylaxis in trauma patients," *Thrombosis*, vol. 2011, Article ID 505373, 11 pages, 2011.

[2] O. Visnjevac, L. Pourafkari, and N. D. Nader, "Role of peri-operative monitoring in diagnosis of massive intraoperative cardiopulmonary embolism," *Journal Of Cardiovascular and Thoracic Research*, vol. 6, no. 3, pp. 141–145, 2014.

[3] A. M. Smeltz, L. M. Kolarczyk, and R. S. Isaak, "Update on perioperative pulmonary embolism management: A decision support tool to aid in diagnosis and treatment," *Advances in Anesthesia*, vol. 35, no. 1, pp. 213–228, 2017.

[4] H. Yusuff, V. Zochios, and A. Vuylsteke, "Extracorporeal membrane oxygenation in acute massive pulmonary embolism: a systematic review," *Perfusion*, vol. 30, no. 8, pp. 611–616, 2015.

[5] L. Sermeus, J. Van Hemelrijck, J. Vandommele, and H. Van Aken, "Pulmonary embolism confirmed by transoesophageal echocardiography," *Anaesthesia*, vol. 47, no. 1, pp. 28-29, 1992.

[6] R. Chang, J. C. Cardenas, C. E. Wade, and J. B. Holcomb, "Advances in the understanding of trauma-induced coagulopathy," *Blood*, vol. 128, no. 8, pp. 1043–1049, 2016.

[7] R. Chang, J. C. Cardenas, C. E. Wade, and J. B. Holcomb, "Advances in the understanding of trauma-induced coagulopathy," in *Blood*, blood-2016-01-636423, 2016.

[8] R. Parakh, V. V. Kakkar, and A. K. Kakkar, "Management of venous thromboembolism," *The Journal of the Association of Physicians of India*, vol. 55, pp. 49–70, 2007.

[9] S. Garvin, O. Stundner, and S. G. Memtsoudis, "Transesophageal echocardiography during cardiac arrest in orthopedic surgery patients: A report of two cases and a review of the literature," *HSS Journal ®*, vol. 9, no. 3, pp. 275–277, 2013.

[10] E. V. Dolmatova, K. Moazzami, T. P. Cocke et al., "Extracorporeal membrane oxygenation in massive pulmonary embolism," *Heart & Lung: The Journal of Acute and Critical Care*, vol. 46, no. 2, pp. 106–109, 2017.

[11] F. Corsi, G. Lebreton, N. Bréchot et al., "Life-threatening massive pulmonary embolism rescued by venoarterial-extracorporeal membrane oxygenation," *Critical Care*, vol. 21, no. 1, p. 76, 2017.

[12] O. E. Dahl, T. E. Gudmundsen, B. T. Bjørnarå, and D. M. Solheim, "Risk of clinical pulmonary embolism after joint surgery in patients receiving low-molecular-weight heparin prophylaxis in hospital: A 10-year prospective register of 3,954 patients," *Acta Orthopaedica*, vol. 74, no. 3, pp. 299–304, 2003.

[13] A. Gonzalez Della Valle, A. Blanes Perez, Y.-Y. Lee et al., "The clinical severity of patients diagnosed with an in-hospital pulmonary embolism following modern, elective joint arthroplasty is unrelated to the location of emboli in the pulmonary vasculature," *The Journal of Arthroplasty*, vol. 32, no. 4, pp. 1304–1309, 2017.

[14] L. A. Poultsides, A. Gonzalez Della Valle, S. G. Memtsoudis et al., "Meta-analysis of cause of death following total joint replacement using different thromboprophylaxis regimens," *The Journal of Bone & Joint Surgery (British Volume)*, vol. 94, no. 1, pp. 113–121, 2012.

[15] L. A. Cusick and D. E. Beverland, "The incidence of fatal pulmonary embolism after primary hip and knee replacement in a consecutive series of 4253 patients," *The Journal of Bone & Joint Surgery (British Volume)*, vol. 91, no. 5, pp. 645–648, 2009.

[16] A. B. Nathens, M. K. McMurray, J. Cuschieri et al., "The practice of venous thromboembolism prophylaxis in the major trauma patient," *Journal of Trauma - Injury Infection and Critical Care*, vol. 62, no. 3, pp. 557–562, 2007.

[17] S. Leer-Salvesen, E. Dybvik, O. E. Dahl, J.-E. Gjertsen, and L. B. EngesæTer, "Postoperative start compared to preoperative start of low-molecular weight heparin increases mortality in patients with femoral neck fractures," *Acta Orthopaedica*, vol. 88, no. 1, pp. 48–54, 2017.

47

Ketamine Use for Successful Resolution of Post-ERCP Acute Pancreatitis Abdominal Pain

Suneel M. Agerwala, Divya Sundarapandiyan, and Garret Weber

New York Medical College, Valhalla, NY, USA

Correspondence should be addressed to Garret Weber; garret.weber@wmchealth.org

Academic Editor: Alparslan Apan

We report a case in which a patient with intractable pain secondary to post-endoscopic retrograde cholangiopancreatography (ERCP) acute pancreatitis is successfully treated with a subanesthetic ketamine infusion. Shortly after ERCP, the patient reported severe stabbing epigastric pain. She exhibited voluntary guarding and tenderness without distension. Amylase and lipase levels were elevated. Pain persisted for hours despite hydromorphone PCA, hydromorphone boluses, fentanyl boluses, and postprocedure anxiolytics. Pain management was consulted and a ketamine infusion was trialed, leading to a dramatic reduction in pain. This case suggests that ketamine may be a promising option in treating intractable pain associated with ERCP acute pancreatitis.

1. Introduction

While subanesthetic ketamine infusion has been used to manage postoperative pain and opioid resistant pain, as well as acute pain and procedural sedation in the emergency department and in the pediatric population, there has been no study examining its use in ERCP pancreatitis in the adult population. We present a novel case in which intractable post-ERCP acute pancreatitis pain in an adult patient was successfully managed using a subanesthetic dose of ketamine infusion.

2. Case Description

The pain management service was consulted for a 24-year-old female with past medical history notable for polycystic ovarian syndrome. She presented with intractable abdominal pain, status post-endoscopic retrograde cholangiopancreatography (ERCP), for suspected choledocholithiasis/post-cholecystectomy syndrome. Six weeks earlier, the patient underwent elective cholecystectomy and was discharged home uneventfully, with pain well controlled on oral analgesics. On the day prior to admission, the patient awoke with severe abdominal pain and presented to the emergency department. Her pain was reported as 10/10 on the numerical rating scale in severity and was described as sharp, located in her mid-abdomen above the umbilicus, radiating to the right upper quadrant and back, and accompanied by nausea. She was then admitted as an inpatient for further workup.

On hospital day #1 her pain was treated with morphine sulfate IV 3 mg q4h prn. She received four doses. On hospital day #2 the patient complained of persistent pain and her pain regimen was switched to Hydromorphone IV 0.2 mg q4h PRN. She was given 2 doses on hospital day #2. Abdominal imaging, which included right upper quadrant ultrasound and abdominal CT, revealed intrahepatic and extrahepatic bile duct dilatation, which was suspicious for possible biliary stones. Amylase and lipase were within normal limits. The primary team decided to pursue ERCP given the inconclusive workup.

Prior to the ERCP, the patient was given Hydromorphone IV 0.5 mg. She then underwent general anesthesia with endotracheal tube, with an uneventful anesthetic course. Anesthesia was induced with propofol and lidocaine and maintained with propofol boluses. She was also given a total of 100 mcg of fentanyl. Her ERCP showed diffuse common bile duct dilation of 12 mm and a possible amorphous filling defect in the common bile duct. The common bile duct was ballooned, a sphincterotomy was performed, and the pancreatic duct was stented. She was then extubated and brought to the PACU.

In the PACU, the patient complained of severe, excruciating, stabbing epigastric pain and demonstrated voluntary guarding and tenderness without distension. Amylase and lipase levels were elevated to 199 and 121, respectively, and her pain was attributed to post-ERCP acute pancreatitis. The anesthesia service immediately ordered Hydromorphone IV 2 mg, fentanyl 100 mcg, and midazolam 2 mg. With her pain still uncontrolled, approximately 1 hour later, while still in the PACU, the patient was given over the next hour one additional dose each of midazolam 2 mg, fentanyl 100 mcg, and hydromorphone 2 mg. Hydromorphone PCA with demand dosing 0.2 mg every 10 minutes was then started. The patient's pain remained uncontrolled over the next three hours, so an additional nurse-administered hydromorphone bolus was given. The pain management service was consulted at this point.

Given the patient's persistent pain despite hydromorphone PCA, hydromorphone boluses, fentanyl boluses, and postprocedural anxiolytics, a decision was made to start ketamine infusion (3 mcg/kg/min) at low dose for analgesia. The patient then experienced significantly improved pain which allowed her to leave the PACU stably and comfortably. This was accompanied by a reduction in PCA use overnight requiring only one demand dose and no additional nurse-administered boluses. The next morning she expressed that the pain had resolved to a feeling of mild soreness. On hospital day #4, the ketamine drip was discontinued and pain was controlled to a minimum. On hospital day #5, her labs had normalized, she was tolerating diet, and was discharged home.

3. Discussion

Current management for pain secondary to acute pancreatitis includes NSAIDs, acetaminophen, and opioids [1]. We present a case where traditional management for this type of pain was insufficient for analgesia and where a subanesthetic ketamine infusion was used to successfully alleviate pain.

A recent cohort study in pediatric pain management examined the use of low-dose ketamine infusion in the treatment of acute pain for multiple different diagnoses. The study showed reduction in pain scores after ketamine infusion for a pooled "inflammatory diseases" group that included patients with Crohn's disease and pancreatitis, in general, but did not delineate between the two diseases [2]. To our knowledge, our case study is the first report of ketamine used as an analgesic to treat intractable post-ERCP, specific, pancreatitis pain in the adult population.

The incidence of post-ERCP pancreatitis (PEP) is estimated to be 3.47%. Risk factors include female gender, young age, sphincter of Oddi dysfunction, absence of chronic pancreatitis, and history of prior PEP. Prevention in high-risk patients includes pharmacologic prophylaxis using anti-inflammatory medication and improved endoscopic techniques, such as stenting and faster biliary cannulation time [3].

In order to diagnose acute pancreatitis, two of the main three features must be confirmed. These features are abdominal pain typical for acute pancreatitis, serum amylase/lipase greater than 3 times the upper normal limit, and evidence of acute pancreatitis on CT scan. Initial assessment of severity is important for planning proper management. Mild acute pancreatitis is defined by lack of organ failure, moderate severity includes transient (<48 hr) organ failure, and severe is characterized by persistent (>48 hr) organ failure [4].

Analgesia does not modify the course or outcome of acute pancreatitis but supports patient comfort and patient-reported outcomes. Opioids, commonly used to treat pain in acute pancreatitis, work on the mu receptor pathway, both peripherally and centrally, to modulate the nociceptive response and perception of pain [5].

Classically, ketamine has been used for procedural sedation and postoperative pain. When given at anesthetic doses ketamine causes analgesia, amnesia, and sedation while having relatively little effect on respiration and overall hemodynamics [6]. At subanesthetic doses, the drug has been found to be effective in achieving analgesia in opioid resistant patients [7].

Ketamine's therapeutic effects have long been attributed to its ability to reversibly block the activity of N-methyl-D-aspartate (NMDA) receptors (NR). NR hyperactivity leads to sensitization to noxious stimuli and desensitization to opioids. Thus, blocking this pathway has dramatic effects on analgesia and opioid unresponsiveness. In chronic pain states, central and peripheral sensitization of pain pathways can cause the experience of pain to decouple from an appropriate stimulus. NRs are implicated in the plasticity that leads to sensitization, and blocking this plasticity with ketamine may help in chronic pain states. In the same way opioid receptors may be attenuated through NR-dependent mechanisms, leading to opioid tolerance. Blockade of this pathway may prevent, reduce, or delay desensitization to opioids [8, 9].

There are other pathways that may contribute to the analgesic effects of ketamine. An increase in substance P receptors has been implicated in greater pain sensitivity and loss of substance P receptors in less pain sensitivity. Ketamine is known to have a direct inhibitory effect on substance P receptors. There is some indication that ketamine may reduce the release of substance P into the synapse. Dopaminergic pathways may contribute as well. Ketamine has been shown to increase dopamine signaling, and preliminary evidence has shown that this is involved in pain reduction. Muscarinic acetylcholine receptor agonists may increase pain sensitivity thresholds, and ketamine may have some direct regulatory effects on those receptors. Serotonergic pathways may have pronociceptive roles, and ketamine may have an additional role in modulation [9].

Ketamine's analgesic effects were shown to be beneficial in many settings. Using ketamine in conjunction with morphine was shown to be superior for pain management in the postoperative setting, compared to morphine alone [7]. Ketamine has also been used in the emergency department for acute pain, where it showed similar analgesic effects to morphine [10]. A recent randomized, double-blind, placebo-controlled trial showed that after a subanesthetic infusion of ketamine over 15 minutes, patients reported significant decrease in pain scores for the first 30 minutes when compared to placebo infusions [11]. Another study showed increased analgesia of ketamine infusion when compared to placebo over a 2-hour period [12].

One shortcoming is the monitoring necessary to treat a patient with a subanesthetic ketamine drip. At our institution, the patient was required to stay in the PACU for 24 hours because of state regulations that require a higher level of monitoring for patients with a ketamine drip [13]. Additionally, she was transferred from the PACU to a higher acuity stepdown unit before being transferred to a lower acuity floor. These rules may vary by state, but the additional resources for monitoring may be prohibitive for some institutions.

In summary, while ketamine has been used to manage postoperative pain, opioid resistant pain, and acute pain in the emergency department, evidence for its use to treat pain associated with an acute pancreatitis is limited. In our patient with severe post-ERCP pain associated with acute pancreatitis, opioids and coanalgesics were unable to control her pain. The addition of a subanesthetic ketamine drip offered quick and long-lasting analgesia. This could have been due to the ability of ketamine to modify the effects of opioids or the direct effect of ketamine itself on the nociceptive system. The patient was able to comfortably recover from her acute event, being discharged home with no complications. Further studies on the safety and the appropriate level of monitoring at subanesthetic dosing should be investigated to allow for further use outside of a highly monitored unit.

Authors' Contributions

Suneel M. Agerwala participated in literature review, researching case information, writing case description, writing discussion, and writing abstract. Divya Sundarapandiyan was involved in literature review, researching case information, writing case description, writing discussion, and organizing references. Dr. Garret Weber managed treatment of patient, guided literature review, guided research of case information, guided writing of case description, and guided writing of discussion.

References

[1] B. Gülen, A. Dur, M. Serinken, Ö. Karcioğlu, and E. Sönmez, "Pain treatment in patients with acute pancreatitis: A randomized controlled trial," *Turkish Journal of Gastroenterology*, vol. 27, no. 2, pp. 192–196, 2016.

[2] K. A. Sheehy, C. Lippold, A. L. Rice, R. Nobrega, J. C. Finkel, and Z. M. Quezado, "Subanesthetic ketamine for pain management in hospitalized children, adolescents, and young adults: a single-center cohort study," *Journal of Pain Research*, vol. Volume 10, pp. 787–795, 2017.

[3] N. M. Szary and F. H. Al-Kawas, "Complications of endoscopic retrograde cholangiopancreatography: How to avoid and manage them," *Gastroenterology and Hepatology*, vol. 9, no. 8, pp. 496–504, 2013.

[4] C. S. Dupuis, V. Baptista, G. Whalen et al., "Diagnosis and management of acute pancreatitis and its complications," *Gastrointestinal Intervention*, vol. 2, no. 1, pp. 36–46, 2013.

[5] X. Basurto Ona, D. Rigau Comas, and G. Urrútia, "Opioids for acute pancreatitis pain," *The Cochrane database of systematic reviews*, vol. 26, 2013.

[6] R. J. Strayer and L. S. Nelson, "Adverse events associated with ketamine for procedural sedation in adults," *The American journal of emergency medicine*, vol. 26, no. 9, pp. 985–1028, 2008.

[7] A. A. Weinbroum, "A single small dose of postoperative ketamine provides rapid and sustained improvement in morphine analgesia in the presence of morphine-resistant pain," *Anesthesia and Analgesia*, vol. 96, no. 3, pp. 789–795, 2013.

[8] S. K. Lee, "The use of ketamine for perioperative pain management," *Korean Journal of Anesthesiology*, vol. 63, no. 1, pp. 1-2, 2012.

[9] G. J. Iacobucci, O. Visnjevac, L. Pourafkari, and N. D. Nader, "Ketamine: an update on cellular and subcellular mechanisms with implications for clinical practice," *Pain Physician*, vol. 20, no. 2, pp. E285–E301, 2017.

[10] T. W. Barrett and D. L. Schriger, "Move over morphine: is ketamine an effective and safe alternative for treating acute pain? journal club," *Annals of emergency medicine*, vol. 67, no. 2, pp. 289–294, 2015.

[11] B. Sin, T. Tatunchak, M. Paryavi et al., "The use of ketamine for acute treatment of pain: a randomized, double-blind, placebo-controlled trial," *The Journal of Emergency Medicine*, vol. 52, no. 5, pp. 601–608, 2017.

[12] F. L. Beaudoin, C. Lin, W. Guan, and R. C. Merchant, "Low-dose Ketamine Improves Pain Relief in Patients Receiving Intravenous Opioids for Acute Pain in the Emergency Department: Results of a Randomized, Double-blind, Clinical Trial," *Academic Emergency Medicine*, vol. 21, no. 11, pp. 1194–1202, 2014.

[13] B. Zittel, "Practice Information: IV Drug Administration of Ketamine for the Treatment of Intractable Pain," NYSed.gov, June 2011, http://www.op.nysed.gov/prof/nurse/nurse-iv-ketamine.htm.

48

An Unusual Lacerated Tracheal Tube during Le Fort Surgery: Literature Review and Case Report

Preeta George,[1] John E. Fiadjoe,[2] and Allan F. Simpao[2]

[1]St. Louis Children's Hospital, Washington University, 1 Children's Pl., St. Louis, MO 63108, USA
[2]Perelman School of Medicine at the University of Pennsylvania and the Children's Hospital of Philadelphia, 3401 Civic Center Blvd., Philadelphia, PA 19104, USA

Correspondence should be addressed to Allan F. Simpao; simpaoa@email.chop.edu

Academic Editor: Alparslan Apan

Maxillofacial surgeries can present unique anesthetic challenges due to potentially complex anatomy and the close proximity of the patient's airway to the surgical field. Damage to the tracheal tube (TT) during maxillofacial surgery may lead to significant airway compromise. We report the management of a patient with a partially severed TT during Le Fort surgery for midfacial hypoplasia and management strategies based on peer-reviewed literature. This case illustrates the clinical clues associated with a damaged TT and explores the challenges of managing this potentially catastrophic issue.

1. Introduction

Maxillofacial surgeries can present numerous challenges to anesthesiologists due to the potential for complex facial anatomy and the close proximity of the tracheal tube (TT) to the surgical field. Damage to the TT during maxillofacial surgery can lead to airway compromise; thus, anesthesia providers should have a strategy in place to prevent or mitigate such events. In this case, we report the intraoperative management of a patient with a partially severed nasal TT during a Le Fort surgery.

2. Case Description

A 17-year-old, 56 kg male with midface hypoplasia presented for an elective Le Fort-1 advancement surgery with bilateral malar osteotomies. His prior medical history was unremarkable. On physical examination, the patient had a Mallampati-2 airway, and his mental-hyoid distance, mouth opening, and mandibular subluxation were normal. Anesthesia was induced with sevoflurane and oxygen, obtained peripheral IV access, and applied oxymetazoline to both nares prior to smooth nasotracheal intubation with a 6.5 cuffed TT. The TT cuff was inflated with 3 mL of air; auscultation, squeezing

of the pilot balloon, and palpation of the patient's neck confirmed the TT cuff's proper inflation and position.

The surgeon placed a throat pack and started the procedure. While performing a left maxillotomy, the surgical team expressed concern that the TT may have been cut because of visible bubbling of gas from the nose after resection of the left lateral nasal wall. The surgeon placed the patient's head in the neutral position while the situation was assessed. The anesthesia team inspected the TT, confirmed that cephalad migration had not occurred, and discovered that the pilot balloon did not sustain inflation. The team called for help, requested additional equipment (difficult airway cart, surgical airway kit), and prepared for a possible reintubation through a bloody field. However, at this point the patient's vital signs, capnograph waveform, and the ventilator's flow-volume loop patterns had all stabilized. After a brief discussion, the intraoperative team agreed to proceed.

Shortly thereafter, when the surgeons turned the patient's head away from the midline neutral position, the anesthesia machine warned of a circuit leak and air bubbles were again observed in the surgical field. The patient's head was immediately returned to the midline position and the leak again disappeared completely. The anesthesia team surmised that the

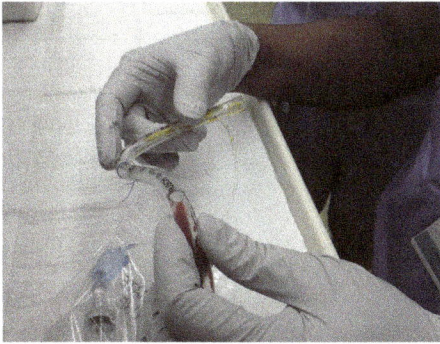

FIGURE 1: Inspection of the lacerated tracheal tube following the safe emergence and extubation of our patient. Note the widened aperture during bending of the tracheal tube and the severed pilot balloon tubing.

tracheal tube was partially severed, resulting in an aperture that opened when the head was turned away from midline.

The surgeons stated that the remainder of the case could be performed satisfactorily in the midline position. The patient's ventilation remained completely stable for several minutes, so the decision was made to proceed cautiously with the in situ TT. A tube exchange was eschewed because of the successful conservative measures and the concern of airway loss during an exchange. The remainder of the surgery was uneventful, and we extubated the patient without incident. The patient was transported safely to the postanesthesia care unit where he experienced a full recovery. Inspection of the TT revealed a cut across half of the tube's diameter; the pilot balloon tubing had been severed completely (Figure 1).

3. Discussion

Tracheal tube damage during maxillofacial surgery is a potentially catastrophic complication. In some cases, conservative measures such as tube stabilization and laryngeal packing provide adequate ventilatory conditions to complete a surgical case [1, 2]. The definitive solution is to replace the damaged TT, yet reintubation may be difficult due to poor visibility, bleeding, and badly defined tissue planes [3]. Replacing the TT interrupts ventilation, risks aspiration, and can be cumbersome during surgeries of the head, neck, and thorax; furthermore, TT changers and fiberoptic bronchoscopes are not failsafe [4].

Table 1 lists prior reports of damaged TTs during Le Fort procedures as well as the challenges presented by different management strategies. Schwartz et al. described an inability to withdraw the TT more than a few millimeters, where the lacerated end of the tube had formed a barb that caught on a bone snag; their patient was extubated successfully after the lacerated TT was sealed with cement prior to removal [5]. In another case report, a completely severed, wire-reinforced TT obstructed the airway, thereby requiring a surgical airway [6]. Valentine and Kaban reported a case where the pilot tube was severed and the heat from the surgical drill occluded the distal

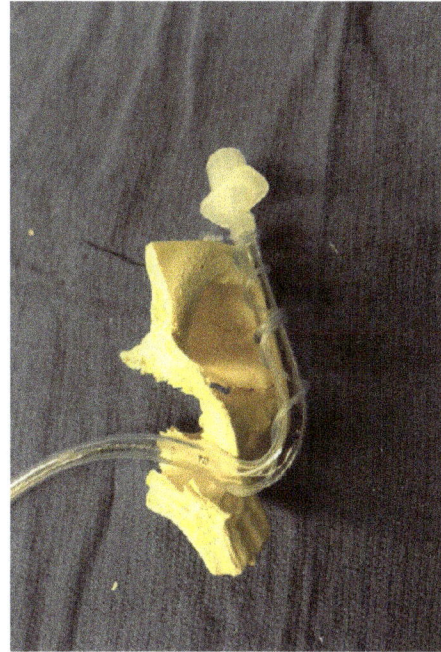

FIGURE 2: A side and sagittal view of a nasal tracheal tube and its passage through a model of the bony structures of the face.

pilot balloon inflation line resulting in a permanently inflated cuff, which complicated the removal of the TT [7].

Anesthesiologists should anticipate TT damage during maxillofacial surgery and take precautionary measures if possible. For a unilateral maxillotomy, intubation via the contralateral nares will reduce the risk of TT damage. The surgeons' use of a nasal septum osteotome with blunt horns may deflect a TT and reduce the likelihood of damage [2]. Intraoperative radiographic imaging may be a useful tool for maxillofacial procedures that require pterygomaxillary disjunction with malar osteotomies. Although this has been neither reported nor studied, this may be a useful guide during the maxillotomy phase of Le Fort surgery to help prevent this complication. The team can then appreciate the proximity of the tracheal tube to the maxilla, and the surgeon can use this information to guide the placement of the osteotomy to avoid TT damage.

If damage to TT occurs during surgery, then a swift assessment of airway patency and ventilation should drive the decision to reestablish the airway. This includes examining the TT depth and auscultating the chest and direct laryngoscopy, if possible [15]. Repositioning the patient's head may improve ventilation in the case of a partially severed tube. Per El-Orbany and Salem [15], a thorough risk/benefit analysis should be performed. Factors that should be considered in this analysis process include the following: (1) length of time for which the patient will require mechanical ventilation; (2) patient's history of a difficult airway or poor laryngeal visualization; (3) the leaked volume and its effect on patient's ventilation; (4) risk of aspiration; (5) tolerance to brief periods of ventilation interruption; (6) expected response to laryngoscopy and intubation; (7) cervical spine status

TABLE 1: Case reports of damaged tracheal tubes (TTs) during maxillofacial surgery.

Author	Journal/year	Complication	Management
Nair and Balagopal	Indian J Anaesth. 2012 [8]	Partial transection of TT	Unable to ventilate, reintubated over a gum elastic boogie
Ladi and Aphale	Indian J Anaesth. 2011 [6]	Complete TT transection	Flexometallic tube, difficulty removing distal end, emergent tracheostomy
Jain et al.	Indian J Anaesth. 2008 [9]	Partial transection of TT	Unable to ventilate, intubated over a tube exchanger
Bang et al.	Korean J Anesthesiol. 2007 [10]	Partial transection of TT	Continued with a throat pack
Adke and Mendonca	Anaesthesia. 2003 [11]	Partial transection of TT	Noticed after extubation, no leak, intraoperatively
Bidgoli et al.	Eur J Anaesthesiol. 1999 [3]	Partial transection of TT	Unable to ventilate, a nasogastric tube was inserted through the transected TT, which was used as a guide to reintubate
Ketzler and Landers	J Clin Anesth. 1992 [12]	Near total (95%) transection	Continued with a throat pack
Thyme et al.	J Oral Maxillofac Surg. 1992 [13]	Partial transection with pilot tube damage	Unable to ventilate, reintubated, no details
Valentine and Kaban	J Oral Maxillofac Surg. 1992 [7]	Pilot tube damage, unable to deflate cuff	Waited for 2 hrs and for deflation of cuff to extubate
Fagraeus et al.	Anesth Analg. 1980 [14]	Partial transection with pilot tube damage	Unable to deflate cuff, unable to ventilate, aspiration of bloodreintubated without difficulty

and presence of hard neck collar or halo fixation; and (8) patient's position (supine versus prone or rotated away from anesthesia workstation) [15]. The TT should be exchanged if ventilation and oxygenation are inadequate. Maintaining a sterile field may be challenging; however, a sterile endoscope may allow inspection of the tube prior to exchange if feasible. Emergency airway equipment should be readily available, including a tube exchanger, a video laryngoscope, and a surgical airway kit. The team should prepare for potential difficulty when removing the damaged TT and be ready to perform invasive surgical airway access. A smaller-sized TT can be inserted through a damaged TT to stem a crisis and improve surgical conditions prior to a reintubation attempt [16].

Our case illustrates the challenges of managing a damaged TT midway through a maxillotomy procedure. In our case, we chose to proceed without TT exchange due to adequate oxygenation and ventilation with the head in neutral position. Figure 1 shows the partially severed TT, damaged pilot balloon tubing, and deflated TT cuff from this case. The proximity of the TT to the maxilla in the anterior and lateral views can be observed in Figures 2 and 3. We surmised that the aperture of the severed tube was approximated with the head in neutral positon. Our concerns for a difficult reintubation and the damaged tube catching on bone outweighed the risks of a reasonably stable, albeit suboptimal airway. We remained vigilant throughout the case for any signs of airway

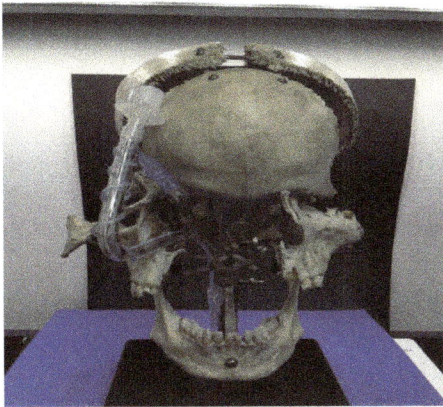

FIGURE 3: A frontal view of a nasal tracheal tube and its passage through a model of the skull and facial bone structures.

compromise and were prepared for a tube exchange and surgical airway placement. Our case illustrates two important clues that should lead anesthesiologists to consider a partially transected TT during Le Fort surgeries: (1) a pilot balloon that fails during the surgery and (2) an intermittent leak that appears and resolves with changes in head position. Either of these signs should prompt immediate investigation of the airway and communication with the surgical team.

Competing Interests

The authors report no relevant competing interests.

References

[1] V. Mayoral Rojals and P. Casals Caus, "Two different solutions to a severed nasotracheal tube during maxillary osteotomy," *Revista Española de Anestesiología y Reanimación*, vol. 49, pp. 201–204, 2002.

[2] J. R. Davies and P. V. Dyer, "Preventing damage to the tracheal tube during maxillary osteotomy," *Anaesthesia*, vol. 58, no. 9, pp. 914–915, 2003.

[3] S. J. H. Bidgoli, L. Dumont, M. Mattys, C. Mardirosoff, and P. Damseaux, "A serious anaesthetic complication of a Lefort I osteotomy," *European Journal of Anaesthesiology*, vol. 16, no. 3, pp. 201–203, 1999.

[4] A. M.-H. Ho and L. H. Contardi, "What to do when an endotracheal tube cuff leaks," *Journal of Trauma-Injury, Infection and Critical Care*, vol. 40, no. 3, pp. 486–487, 1996.

[5] L. B. Schwartz, W. C. Sordill, R. M. Liebers, and W. Schwab, "Difficulty in removal of accidentally cut endotracheal tube," *Journal of Oral and Maxillofacial Surgery*, vol. 40, no. 8, pp. 518–519, 1982.

[6] S. D. Ladi and S. Aphale, "Accidental transection of flexometallic endotracheal tube during partial maxillectomy," *Indian Journal of Anaesthesia*, vol. 55, no. 3, pp. 284–286, 2011.

[7] D. J. Valentine and L. B. Kaban, "Unusual nasoendotracheal tube damage during Le Fort I osteotomy. Case report," *International Journal of Oral and Maxillofacial Surgery*, vol. 21, no. 6, pp. 333–334, 1992.

[8] V. A. Nair and P. G. Balagopal, "Intra-operative endotracheal tube damage: anaesthetic challenges," *Indian Journal of Anaesthesia*, vol. 56, no. 3, pp. 311–312, 2012.

[9] M. Jain, M. Garg, and A. Gupta, "Accidental perforation of endotracheal tube during orthognathic surgery for maxillary prognathism—a case report," *Indian Journal of Anaesthesia*, vol. 52, pp. 205–207, 2008.

[10] E. G. Bang, Y. H. Jeon, and J. G. Hong, "Damage to an endotracheal tube during Lefort I osteotomy-a case report," *Korean Journal of Anesthesiology*, vol. 53, no. 4, pp. 516–519, 2007.

[11] M. Adke and C. Mendonca, "Concealed airway complication during LeFort I osteotomy," *Anaesthesia*, vol. 58, no. 3, pp. 294–295, 2003.

[12] J. T. Ketzler and D. F. Landers, "Management of a severed endotracheal tube during LeFort osteotomy," *Journal of Clinical Anesthesia*, vol. 4, no. 2, pp. 144–146, 1992.

[13] G. M. Thyme, J. W. Ferguson, and F. D. Pilditch, "Endotracheal tube damage during orthognathic surgery," *Journal of Oral and Maxillofacial Surgery*, vol. 21, no. 2, article 80, 1992.

[14] L. Fagraeus, J. C. Angelillo, and E. A. Dolan, "A serious anesthetic hazard during orthognathic surgery," *Anesthesia and Analgesia*, vol. 59, no. 2, pp. 150–153, 1980.

[15] M. El-Orbany and M. R. Salem, "Endotracheal tube cuff leaks: causes, consequences, and management," *Anesthesia and Analgesia*, vol. 117, no. 2, pp. 428–434, 2013.

[16] R. M. Peskin and S. A. Sachs, "Intraoperative management of a partially severed endotracheal tube during orthognathic surgery," *Anesthesia Progress*, vol. 33, no. 5, pp. 247–251, 1986.

49

Case Report of a Massive Thigh Hematoma after Adductor Canal Block in a Morbidly Obese Woman Anticoagulated with Apixaban

Katherine L. Koniuch ⓘ, Bradley Harris, Michael J. Buys, and Adam W. Meier

University of Utah Department of Anesthesiology, USA

Correspondence should be addressed to Katherine L. Koniuch; kate.koniuch@hsc.utah.edu

Academic Editor: Ehab Farag

Hematoma formation after peripheral nerve block placement is a rare event. We report a case of a morbidly obese patient who was anticoagulated with apixaban and developed a massive thigh hematoma after an ultrasound-guided adductor canal block. Despite continuous visualization of the block needle, an unrecognized vascular injury occurred leading to a 14-cm hematoma in the anterolateral thigh. Morbid obesity warrants additional risk consideration when placing nerve blocks in an anticoagulated patient. In addition, early recognition and expert consultation are both important in the management of block-related hematomas.

1. Introduction

Peripheral nerve blocks provide effective postoperative analgesia for extremity surgeries [1] and have been associated with few complications [2]. In morbidly obese patients taking anticoagulants near the time of surgery, there may be increased risk of bleeding or hematoma formation which should be considered based on the 2018 American Society of Regional Anesthesia (ASRA) guidelines for Regional Anesthesia in the Patient Receiving Antithrombotic or Thrombolytic Therapy [3]. In this case report, we describe a morbidly obese patient taking apixaban whose postoperative course was complicated by a massive thigh hematoma that developed after an adductor canal block. We detail the factors that may have contributed to this complication, how it could have been avoided, and how the hematoma was managed.

2. Case Description

The patient involved provided written consent for reporting of this case.

A 63-year-old woman with medical history of super morbid obesity (BMI 54) and atrial fibrillation for which she was anticoagulated with apixaban presented for an open reduction internal fixation (ORIF) of an ankle fracture. Significant medical history included diabetes mellitus type 2, obstructive sleep apnea, chronic obstructive pulmonary disease, and diastolic heart failure. The patient's last dose of apixaban was 48 hours prior to surgery. Other than moderate anemia (hemoglobin 8.8 g/dL), all laboratory studies, including a coagulation profile, were normal.

Prior to surgery, the patient was offered a sciatic nerve catheter and an adductor canal block as part of a multimodal postoperative analgesia strategy. Because of her many, serious medical conditions, we concluded that a peripheral nerve block offered the best opportunity to provide satisfactory postoperative analgesia. Specifically, we were concerned that the postoperative pain management primarily with opioid medications would pose increased cardiopulmonary risk to the patient. We were careful to explain the risks associated with peripheral nerve blocks, including the risk of bleeding and hematoma formation, and verbal consent was obtained.

The surgery was performed under general anesthesia and her intraoperative course was uncomplicated. Upon arrival to the recovery room, our acute pain service was contacted to evaluate her for peripheral nerve blockade. We positioned the patient in the lateral decubitus position and placed a sciatic nerve catheter. Though technically challenging due to body habitus, this sciatic nerve block was performed successfully and without any complication. The patient was then positioned supine for the adductor canal block. The leg was externally rotated and the knee slightly flexed for optimal positioning. A high-frequency linear array ultrasound transducer was applied to the mid-thigh in short-axis and the adductor canal was identified. Imaging was again challenging given the patient's habitus, but with firm compression of the ultrasound transducer, the important anatomical structures were clearly identified. The superficial femoral artery (SFA) was visualized dorsal to the sartorius muscle and a hyperechoic structure anterolateral to the artery was identified as the adductor canal and saphenous nerve [4, 5]. The skin adjacent to the probe was cleansed with a chlorhexidine and alcohol solution. A 20-gauge × 4-inch beveled, echogenic needle was inserted using an in-plane technique. The needle was visualized continuously as it coursed between the vastus medialis and sartorius toward the adductor canal. The needle was positioned lateral to the SFA within the canal and a bolus of 20 ml of 0.25% bupivacaine with 5 mcg/ml epinephrine was administered with negative heme aspiration checks after every 5 ml injection. Spread of local anesthetic within the adductor canal was clearly observed under ultrasound visualization. There was no evidence of intravascular injection of epinephrine while monitoring the patient. Upon needle withdrawal, brisk bleeding was noted at the skin insertion site but with direct manual pressure for approximately 60 seconds, bleeding ceased completely.

Shortly after the blocks were performed, the patient reported complete resolution of her ankle pain and was transferred to her hospital room. Approximately 6 hours after surgery, the patient reported new anterior thigh pain on the operative leg, which was treated by her nurse with intravenous hydromorphone. Roughly 13 hours after surgery, the patient's nurse finally contacted the orthopedic surgery team due to unmanageable mid-thigh pain. The orthopedics team initially believed the pain was due to tourniquet compression pain which occurred during surgery. Upon further physical examination, a hematoma was noted in the anterolateral mid-thigh. Vital signs were within normal ranges and distal pulses were intact. A CT scan with contrast was ordered and revealed a 14-cm hematoma in the right thigh (Figure 1). Lab studies showed a drop in hemoglobin from 8.8 g/dL preoperatively to 6.9 g/dL the morning of postoperative day (POD) 1. Coagulation studies at that time were within normal limits including partial thromboplastin time, prothrombin time, and international normalized ration, as well as platelet count. The patient's primary medicine service transfused 1 unit of packed red blood cells, which improved her hemoglobin to 7.6 g/dL.

Interventional radiology was consulted on the morning of POD 1 for management recommendations for the hematoma. A CT angiogram was performed revealing active extravasation from a small superficial branch of the SFA (Figure 2). Embolization with coil and gel foam was performed and compressive dressings were used to apply direct pressure. Throughout the day, the patient's hemoglobin remained stable and the hematoma showed no evidence of further expansion.

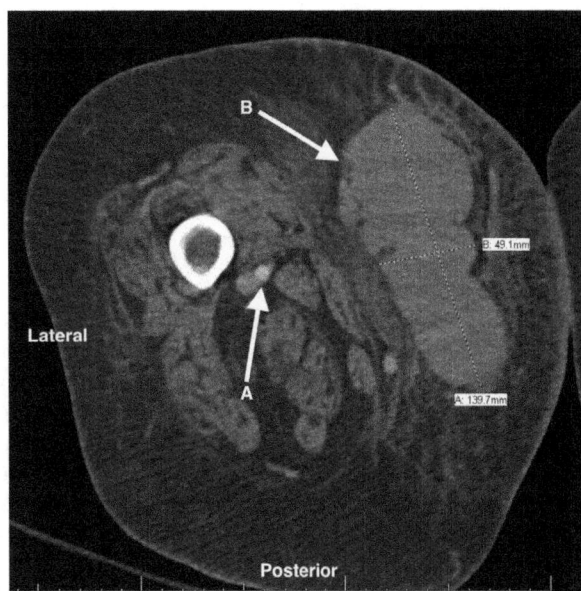

Figure 1: CT of the patient's right thigh showing the superficial femoral artery (A) and 5 × 14 cm hematoma (B).

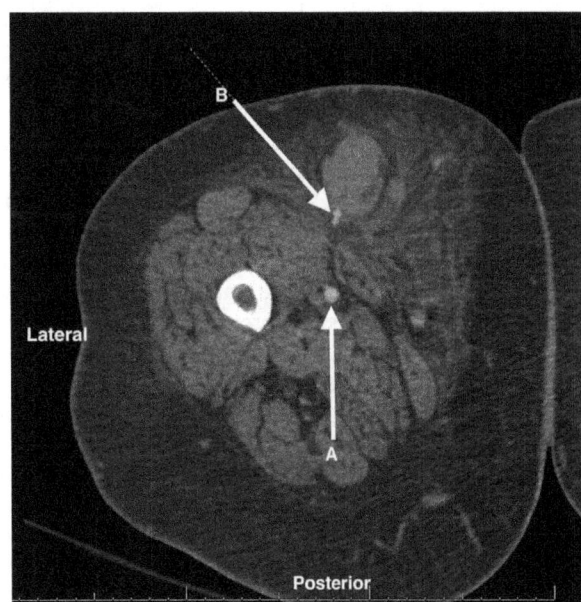

Figure 2: CT angiogram of the patient's right thigh showing the superficial femoral artery (A) and active extravasation from a small branch of the SFA (B).

On POD 2, further consultation from the vascular surgery and interventional radiology teams was sought for possible hematoma evacuation versus drain placement given the massive size. Vascular surgery recommended conservative management with application of direct pressure. Interventional radiology, however, recommended placement of a drain within the hematoma. A pigtail catheter was placed and fluid cultures were obtained. Minimal output from the drain was observed, so beginning on POD 3, tissue plasminogen activator (TPA) was administered through the catheter daily to facilitate hematoma drainage. Follow-up ultrasound on POD 6 showed a persistent hematoma despite TPA administration. Hematoma cultures resulted negative for infection. On POD 7, she was discharged to a rehabilitation facility with the drain in place and care team instructions to flush 5-10 ml saline twice daily until evaluation with interventional radiology one week later.

On POD 14, the drain was inadvertently pulled out requiring a return visit to interventional radiology and drain replacement. On POD 19, the hematoma cavity had decreased to an acceptable size so the drain was removed. One week later, on POD 26, she returned to interventional radiology due to increased pain and swelling at the hematoma site. A recurrent fluid collection was noted on ultrasound examination so the drain was replaced a third time and aspirated fluid was sent for culture, which grew staphylococcus aureus. She was treated for hematoma superinfection with a five-day course of levofloxacin and when she returned two weeks later, the abscess had resolved and the drain was removed.

3. Discussion

This case demonstrates important points regarding regional anesthesia in an anticoagulated, morbidly obese patient. First, morbid obesity represents an additional risk factor when considering a superficial peripheral nerve block on an anticoagulated patient. Second, there is a paucity of case reports detailing the complication of hematoma formation due to a peripheral nerve block. Third, the subsequent management of the hematoma after peripheral nerve block is not well reported in the literature and presents a considerable challenge, especially in patients with multiple comorbidities.

Peripheral nerve blocks can provide excellent analgesia for patients having ankle surgery [6]. In a morbidly obese patient, a nerve block may significantly reduce the need for opioid administration [7, 8]. This can provide great benefit for patients at risk for postoperative opioid-induced hypoventilation. When considering the risks and benefits of a nerve block for our patient, opioid reduction was a clear benefit. Throughout her hospital course, she never received opioids for ankle pain while nerve blocks were in effect. Thus we believe there was a clear analgesic benefit to regional anesthesia.

For this patient, however, the risk of bleeding due to her anticoagulation status was also concerning. Although vascular injuries resulting from peripheral nerve blocks are rare complications [2, 7, 9, 10], this case demonstrates the significant morbidity that may occur. The recently updated (2018) ASRA guidelines recommend "management based on site compressibility, vascularity, and consequences of bleeding." [3] While an adductor canal block is considered to be superficial, we feel it is more appropriately categorized as a deep block in a morbidly obese patient because compressibility is more difficult if inadvertent vascular puncture were to occur. In addition, given the potential for massive bleeding into the thigh, additional consideration should be made for procedures on the upper leg. Anticoagulation

recommendations for deep peripheral blocks are the same as neuraxial techniques—the ASRA guidelines recommend waiting 72 hours after the last dose of apixaban for block placement [3]. Although it had only been 48 hours since our patient's last dose, we felt the benefit of opioid reduction would outweigh the risk of vascular injury or significant bleeding.

In this case, the anesthesiologist performing the adductor canal block was an experienced regional anesthesiology fellow who had performed adductor canal blocks in this same manner many times before. A fellowship-trained regional anesthesiologist supervised the nerve block placement. Direct visualization of the needle and of the neurovascular structures was uninterrupted. We believe the vascular injury likely occurred when the needle passed through the superficial branch of SFA as the ultrasound probe was compressing it. This small branching artery was never recognized on ultrasound imaging. Although the vascular injury may not have been easily avoided regardless of the patient's coagulation status, waiting an additional 24 hours to perform the block (72 hours after her last apixaban dose) may have decreased the extent of hematoma formation. While this may have made no difference in her clinical outcome, perhaps it can be used to better guide risk versus benefit discussions in morbidly obese patients who are anticoagulated before receiving a peripheral nerve block.

Another factor that contributed to the significant morbidity in this case was the management of the hematoma after it was recognized. The patient underwent multiple procedures to drain the hematoma and required return to the hospital for drain replacement, and ultimately her course was complicated by an infection of the hematoma cavity. Despite a thorough literature search, we were unable to find clear recommendations as to the management of extremity hematomas. We believe that a more conservative approach of close monitoring instead of drain placement would have resulted in an acceptable outcome without additional procedures, increased cost, a prolonged hospital stay, and increased risk of infection.

Disclosure

Katherine L. Koniuch is first author. Bradley Harris and Michael J. Buys are coinvestigators. Adam W. Meier is principal investigator.

Authors' Contributions

Katherine L. Koniuch wrote, edited, and submitted this article. Bradley Harris and Michael J. Buys helped in compiling and editing this article. Adam W. Meier helped in compiling, editing, and submitting this article.

References

[1] H. B. Joe, H. S. Choo, J. S. Yoon, S. E. Oh, J. H. Cho, and Y. U. Park, "Adductor canal block versus femoral nerve block combined with sciatic nerve block as an anesthetic technique for hindfoot and ankle surgery: A prospective, randomized noninferiority trial," *Medicine (United States)*, vol. 95, no. 52, Article ID e5758, 2016.

[2] T. Huo, L. Sun, S. Min et al., "Major complications of regional anesthesia in 11 teaching hospitals of China: a prospective survey of 106,569 cases," *Journal of Clinical Anesthesia*, vol. 31, pp. 154–161, 2016.

[3] T. T. Horlocker, E. Vandermeulen, S. L. Kopp, W. Gogarten, L. R. Leffert, and H. T. Benzon, "Regional Anesthesia in the Patient Receiving Antithrombotic or Thrombolytic Therapy: American Society of Regional Anesthesia and Pain Medicine Evidence-Based Guidelines (Fourth Edition)," *Regional Anesthesia and Pain Medicine*, vol. 43, no. 3, pp. 263–309, 2018.

[4] J. Lund, M. T. Jenstrup, P. Jæger, A. M. Sørensen, and J. B. Dahl, "Continuous adductor-canal-blockade for adjuvant post-operative analgesia after major knee surgery: Preliminary results," *Acta Anaesthesiologica Scandinavica*, vol. 55, no. 1, pp. 14–19, 2011.

[5] N. A. Hanson, C. J. Allen, L. S. Hostetter et al., "Continuous ultrasound-guided adductor canal block for total knee arthroplasty: a randomized, double-blind trial," *Anesth & Analg*, vol. 118, no. 6, pp. 1370–1377, 2014.

[6] P. F. White, T. Issioui, G. D. Skrivanek, J. S. Early, and C. Wakefield, "The Use of a Continuous Popliteal Sciatic Nerve Block After Surgery Involving the Foot and Ankle: Does It Improve the Quality of Recovery?" *Anesthesia & Analgesia*, vol. 97, no. 5, pp. 1303–1309, 2003.

[7] X. Capdevila, P. Pirat, S. Bringuier et al., "Continuous peripheral nerve blocks in hospital wards after orthopedic surgery: a multicenter prospective analysis of the quality of postoperative analgesia and complications in 1,416 patients," *Anesthesiology*, vol. 103, no. 5, pp. 1035–1045, 2005.

[8] J. R. Soberón, C. McInnis, K. S. Bland et al., "Ultrasound-guided popliteal sciatic nerve blockade in the severely and morbidly obese: a prospective and randomized study," *Journal of Anesthesia & Clinical Research*, vol. 30, no. 3, pp. 397–404, 2016.

[9] C. W. Njathi, R. L. Johnson, R. S. Laughlin, D. R. Schroeder, A. K. Jacob, and S. L. Kopp, "Complications after Continuous Posterior Lumbar Plexus Blockade for Total Hip Arthroplasty: A Retrospective Cohort Study," *Regional Anesthesia and Pain Medicine*, vol. 42, no. 4, pp. 446–450, 2017.

[10] T. C. Stan, M. A. Krantz, D. L. Solomon, J. G. Poulos, and K. Chaouki, "The incidence of neurovascular complications following axillary brachial plexus block using a transarterial approach: A prospective study of 1,000 consecutive patients," *Regional Anesthesia*, vol. 20, no. 6, pp. 486–492, 1995.

50

Pneumomediastinum and Bilateral Pneumothoraces Causing Respiratory Failure after Thyroid Surgery

Michael Koeppen,[1] Benjamin Scott,[2] Joseph Morabito,[2] Matthew Fiegel,[2] and Tobias Eckle[2]

[1]*Anesthesiology, Ludwig Maximilian University of Munich, Munich, Germany*
[2]*Anesthesiology, University of Denver School of Medicine, Aurora, CO, USA*

Correspondence should be addressed to Tobias Eckle; tobias.eckle@ucdenver.edu

Academic Editor: Audun Stubhaug

We report the first case of severe respiratory failure after thyroid surgery requiring venovenous extracorporeal membrane oxygenation (vvECMO). The patient was a 41-year-old woman with metastatic thyroid cancer. She underwent thyroidectomy, including left lateral and bilateral central neck dissection. During surgery, the patient developed pneumomediastinum with bilateral pneumothoraces. Despite early treatment with bilateral chest tubes and no evidence of a tracheal perforation, the patient developed severe respiratory failure after extubation on the intensive care unit. Because pneumothorax and pneumomediastinum might be more common than reported, and considering increasing cases of thyroid surgery, staff should remain vigilant of pulmonary complications after thyroid surgery.

1. Introduction

The incidence of thyroid cancer has more than tripled since 1975 and, in women, it is the cancer with the fastest-growing number of new cases [1]. The treatment includes thyroidectomy, a very common surgical procedure with approximately 100,000 cases each year in the United States [2]. In fact, a recent study among patients in the United States diagnosed with thyroid cancer from 1974 to 2013 found that the overall incidence of thyroid cancer increased by 3% annually, with increases in the incidence and mortality rate [3]. These findings show a true increase in the occurrence of thyroid cancer in the United States. Inevitably, this may increase the number of complications from thyroid surgery and the number of anesthesiologists caring for patients undergoing thyroid surgery. Complications considered "rare" now might become more common in the future. Here, we report a patient who developed bilateral pneumothoraces and pneumomediastinum during thyroid surgery with neck dissection. After postsurgical extubation, the patient deteriorated. The bilateral pneumothoraces worsened despite bilateral chest tubes, ultimately leading to severe respiratory failure that required ECMO treatment. Rapid initiation of therapy facilitated

a fast recovery and the patient was discharged. Following a thorough literature review, we identified only a few published reports of pneumothorax after thyroid surgery. However, one series of 300 cases suggests a higher incidence rate [4].

2. Case Description

A 41-year-old, 75 kg, 150 cm (body mass index of 33), woman with thyroid cancer metastatic to the bilateral neck underwent thyroidectomy, including left lateral and bilateral central neck dissection. No chemotherapy or radiation therapy was employed as an adjunctive prior to surgery. Her medical history included well-controlled arterial hypertension and diabetes mellitus type 2. She was a nonsmoker and denied any history of cardiac or pulmonary disease. The physical exam prior to surgery was unremarkable. The initial CT scan of the neck showed no abnormalities of the trachea (Figure 1). The preoperative vital signs were as follows: blood pressure 121/81 mmHg, heart rate 91/min, respiratory rate of 16/min, temperature 37.4 Celsius, and a SpO_2 of 96% on room air.

Standard anesthesia monitoring (ECG, SpO_2, $ETCO_2$, and NIBP [IBP added after 4 hours of surgery]) was established and maintained throughout the procedure. After

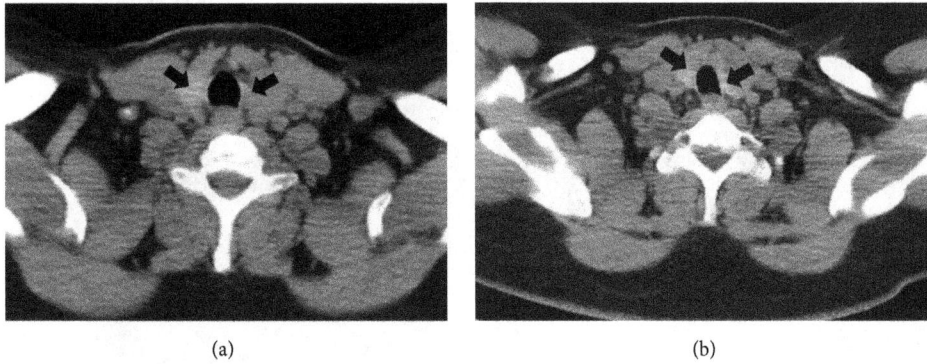

FIGURE 1: Preoperative CT scan of the neck. The preoperative CT scan of the neck shows no abnormalities. Shown are two different levels (a, b). Black arrows indicate thyroid tissue.

intravenous pretreatment with midazolam 2 mg and fentanyl 0.15 mg, general anesthesia was induced using propofol 200 mg, followed by 80 mg succinylcholine to facilitate intubation. We maintained anesthesia using desflurane inhalation and remifentanil infusion (0.2 μg/kg/min). To minimize the risk of recurrent laryngeal nerve damage, we used an electromyogram endotracheal tube (EMG-ETT, Medtronic), placed using a video laryngoscope and inflated the cuff to a pressure of 25 cm H_2O. Then, guaranteed volume, pressure-controlled ventilation was established and we maintained the end-tidal CO_2 ($ETCO_2$) levels at 35 mmHg with tidal volumes (TV) of 350 ml and a respiratory rate of 15/min. The adjustable pressure limiting valve was set to 5 cm H_2O and average peak inspiratory pressures (PIP) and mean airway pressures (AP mean) were 22 cm H_2O and 12 cm H_2O, respectively.

During positioning, the patient coughed (TV 139 ml, PIP 37 cm H_2O, AP mean 16 cm H_2O) and received 50 mg propofol (i.v.). During cervical lymph node dissection and thymus removal, the care team noted a gurgling and bubbling sound radiating from the thorax. We checked the cuff pressure and tube position using a video laryngoscope, but no abnormalities were found. Three hours into the surgery the thyroid was unroofed and the thyroid ligament was dissected. In addition, all the lymphatic tissue from the carotid and innominate artery towards the midline was cleared out. In addition, the esophagus nerve and the side of the trachea from the thyroid cartilage down to the innominate artery just below the sternum were skeletonized. Again, a cycle of gurgling and bubbling of air into the neck occurred and the patient became difficult to ventilate. The patient slightly desaturated (SpO_2 91%) and low tidal volume alarms were noticed. The FiO_2 was set to 1.0 and the patient was manually ventilated. During manual ventilation decreased resistance was noted and TVs were as low as 42 ml, PIPs were as low as 11 cm H_2O, and AP mean was as low as 7 cm H_2O. The $ETCO_2$ was 30 mmHg due to increased manual ventilation rates (30/min). To check for an airway leak, the surgical team poured normal saline over the surgical field and observed bubbles in the saline but could not identify any lacerations of the trachea or pleural defects. As ventilation remained difficult with TVs constantly dropping and requiring consecutive recruitment maneuvers

over the next 30 minutes, a bronchoscopy was performed. The cuff was deflated and the ET tube was withdrawn until the vocal cords became visible. Ventilation was paused and the bronchoscopy was performed which showed a normal looking tracheal and lobar bronchial mucosa. However, the distal trachea and left mainstem bronchus appeared dynamically collapsed. Subsequent intraoperative chest X-ray revealed a small left-sided pneumothorax and a mild pneumomediastinum (Figure 2). The surgeon placed a chest tube to relieve the pneumothorax. Several hours later, the patient once again became difficult to ventilate and a second chest X-ray was performed to verify the correct position of the chest tube. While the left pneumothorax had decreased in size, a new right pneumothorax had developed (Figure 2) and a second chest tube was placed. After parathyroidectomy, near total thyroidectomy, bilateral central neck dissection, and left lateral neck dissection the surgery was aborted after 11.5 hours secondary to recurrent unstable clinical status. The patient was transferred, intubated, and hemodynamically stable, to the intensive care unit. On postoperative day 1, the patient met extubation criteria. Postextubation chest X-ray showed proper chest tube position, but the pneumothoraces had increased (Figure 3). In the hours following extubation, the patient stated shortness of breath and experienced labored breathing and pressure in the chest. The heart rate [104/min] and the systolic blood pressure became elevated [180 mmHg], and the SpO_2 dropped to 80% with a respirator rate of 41/min, indicating acute hypoxic respiratory failure and requiring reintubation (Figure 4). An echocardiogram showed normal left ventricular function (estimated ejection fraction 55.9%) and a severely dilated right ventricle with mild right ventricular hypertrophy. With poor oxygenation (PaO_2 60 mmHg, FiO_2 0.8) in the absence of cardiac failure, the care team diagnosed a severe respiratory distress syndrome (ARDS) based on the Berlin definition ($PaO_2/FiO_2 < 100$ and PEEP 5+, Figure 4) [5]. Following intubation sequential bronchoscopies revealed no evidence for a tracheal injury. As hypercarbic respiratory failure worsened ($PaCO_2$ 71 mmHg, pH 7.1, RR 35/min, PEEP 20 cm H_2O, plateau pressure 32 cm H_2O, Vt 6.5 ml/kg, I : E ratio 1 : 1, and Adaptive Support Ventilation [Hamilton G5]) with SpO_2s in the 80s (FiO_2 1.0, O_2 saturation mixed venous

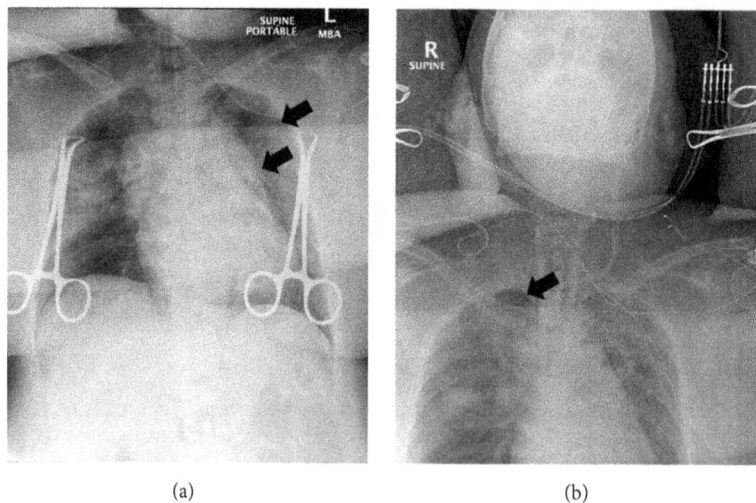

(a)

(b)

FIGURE 2: X-rays during surgery showing pneumomediastinum and pneumothorax. First intraoperative chest X-ray revealed a small left-sided pneumothorax and a mild pneumomediastinum ((a) black arrows). Second intraoperative chest X-ray found that the left pneumothorax had decreased in size; however, a new right pneumothorax had developed ((b) black arrows).

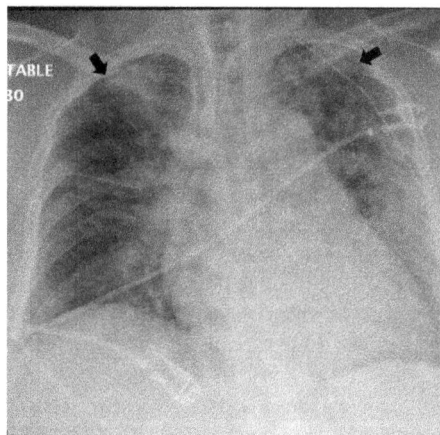

FIGURE 3: X-ray on postoperative day 1 after extubation. The patient was extubated on postoperative day 1 as he met extubation criteria. Shown is the X-ay after extubation, indicating that the bilateral pneumothoraces had increased despite bilateral chest tubes.

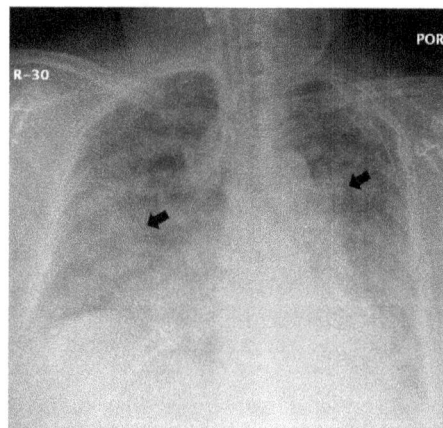

FIGURE 4: Respiratory failure on postoperative day 2. Shown is the chest X-ray with bilateral patchy opacities (black arrows) after urgent reintubation. Together with a normal left ventricular function and poor oxygenation (PaO_2 60 mmHg, FiO_2 0.8, Horowitz quotient of 75), an acute respiratory distress syndrome (ARDS) was diagnosed, based on the Berlin definition.

55%), the patient was placed on venovenous extracorporeal membrane oxygenation (vvECMO). Over the following three days the patient's respiratory function improved. VvECMO therapy was discontinued and the patient was subsequently extubated. Follow-up echocardiography found normal heart function with an EF of 73%. We discharged the patient from the hospital on postoperative day 12 in good physical condition. Due to posttraumatic stress disorder, the missing right lateral neck dissection was postponed but successfully performed eight months later.

3. Discussion

Pneumothorax is a known complication of thyroid surgery, reported as early as 1947 [6]. Nevertheless, only a few cases have been published suggesting a low incidence rate [7–10]. In strong contrast to this, one study reported pneumothorax as a complication of thyroid surgery in 1.53% of the cases [4]. Thus, the literature might underreport this problem, maybe because it bears the stigma of an iatrogenic complication.

In our case, bubbling and gurgling radiating from the thorax suggested either an airway injury or a leak around the endotracheal tube (ETT). Direct laryngoscopy and auscultation ruled out a partial extubation (e.g., caused by head movements during thyroid preparation). As the ETT cuff maintained the applied pressure, a cuff leak seemed unlikely. In fact, the majority of airway leaks are not associated with cuff defects [11]. Thus, the bubbling and gurgling were most likely a sign of an airway leak.

When air enters the thoracic cavity or the mediastinum, pneumothorax and pneumomediastinum develop. This requires a direct communication either between the alveoli and the pleural cavity or between the atmosphere and the pleura [12]. This can result from tracheal perforation, which has been reported to occur in 0.06% of thyroidectomy cases [13]. During thyroid surgery two possible sites of tracheal injury exist: at the isthmus, when the thyroid is separated from the trachea, and at the area where the recurrent laryngeal nerve enters the thyroid cartilage during lateral and posterior dissection [13]. An air leak usually causes self-resolving subcutaneous emphysema or a pneumomediastinum. When deep cervical lymph node dissection is performed, the air can track through the cervical fascial planes and create a pressure gradient causing a pleural injury. Also, an inadvertent violation of the pleura during deep lymph node dissection would allow air to enter the pleural cavity. However, the absence of obvious subcutaneous emphysema and no visible tracheal perforation during bronchoscopy complicated the clinical scenario in our patient.

In our case, the thyroid gland was described as "rock" hard and after dissecting the thyroid, the thyroid ligaments, and the deep cervical lymph nodes, gurgling and bubbling of air into the neck and difficult ventilation occurred. The size of the excised thyroid was 7.2 cm from superior to inferior, 6.0 cm from right to left, and 2.0 cm from posterior to anterior and weighing 35 grams. In addition, the papillary thyroid carcinoma had spread to the thymus and several lymph node levels (levels III–V), with the largest metastatic focus at a level V lymph node (1.3 cm). The relative large size and the changed tissue structure of the thyroid indicate a difficult dissection which is also reflected by the time (3 hours) it took to unroof the thyroid. Thus, the difficult "unroofing" of the thyroid in conjunction with a deep cervical lymph node dissection makes traumatic pneumothorax likely.

However, in our patient pneumomediastinum and pneumothorax could have also developed unrelated to surgery. During intraoperative bronchoscopy, we found dynamic airway collapse at the distal trachea and the left main stem bronchus. This finding can imply preexisting and undetected airway disease [14], including tracheomalacia or chronic obstructive pulmonary disease. Both go along with thinning of the airway walls; thus, high airway pressure (e.g., when the patient coughed during positioning) could have caused an airway leak with subsequent pneumothorax and pneumomediastinum, before surgery even started. The relative large and "rock" hard thyroid gland and airway collapse during bronchoscopy indicate that tracheomalacia could have contributed to the clinical scenario. Since the bronchoscope was advanced during exhalation without any ventilation, the mucosal leak was probably collapsed, missing the mucosal defect. Furthermore, we cannot rule out the possibility that the use of the neural integrity monitor (NIM) tube and electromyogram monitoring contributed to the increased risk of injury. These tubes are slightly stiffer than regular endotracheal tubes and, more importantly, EMG monitoring precludes the use of neuromuscular blocking agents. Although the tube placement was uneventful and proper positioning was confirmed by videolaryngoscopy, negative pressure spontaneous ventilation, such as from coughing, might have caused a breach of the pleura apex leading to a pneumothorax. Nevertheless, in this case, the increase in size of the bilateral pneumothoraces, with persisting pneumomediastinum after extubation, rather strongly suggests a perforation of the airway or the fascial planes undetectable by bronchoscopy. Reintubation and ECMO treatment must have contributed to the resolution of the injury as the patient did not require any further tracheal surgery or neck exploration. It remains remarkable that the intraoperative saline test to detect a perforation seemed positive while the more invasive bronchoscopy revealed a normal mucosa which lulled us into a false sense of security. However, flooding the surgical field with saline and observing bubbles mean that both the pulmonary and parietal pleura have been breached in the presence of positive pressure ventilation. Moreover, the fact that the pneumothoraces occurred serially rather than together is a strong indicator that this was surgical trauma-related and related to on-going dissection.

Why the patient developed ARDS postoperatively is unclear, since common causes such as pneumonia, sepsis, or severe trauma were absent. However, the literature reports one case of unexpected severe respiratory failure in a surgical patient in the presence of dynamic airway collapse undetected prior to surgery [15]. Thus, a combination of a preexisting subclinical airway disease (implied by the dynamic airway collapse) and a significant positive fluid balance (+4000 ml) after surgery could have been the cause for the ARDS in our patient. However, while the positive fluid balance was significant after surgery, the fluid balance was already negative (−650 ml) at the time of reintubation. As the patient did not require blood transfusions, TRALI as cause of ARDS can be ruled out.

In conclusion, we report the first case of acute respiratory failure with ECMO treatment following thyroid surgery, complicated by pneumomediastinum and bilateral pneumothoraces. It highlights that anesthesiologists need to be aware of the anatomical routes and the pathogenesis of air trapping in patients undergoing thyroid surgery in particular in cancer-related bilateral neck dissection. Even in the absence of an obvious airway perforation, the care team should critically evaluate the airway before early postoperative extubation. As also suggested by others [4], any unexplained episodes of oxygen desaturation during surgery or in the recovery room need follow-up chest radiography.

Acknowledgments

This study was funded by a departmental support.

References

[1] L. Davies and H. G. Welch, "Current thyroid cancer trends in the United States," *JAMA Otolaryngology—Head & Neck Surgery*, vol. 140, no. 4, pp. 317–322, 2014.

[2] G. H. Sun, S. Demonner, and M. M. Davis, "Epidemiological and economic trends in inpatient and outpatient thyroidectomy in the United States, 1996–2006," *Thyroid*, vol. 23, no. 6, pp. 727–733, 2013.

[3] H. Lim, S. S. Devesa, J. A. Sosa, D. Check, and C. M. Kitahara, "Trends in thyroid cancer incidence and mortality in the United States, 1974–2013," *JAMA*, vol. 317, no. 13, pp. 1338–1348, 2017.

[4] H. K. Eltzschig, M. Posner, and F. D. Moore Jr., "The use of readily available equipment in a simple method for intraoperative monitoring of recurrent laryngeal nerve function during thyroid surgery: initial experience with more than 300 cases," *Archives of Surgery*, vol. 137, no. 4, pp. 452–457, 2002.

[5] V. M. Ranieri, G. D. Rubenfeld, B. T. Thompson et al., "Acute respiratory distress syndrome: the Berlin definition," *JAMA*, vol. 307, pp. 2526–2533, 2012.

[6] B. R. Billimoria, "Bilateral pneumothorax after partial thyroidectomy," *The Lancet*, vol. 249, article 871, no. 6460, 1947.

[7] S. W. Lee, S. H. Cho, J. D. Lee, J. Y. Lee, S. C. Kim, and Y. W. Koh, "Bilateral pneumothorax and pneumomediastinum following total thyroidectomy with central neck dissection," *Clinical and Experimental Otorhinolaryngology*, vol. 1, pp. 49–51, 2008.

[8] L. Bertolaccini, C. Lauro, R. Priotto, and A. Terzi, "It sometimes happens: Late tracheal rupture after total thyroidectomy," *Interactive Cardiovascular and Thoracic Surgery*, vol. 14, no. 4, pp. 500–501, 2012.

[9] B. Slater and W. B. Inabnet, "Pneumothorax: an uncommon complication of minimally invasive parathyroidectomy," *Surgical Laparoscopy, Endoscopy & Percutaneous Techniques*, vol. 15, no. 1, pp. 38–40, 2005.

[10] M. A. Guerrero, C. J. Wray, S. S. Kee, J. C. Frenzel, and N. D. Perrier, "Minimally invasive parathyroidectomy complicated by pneumothoraces: a report of 4 cases," *Journal of Surgical Education*, vol. 64, no. 2, pp. 101–113, 2007.

[11] R. A. Kearl and R. G. Hooper, "Massive airway leaks: An analysis of the role of endotracheal tubes," *Critical Care Medicine*, vol. 21, no. 4, pp. 518–521, 1993.

[12] M. Noppen and T. De Keukeleire, "Pneumothorax," *Respiration*, vol. 76, no. 2, pp. 121–127, 2008.

[13] J. E. Gosnell, P. Campbell, S. Sidhu, M. Sywak, T. S. Reeve, and L. W. Delbridge, "Inadvertent tracheal perforation during thyroidectomy," *British Journal of Surgery*, vol. 93, no. 1, pp. 55–56, 2006.

[14] J. A. Gorden and A. Ernst, "Endoscopic management of central airway obstruction," *Seminars in Thoracic and Cardiovascular Surgery*, vol. 21, no. 3, pp. 263–273, 2009.

[15] M. R. Lyaker, V. R. Davila, and T. J. Papadimos, "Excessive dynamic airway collapse: an unexpected contributor to respiratory failure in a surgical patient," *Case Reports in Anesthesiology*, vol. 2015, Article ID 596857, 5 pages, 2015.

51

Ultrasound-Guided Femoral and Sciatic Nerve Blocks for Repair of Tibia and Fibula Fractures in a Bennett's Wallaby (*Macropus rufogriseus*)

Paolo Monticelli,[1] Luis Campoy,[2] and Chiara Adami[1]

[1]*Department of Clinical Sciences and Services, Royal Veterinary College, University of London, Hatfield, Hertfordshire AL97TA, UK*
[2]*Department of Anesthesiology and Analgesia, College of Veterinary Medicine, Cornell University, Ithaca, NY 14853, USA*

Correspondence should be addressed to Paolo Monticelli; pmonticelli@rvc.ac.uk

Academic Editor: Ehab Farag

Locoregional anesthetic techniques may be a very useful tool for the anesthetic management of wallabies with injuries of the pelvic limbs and may help to prevent capture myopathies resulting from stress and systemic opioids' administration. This report describes the use of ultrasound-guided femoral and sciatic nerve blocks in Bennett's wallaby (*Macropus rufogriseus*) referred for orthopaedic surgery. Ultrasound-guided femoral and sciatic nerve blocks were attempted at the femoral triangle and proximal thigh level, respectively. Whilst the sciatic nerve could be easily visualised, the femoral nerve could not be readily identified. Only the sciatic nerve was therefore blocked with ropivacaine, and methadone was administered as rescue analgesic. The ultrasound images were stored and sent for external review. Anesthesia and recovery were uneventful and the wallaby was discharged two days postoperatively. At the time of writing, it is challenging to provide safe and effective analgesia to Macropods. Detailed knowledge of the anatomy of these species is at the basis of successful locoregional anesthesia. The development of novel analgesic techniques suitable for wallabies would represent an important step forward in this field and help the clinicians dealing with these species to improve their perianesthetic management.

1. Introduction

In this report we describe the use of ultrasound-guided femoral and sciatic nerve blocks in a wallaby undergoing surgical fixation of tibial and fibular fractures. This technique [1] is commonly used in our referral hospital for patients undergoing orthopaedic surgeries involving the stifle joint or structures located distal to it. Its analgesic efficacy has been demonstrated in various animal species, including dogs, goats, pet rabbits, and raptors [2–5].

It is reasonable to assume that, similarly to other animal species, also wallabies would benefit from femoral-sciatic block as a part of the management of the pelvic limb surgeries. Furthermore, Macropods have unique physiological features which make locoregional anesthesia a particularly attractive option for the treatment of perioperative pain. As wild animal species, they are prone to develop a life-threatening condition known as capture myopathy, of which opioids

administration and stressors, such as physical restraint and poorly managed pain, are well-recognised triggering factors [6, 7]. Within the last decades, a lot of research has been done with the purpose of developing novel techniques to minimise the stress response and its fatal sequels [8, 9], and it has been demonstrated that the choice of the anesthetic technique does play a major role in decreasing the incidence of these events [8]. As a matter of fact, successful locoregional anesthesia is likely to have a sparing effect on intraoperative requirement of opioids, which are believed to be implicated in the pathogenesis of rhabdomyolysis possibly through vasospasm, hyperpyrexia, and direct myofibrillar damage [6]. Similarly, poorly managed pain and the resulting stress would cause decreased muscular perfusion, lactic acidosis, and adenosine triphosphate depletion through a prolonged adrenergic stimulation [6, 7, 9].

When selecting a locoregional anesthetic technique for wallabies, some species-specific consideration should be taken into account. One advantage of peripheral nerve blocks over neuroaxial anesthesia is the unilateral versus bilateral motor blockade, an aspect particularly desirable in wild Macropods, whose early regain of pelvic limbs' motor function is of primary importance to minimise the stress response and to increase the chance of postsurgical survival. In the light of these considerations, sciatic-femoral block was regarded by the authors as a suitable option to provide analgesia to the wallaby object of this report, undergoing surgical treatment of comminuted tibial and fibular fractures.

The aim of this report was to describe the technical aspects of this locoregional technique and to discuss the encountered challenges, when applied to wallabies.

2. Case Presentation

Two-month-old female entire pet Bennett's wallaby (*Macropus rufogriseus*) weighing 4 Kg was referred to the Queen Mother Hospital for Animals (QMHA) for diagnosis and treatment of sudden onset-left pelvic limb lameness. A protective bandage had been applied by the referral veterinarian and buprenorphine (20 mcg/kg) was administered intramuscularly (IM) every 8 hours. The wallaby was scheduled for diagnostic imaging and possibly surgery on the following day.

The wallaby was ambulatory on presentation and appeared bright, alert, and responsive. Resting heart rate was 144 beats/min with regular rhythm. Thoracic auscultation was unremarkable with a respiratory rate of 28 breaths/min. Preanesthetic blood work results were not available. The radiographic exam, performed in the anaesthetised animal, showed a complete, mild comminuted fracture of the distal physis of the tibia affecting the distal part of the adjacent metaphysis. The fracture was slightly displaced craniolaterally. A complete, short oblique fracture of the distal third of the fibula was also visible. Moderate swelling extending along the crus was also present. It was decided to proceed with surgical fracture fixation and cast application.

Food and drinking water were withdrawn immediately before anesthesia. The wallaby was tail restrained [10] to allow injection of 50 mcg/kg of dexmedetomidine and 5 mg/kg of ketamine in the left quadriceps. Onset of anesthesia was approximately 5 minutes from injection. Thereafter, a 22-gauge catheter was inserted in the right cephalic vein and the wallaby was positioned in dorsal recumbency with the neck extended to allow endotracheal (ET) intubation. The latter was accomplished with a 3.0 mm ID cuffed ET-tube, inserted orotracheally under direct laryngoscopy through an "over the catheter" technique. The ET-tube was then connected to modified Ayre's T-piece and the fresh gas flow rate was adjusted in order to prevent carbon dioxide rebreathing. The inspired fraction of oxygen (F_iO_2) was 1. Anesthesia was maintained with sevoflurane vaporised in oxygen (end-tidal: 1.5–2.0%). Crystalloids (Lactated Ringer's) were infused intravenously (IV) at a rate of 5 mL/kg/h. A multiparametric module (S/5 Datex-Ohmeda) was used to continuously monitor physiological parameters, which were manually recorded at a 5-minute interval. The systolic, mean, and diastolic arterial blood pressure (SAP, MAP, and DAP, resp.) were measured noninvasively (oscillometry

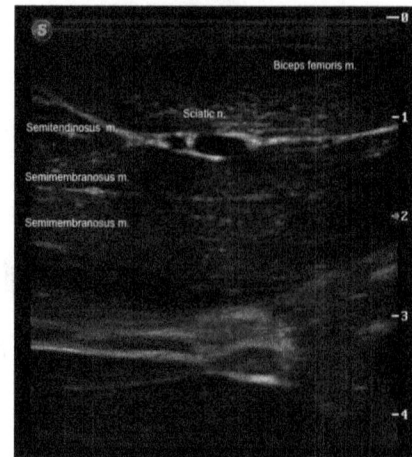

FIGURE 1: Sciatic nerve: ultrasonographic short axis view image of the sciatic nerve of a wallaby (*Macropus rufogriseus*). The sciatic nerve can be identified as a hypoechoic double-ellipsoid structure located deep to the fascia of the *biceps femoris* muscle and cranial and superficial to the two bellies of the semimembranosus muscle, respectively. S is caudal.

technique), with a size 4-cuff placed at the base of the tail over the coccygeal artery. During the anesthetic, the wallaby was allowed to breathe spontaneously with a respiratory rate ranging from 20 to 30 breaths/min. No further rescue analgesics were required during surgery. Intraoperatively, moderate bradycardia (65 beats/min) and associated hypotension (MAP 45 mmHg) occurred approximately 45 minutes after anesthetic induction and were initially treated with IV glycopyrronium (10 mcg/kg). Due to the lack of response in heart rate and persistent hypotension, a dopamine infusion was commenced 10 minutes later at a rate of 5 mcg/kg/min. Subsequently, heart rate returned to baseline values and MAP increased to 75 mmHg and both variables were maintained at physiological values until the end of the procedure.

In order to provide perioperative analgesia, an ultrasound- (US-) guided combined femoral and sciatic nerve block was attempted as previously described by Campoy and colleagues in the dog [1]. An ultrasonographer (S9v, Sonoscape, China) equipped with a 25 mm linear-array transducer (10–6 MHz) was used.

Briefly, the sciatic nerve block was performed with the wallaby in lateral recumbency and the affected limb positioned uppermost. The ischiatic tuberosity and the greater trochanter were identified by palpation and used as anatomical landmarks. The transducer was then positioned immediately distal to these landmarks, on a transverse plane with respect to the long axis of the femur in an attempt to obtain a short axis view of the sciatic nerve. The sciatic nerve was identified as a hypoechoic rounded structure (Figure 1) located between the hyperechoic fascias of the *biceps femoris*, the abductor, and the two bellies of the semimembranosus muscles. Subsequently, a 22 G, 63 mm Quincke spinal needle was advanced "in-plane" from the caudal aspect of the thigh towards the nerve. Once the needle could be visualised in the proximity to the sciatic nerve, an aspiration test was

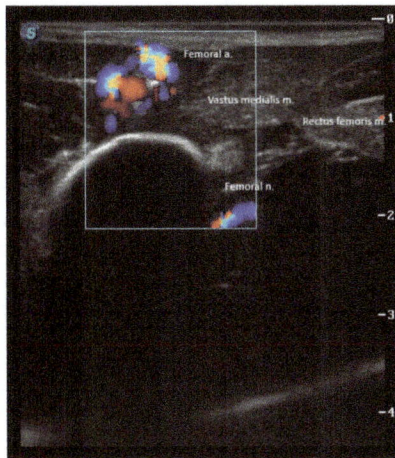

FIGURE 2: Femoral nerve: ultrasonographic view of the inguinal area of a wallaby (*Macropus rufogriseus*). The transducer was positioned on a transverse plane with respect to the long axis of the femur to obtain a short axis view of the femoral nerve. The femoral nerve can be identified as a hyperechoic rounded structure cranial to the femur, caudal to the *rectus femoris* muscle, and deep to the femoral artery and *vastus medialis* muscle. S is caudal.

performed to rule out intravascular location of the tip of the needle. Ropivacaine 0.75% was injected at a volume of 0.05 mL/kg. The correct perineural position of the needle was confirmed by the observation of even spread of the local anesthetic around the sciatic nerve.

The ultrasonographic identification of the femoral nerve was more challenging. As a consequence, additional nerve stimulator guidance was used.

Briefly, with the animal in right lateral recumbency, the left pelvic limb was abducted 90° and slightly extended caudally, and the transducer was positioned on a transverse plane with respect to the long axis of the femur in order to obtain a short axis view of the femoral nerve. The femoral artery was located by pulse palpation within the femoral triangle. The femoral nerve, as previously described in the dog [1], should be typically identified as a hyperechoic nodular structure located cranial and deep to the femoral artery and the fascia iliaca and caudal to the *rectus femoris* muscle. However, this did not seem to be the case and the targeted nerve could not be clearly identified on an initial attempt. A transient, weak motor response, characterised by extension of the knee and contraction of the quadriceps muscle, could only be evoked at currents greater than 1 mA. The block was aborted and 0.1 mg/kg of methadone was administered IV. Before transferring the patient to the surgery theatre, the ultrasound images of the femoral triangle were stored and sent off seeking a second opinion (Figure 2).

The fracture was reduced via a combined medial and lateral approach. A 0.8 mm K wire was placed as an intramedullary pin within the fibula maintaining limb alignment. Following fibular intramedullary pinning, a 1.2 mm K wire was driven from the medial malleolus across the fracture line to engage the transcortex of the tibia.

General anesthesia lasted 4 hours. Postoperative radiographs demonstrated appropriate fracture reduction and implant positioning. After a cast was applied to the operated limb, the wallaby was transferred to recovery for the early postoperative care.

Despite the use of both active and passive warming devices (two Bair Huggers plus an isolating blanket between the patient and the operating table) throughout anesthesia, moderate hypothermia (rectal temperature: 32.4°C) was observed [9, 11]. Active warming was continued during the early recovery period and the wallaby started eating grass as soon as its rectal body temperature reached 36.5°C, which happened one hour after tracheal extubation. Buprenorphine, 20 mcg/kg, was administered IV 4 hours after the administration of intraoperative methadone. No motor block was observed in the immediate postoperative period.

Physical and radiographic examination performed 6 weeks after surgery revealed a good clinical condition of the wallaby, with normal orthopaedic and neurological function of the operated limb.

3. Discussion

This report describes the challenges encountered when applying the technique described to perform femoral-sciatic nerve block in dogs to a wallaby, undergoing hind limb orthopaedic surgery.

Whilst ultrasonographic identification of the sciatic nerve could be achieved easily, although both operators were familiar with the use of these locoregional techniques in dogs, blocking the femoral nerve in this wallaby was more challenging than expected. A careful, more attentive analysis of the stored ultrasound images carried out at a later stage revealed the slightly different location of the femoral nerve compared with that in the dog. It is difficult to formulate a convincing hypothesis to explain this finding. One possibility may be that the unique hopping locomotion of marsupials implies peculiar geometry of the hind legs, which is accomplished by a different spatial and anatomical arrangement of its related muscles, tendons, and nerves compared to quadrupeds. During hopping, the muscles that deliver the main driving force and those involved in retraction are grouped around the hip, whereas the muscles of the lower, more distal areas store the elastic energy during landing at the end of a hop [12, 13]. Additionally, a marsupial lands all the large muscles of the hind legs which are in an active state simultaneously, unlike in quadrupeds in which the muscles in one leg are relaxed whilst those in the other leg are contracting [12, 13]. These unique anatomical, geometrical, and physiological features of the pelvic limbs of wallabies may explain the slightly different spatial arrangement of the femoral nerve compared to dogs. Nevertheless, it is worth emphasising that the same anatomical features were still preserved. The location of the femoral nerve was still deep to the sartorius muscle, femoral artery, and *vastus medialis* muscle and caudal to the *rectus femoris*. The fact that the *vastus medialis* could be identified on the ultrasound images may indicate a slightly distal location of the transducer compared to the classical approach as described in dogs or alternatively an overdeveloped *vastus medialis* extending more proximally than in the dog. The former theory may agree with the fact that when the targeted structure was electrically stimulated, only currents greater than 1 mA could elicit a mild response of the quadriceps. This seems to indicate that the nerve identified at this location was the saphenous rather than the femoral nerve. In retrospect, the administration of local anesthetic around any of these nerves would have likely yielded a successful blockade.

With respect to the sciatic nerve block performed in the wallaby, the administration of preoperative methadone makes any consideration regarding the analgesic efficacy of the block a speculation. To the best of the authors' knowledge, there are no published data about the pharmacological properties of methadone in *Macropus rufogriseus*. Nevertheless, methadone was administered to the wallaby only once and at a dose lower than the one generally recommended for dogs. Based on our clinical experience, it is unlikely that methadone, used as sole anesthetic at such low dose, would result in satisfactory analgesia in dogs undergoing invasive orthopaedic procedures. Furthermore, the wallaby had a comminuted fracture whose surgical fixation required considerable manipulation of bones and soft tissues, which presumably resulted in intense nociceptive stimulation. This seems to suggest that, to some extent, the sciatic nerve block contributed to providing analgesia to the wallaby during surgery. However, the paucity of scientific literature focusing on analgesia in Macropods, together with the lack of validated scales for recognition of pain in these species, makes proper assessment and treatment of pain a goal very difficult to achieve.

Also the pharmacokinetics and the pharmacodynamics of local anesthetic agents are largely unknown in marsupials. In the wallaby object of this report, it was decided to use ropivacaine for the sciatic nerve block, owing to its favourable pharmacological profile in both humans and dogs, and no adverse effects were observed. Ropivacaine is a long-lasting amino amide whose efficacy is comparable to the one of bupivacaine but with a lower propensity to produce motor block [14] and cardiovascular or neurological toxicity [15]. These features make ropivacaine a more attractive option than bupivacaine in animal species in which there is paucity of literature and an early regain of motor function of the hind limbs is of crucial importance.

In conclusion, with some limitations, this case report highlights the potential usefulness of locoregional anesthetic techniques in wallabies undergoing pelvic limb surgery. The peculiar anatomy of the nerves and muscles of the hind limbs of marsupials should be taken into account when attempting sciatic and femoral nerve blocks. The ultrasonographic study of the area may represent a first step for the development of species-specific locoregional techniques to be used in wallabies.

Competing Interests

The authors declare that they have no competing interests.

Acknowledgments

The authors would like to thank Professor Alex Davies for his kind advice.

References

[1] L. Campoy, A. J. Bezuidenhout, R. D. Gleed et al., "Ultrasound-guided approach for axillary brachial plexus, femoral nerve, and sciatic nerve blocks in dogs," *Veterinary Anaesthesia and Analgesia*, vol. 37, no. 2, pp. 144–153, 2010.

[2] C. Adami, A. Bergadano, R. M. Bruckmaier, M. H. Stoffel, M. G. Doherr, and C. Spadavecchia, "Sciatic-femoral nerve block with bupivacaine in goats undergoing elective stifle arthrotomy," *The Veterinary Journal*, vol. 188, no. 1, pp. 53–57, 2011.

[3] J. Aguiar, G. Mogridge, and J. Hall, "Femoral fracture repair and sciatic and femoral nerve blocks in a guinea pig," *Journal of Small Animal Practice*, vol. 55, no. 12, pp. 635–639, 2014.

[4] D. d'Ovidio, S. Rota, E. Noviello, A. Briganti, and C. Adami, "Nerve stimulator-guided sciatic-femoral block in pet rabbits (*Oryctolagus cuniculus*) undergoing hind limb surgery: a case series," *Journal of Exotic Pet Medicine*, vol. 23, no. 1, pp. 91–95, 2014.

[5] D. d'Ovidio, E. Noviello, and C. Adami, "Nerve stimulator-guided sciatic-femoral nerve block in raptors undergoing surgical treatment of pododermatitis," *Veterinary Anaesthesia and Analgesia*, vol. 42, no. 4, pp. 449–453, 2015.

[6] F. Y. Khan, "Rhabdomyolysis: a review of the literature," *Netherlands Journal of Medicine*, vol. 67, no. 9, pp. 272–283, 2009.

[7] J. Paterson, "Capture myopathy," in *Zoo Animal and Wildlife Immobilization and Anesthesia*, G. West, D. Heard, and N. Caulkett, Eds., pp. 171–179, Wiley Blackwell, 2nd edition, 2014.

[8] T. Bouts, N. Harrison, K. Berry, P. Taylor, A. Routh, and F. Gasthuys, "Comparison of three anaesthetic protocols in Bennett's wallabies (*Macropus rufogriseus*)," *Veterinary Anaesthesia and Analgesia*, vol. 37, no. 3, pp. 207–214, 2010.

[9] L. Vogelnest and T. Portas, "Macropods," in *Medicine of Australian Mammals*, L. Vogelnest and R. Woods, Eds., pp. 133–227, CSIRO Publishing, Collingwood, Australia, 2008.

[10] P. Holtz, "Marsupials," in *Zoo Animal and Wildlife Immobilization and Anesthesia*, G. West, D. Heard, and N. Caulkett, Eds., pp. 521–528, Wiley Blackwell, 2nd edition, 2014.

[11] S. Jackson, "Macropods," in *Australian Mammals, Biology and Captive Management*, S. Jackson, Ed., pp. 245–293, CSIRO, Collingwood, Australia, 2003.

[12] R. M. Alexander and A. Vernon, "The mechanics of hopping by kangaroos (Macropodidae)," *Journal of Zoology*, vol. 177, no. 2, pp. 265–303, 1975.

[13] R. V. Baudinette, "The biomechanics and energetics of locomotion in Macropodidae," in *Kangaroos, Wallabies and Rat-Kangaroos*, G. Grigg, P. Jarman, and I. Hume, Eds., pp. 245–253, Surrey Beatty, Sydney, Australia, 1989.

[14] D. Simpson, M. P. Curran, V. Oldfield, and G. M. Keating, "Ropivacaine: a review of its use in regional anaesthesia and acute pain management," *Drugs*, vol. 65, no. 18, pp. 2675–2717, 2005.

[15] H. S. Feldman, G. R. Arthur, and B. G. Covino, "Comparative systemic toxicity of convusant ans supraconvulsant doses of intravenous ropivacaine, bupivacaine, and lidocaine in conscious dogs," *Anesthesia and Analgesia*, vol. 69, pp. 794–801, 1989.

52

Use of Awake Flexible Fiberoptic Bronchoscopic Nasal Intubation in Secure Airway Management for Reconstructive Surgery in a Pediatric Patient with Burn Contracture of the Neck

Tolga Totoz,[1] **Kerem Erkalp** (ID),[2] **Sirin Taskin,**[3] **Ummahan Dalkilinc,**[2] **and Aysin Selcan**[2]

[1]*Department of Anesthesiology and Reanimation, Nisantasi University, Istanbul Safak Hospital, Turkey*
[2]*Department of Anesthesiology and Reanimation, Health Sciences University,*
 Istanbul Bagcilar Training and Educational Hospital, Turkey
[3]*Department of Anesthesiology and Reanimation, Health Sciences University,*
 Istanbul Haydarpasa Sample Training and Research Hospital, Turkey

Correspondence should be addressed to Kerem Erkalp; keremerkalp@hotmail.com

Academic Editor: Pavel Michalek

Although the use of awake flexible fiberoptic bronchoscopic (FFB) intubation is a well-recognized airway management technique in patients with difficult airway, its use in smaller children with burn contractures or in an uncooperative older child may be challenging. Herein, we report successful management of difficult airway in a 7-year-old boy with burn contracture of the neck, by application of FFB nasal intubation in a stepwise approach, first during an initial preoperative trial phase to increase patient cooperation and then during anesthesia induction for the reconstructive surgery planned for burn scars and contractures. Our findings emphasize the importance of a preplanned algorithm for airway control in secure airway management and feasibility of awake FFB intubation in a pediatric patient with burn contracture of the neck during anesthesia induction for reconstructive surgery. Application of FFB intubation based on a stepwise approach including a trial phase prior to operation day seemed to increase the chance of a successful intubation in our patient in terms of technical expertise and increased patient cooperation and tolerance by enabling familiarity with the procedure.

1. Introduction

Secure airway management is crucial in reconstructive surgeries involving patients with burn contracture of the neck [1, 2], while it is a challenge to the anesthesiologist due to anticipation of difficult intubation with likelihood of profound anatomical variation that may not readily be appreciated even during preoperative assessment [1–3].

Awake intubation is considered a safe approach in the airway management of a patient with burn contracture of the neck, particularly for cases presenting with the combination of difficult laryngoscopy as well as difficult mask ventilation [2, 4, 5]. Hence, awake endotracheal intubation remains at the top of the decision algorithm in the recently updated practice guidelines for management of the difficult airway by American Society of Anesthesiology (ASA), although no specific technique or tool has been suggested for accomplishing this task [6].

Fiberoptic-guided tracheal intubation remains the gold standard for pediatric difficult airways and is an essential skill for anyone practicing pediatric anesthesia [7–10]. Awake flexible fiberoptic bronchoscopic (FFB) intubation is a well-recognized airway management technique in patients with difficult airway [4], while its use in smaller children with burn contractures or in an uncooperative older child may be challenging and necessitate inhalational induction technique [2, 11, 12].

Being a cornerstone of safe anesthetic practice in managing patients with identified difficult airway, awake intubation enables prevention of the disastrous consequences of a potential "cannot intubate and cannot oxygenate" scenario, while necessitating a preplanned strategy for intubation and patient preparation regarding explanation of the proposed procedure, sedation, administration of antisialogogues, and regional anesthesia of the airway [2, 4].

Herein, we report successful management of difficult airway in a 7-year-old boy with burn contracture of the neck, by application of awake FFB nasal intubation in a stepwise approach, first during an initial preoperative trial phase to increase patient cooperation and then during anesthesia induction for the reconstructive surgery planned for burn scars and contractures.

2. Case Report

A 7-year-old Syrian boy with war-related burn injury was referred to our hospital for reconstructive surgery for burn scars and contractures on his face, neck, and body. A consultation with anesthesia department was held by plastic and reconstructive surgery clinic for the preanesthesia evaluation. Patient was conscious and oriented on examination. He had severe scar contractures involving neck, face, anterior chest, and both shoulders leading to restricted mouth opening, no neck extension, and stooped posture with chin and chest fused together by scars and the neck and head contracted in flexed position. The width from upper incisor to lower teeth was approximately 15 mm and Mallampati class was 3, while thyromental and sternomental distance could not be evaluated due to neck and head being contracted in flexed position. Cardiac, thoracic, and laboratory investigations revealed normal findings. Detailed history of the patient obtained from the parents by the help of a translator revealed that the child had been posted for the reconstructive surgery in another university hospital, while the operation was cancelled due to failure to maintain mask ventilation even after pain relief and induction of anesthesia. The previous anesthesiologist had given two attempts after induction of anesthesia but failed at intubation. Then child was awakened. The day after, he was transferred to our hospital for difficult airway approach and the operation. Awake FFB nasal intubation was planned because of the past history of "cannot intubate and cannot oxygenate" scenario. The necessity and details of the procedure were explained to the patient and his family by the help of a translator. After a 6-hour fasting period, the patient was admitted to our intensive care unit (ICU), accompanied by a family member and translator. Following the routine (NIBP, HR, StO$_2$) monitorization (Nihon Kohden, Japan), patient has been informed again about the details and steps of the procedure with the help of the translator. Premedication and sedation were not applied because of the patient's status. During the initial trial phase, nasal drop of xylometazoline 0.1% was instilled for vasoconstriction in both nostrils. Three puffs of 10% lidocaine were implemented for topical anesthesia. Through a nasal cannula, oxygen was administered at 5 L/min through the left side. Tip of the fiberoptic bronchoscope (FOB, 2.8 mm, Karl Storz-Endoskope, Germany)

was inserted into the contralateral nostril. Endoscopy was performed. When the vocal cords were visible, the trial procedure was ended. It was explained to the patient and his family that the same procedure would be repeated on the day of surgery as followed by intubation and induction of general anesthesia. On the day of operation, two days after the initial trial, patient was taken to the surgery room and monitored (Infinity Delta Dräger, Lübeck, Germany) routinely (NIBP, HR, SatO$_2$). A nasal drop of xylometazoline 0.1% was instilled for vasoconstriction. Three puffs of 10% lidocaine spray were implemented for topical anesthesia. It directly sprayed onto the mucosa of the mouth, pharynx, and tongue. Through a nasal cannula, oxygen was administered at 5 L/min through the left nostril. Endoscopy was performed through the right nostril. Two ml of 2% lignocaine was sprayed through the FOB on to the glottis after the vocal cords were seen. The FOB's tip was then passed into the trachea through the laryngeal opening and was stopped just above the carina. Lubricated 5.0 nasotracheal tube was railroaded over the FOB. After three ventilations, position of nasotracheal tube was confirmed by the FOB. Successful tracheal intubation had been achieved while maintaining spontaneous ventilation and was monitored by capnography. Propofol, fentanyl, and rocuronium were used for induction of general anesthesia via intravenous route and maintained with remifentanil 0.1 μg/kg/min and sevoflurane in oxygen (Primus workstation Dräger, Lübeck, Germany). The operation lasted for approximately four hours. The contractures on neck and left axilla were released and graft was placed. The intraoperative course was uneventful. The patient was extubated after complete recovery of consciousness, adequate spontaneous breathing, preventive reflex, and muscle strength [13] (Figure 1).

3. Discussion

Our findings indicate feasibility of awake FFB nasal intubation in a 7-year-old boy with burn contracture of the neck accompanied with restricted mouth opening, no neck extension, and fixed flexion deformity, during anesthesia induction for reconstructive surgery for burn scars and contractures.

Restricted mouth opening, Mallampati class (>2), lack of neck movement, and inability to evaluate thyromental and sternomental distance due to flexed position of neck and head in our patient signify a difficult airway and emphasize that certain airway assessment parameters useful in evaluation of a difficult airway are not applicable in patients with burn contracture of the neck [2, 14].

Given patient's history of difficult tracheal intubation and/or mask ventilation, our findings support the consideration of alternative rather than standard means of securing an airway as a first-line option in patients with face and neck contracture [1, 2]. Our findings also emphasize the utility of awake FFB nasal intubation in postburn pediatric patients with fixed flexion deformity related nonalignment of the oral, pharyngeal, and laryngeal planes for intubation [2, 4], provided that measures to enable sufficient patient cooperation were implied.

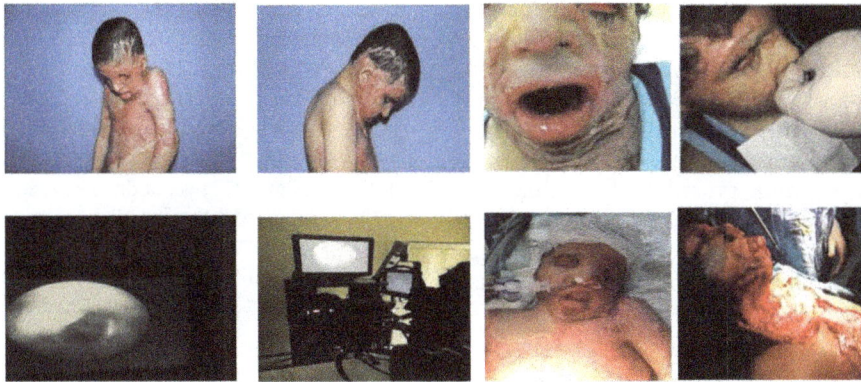

FIGURE 1: Patient's perioperative images.

Although FFB is considered to be the probably most commonly used tool for awake endotracheal intubation in developed countries [4, 15], in accordance with its consideration as the least traumatic and most efficient alternative to direct laryngoscopy in patients with postburn scar contractures of the neck [1, 16, 17], there are other tools available such as Fastrach intubating laryngeal mask airway (ILMA) [4, 18].

In a past study on comparison of safety and efficacy of ILMA and FFB in awake tracheal intubation of patients with difficult airway, FFB was reported to be associated with significantly lower rate of success on the first attempt (58% versus 95%) along with need for multiple attempts in 42% of patient [4]. However, ILMA has been associated with limitations in certain patients such as those with very restricted mouth opening who need a nasal intubation and those aged <10 years or weighing less than 30 kg due to unavailability of pediatric sizes [4, 19, 20]. Hence FFB seemed to be most reasonable option for management of difficult airway via awake intubation in our patient given his young age and the need for a nasal intubation.

FFB intubation with topical anesthesia of the upper airway in an awake or sedated patient is considered by anesthesiologists as the ultimate, safe, nonsurgical technique in difficult airway management [21]. Although, FFB intubation can cause significant circulatory responses in healthy anesthetized children, the circulatory responses to flexible nasal intubation are considered less frequent and shorter-term responses than those to flexible oral intubation [22].

Hence, based on history of an unsuccessful attempt for intubation and mask ventilation under sedation or general anesthesia in our patient, we preferred awake FFB nasal intubation with use of no sedative or anesthetic agent. While, from a physiologic perspective, children have higher rates of oxygen consumption, significantly shortening the period of apnea that can be safely tolerated [23], no hypoxia occurred during the procedure in our patient given that oxygen was applied through the contralateral nostril.

Although application of fiberoptic tracheal intubation through the nasal route rather than the oral route is considered likely to be more straightforward for clinicians with less experience using pediatric bronchoscopes [6], use of FBB in

awake intubation is considered to require significant training and experience to achieve a high success rate [4]. This seems notable given that successful outcome of an awake intubation is considered a net result of different factors including appropriate case selection and good patient preparation to optimize the patient's comfort and compliance as well as technical expertise method of intubation [24].

Awake intubation has been advocated as the safest technique to secure the airway in a cooperative patient for a difficult airway [12, 25]. In this regard, application of FFB nasal intubation based on a stepwise approach including a trial phase prior to operation day seemed to increase the chance of a successful intubation in our patient in terms of improved technical expertise as well as increased patient cooperation and tolerability after familiarity with a procedure limiting the handicaps of a translation-mediated communication.

Our findings support that vigilance and preparedness is the key to success in the postburn patient with crucial role of judicious preoperative airway and scar evaluation to timely recognition of anticipated difficulty with ventilation, intubation, or both in order to develop a preplanned strategy for airway control [1, 2, 14].

Some anesthesiologists have also reserved videolaryngoscopy (VL) for difficult pediatric airway according to the algorithm [26]. On the other hand, FFB intubation is still the gold standard for anticipated difficult airway management in children. Use of VL might have been an alternative [27]. Like our method, awake VL technique also may be considered in children

The limitation of our method is that we did not use short-acting sedatives/opioids, such as remifentanil or midazolam for sedation in this case, because of detrimental effects, such as muscle rigidity, hypoxemia, respiratory arrest, or hemodynamic fluctuations requiring treatment [28], and ketamine or sevoflurane administration during procedure because of awake FFB intubation effort.

In conclusion, our findings emphasize the importance of a preplanned algorithm for airway control in secure airway management and feasibility of awake FFB nasal intubation in a 7-year-old boy with burn contracture of the neck and fixed flexion deformity, during anesthesia induction for reconstructive surgery for burn scars and contractures. Application of FFB intubation via stepwise approach with a trial phase prior to operation day seemed to increase the chance of a successful intubation in our patient in terms of technical expertise and increased patient cooperation and tolerance via familiarity with the procedure. We would also emphasize the importance of preoperative demonstration and explanation of fiberoptic procedure, which is something original and probably resulted in key point for successful maneuver.

Additional Points

Highlights. (i) Use of awake FFB revealed successful airway management in burn contracture of neck. (ii) Preoperative trial FFB seems likely to increase patient cooperation and toleration. (iii) Awake FFB nasal intubation seems feasible in pediatric difficult airway management.

References

[1] T. H. Han, H. Teissler, R. J. Han, J. D. Gaines, and T. Q. Nguyen, "Managing difficult airway in patients with post-burn mentosternal and circumoral scar contractures," *Int J Burns Trauma*, vol. 2, pp. 80–85, 2012.

[2] S. Prakash and P. Mullick, "Airway management in patients with burn contractures of the neck," *Burns*, vol. 41, no. 8, pp. 1627–1635, 2015.

[3] O. Nahlieli, J. P. Kelly, A. M. Baruchin, P. Ben-Meir, and Y. Shapira, "Oro-maxillofacial skeletal deformities resulting from burn scar contractures of the face and neck," *Burns*, vol. 21, no. 1, pp. 65–69, 1995.

[4] S. F. Hanna, M. Mikat-Stevens, J. Loo, R. Uppal, W. S. Jellish, and M. Adams, "Awake tracheal intubation in anticipated difficult airways: LMA Fastrach vs flexible bronchoscope: A pilot study," *Journal of Clinical Anesthesia*, vol. 37, pp. 31–37, 2017.

[5] G. Frova and M. Sorbello, "Algorithms for difficult airway management: A review," *Minerva Anestesiologica*, vol. 75, no. 4, pp. 201–209, 2009.

[6] American Society of Anesthesiologists, "Practice guidelines for management of the difficult airway: an updated report," Anesthesiology 118, 2013.

[7] N. Jagannathan, L. Sequera-Ramos, L. Sohn et al., "Randomized comparison of experts and trainees with nasal and oral fibreoptic intubation in children less than 2 yr of age," *British Journal of Anaesthesia*, vol. 114, no. 2, pp. 290–296, 2015.

[8] C. Sims and B. S. von Ungern-Sternberg, "The normal and the challenging pediatric airway," *Pediatric Anesthesia*, vol. 22, no. 6, pp. 521–526, 2012.

[9] R. A. Sunder, D. T. Haile, P. T. Farrell, and A. Sharma, "Pediatric airway management: current practices and future directions," *Pediatric Anesthesia*, vol. 22, no. 10, pp. 1008–1015, 2012.

[10] M. Weiss and T. Engelhardt, "Proposal for the management of the unexpected difficult pediatric airway," *Pediatric Anesthesia*, vol. 20, no. 5, pp. 454–464, 2010.

[11] J. Fiadjoe and P. Stricker, "Pediatric Difficult Airway Management: Current Devices and Techniques," *Anesthesiology Clinics*, vol. 27, no. 2, pp. 185–195, 2009.

[12] E. Varghese, R. Nagaraj, and R. Shwethapriya, "Comparison of oral fiberoptic intubation via a modified guedel airway or a laryngeal mask airway in infants and children," *Journal of Anaesthesiology Clinical Pharmacology*, vol. 29, no. 1, pp. 52–55, 2013.

[13] M. Sorbello and G. Frova, "When the end is really the end? The extubation in the difficult airway patient," *Minerva Anestesiologica*, vol. 79, no. 2, pp. 194–199, 2013.

[14] J. L. Apfelbaum, C. A. Hagberg, R. A. Caplan et al., "Practice guidelines for management of the difficult airway: an updated report by the American Society of Anesthesiologists Task Force on Management of the Difficult Airway," *Anesthesiology*, vol. 118, no. 2, pp. 251–270, 2013.

[15] O. Langeron, J. Amour, B. Vivien, and F. Aubrun, "Clinical review: Management of difficult airways," *Critical Care*, vol. 10, no. 6, 2006.

[16] B. C. H. Tsui and K. Cunningham, "Fiberoptic Endotracheal Intubation after Topicalization with In-Circuit Nebulized Lidocaine in a Child with a Difficult Airway," *Anesthesia & Analgesia*, vol. 98, no. 5, pp. 1286–1288, 2004.

[17] F. S. Xue, X. Liao, L. CW, X. YC, Q. Y. Yang, and Y. Liu, "Clinical experience of airway management and tracheal intubation under general anesthesia in patients with scar contracture of the neck," *Chin Med J (Engl)*, vol. 121, pp. 989-97, 2008.

[18] A. I. J. Brain, C. Verghese, E. V. Addy, A. Kapila, and J. Brimacombe, "The intubating laryngeal mask. II: a preliminary clinical report of a new means of intubating the trachea," *British Journal of Anaesthesia*, vol. 79, no. 6, pp. 704–709, 1997.

[19] O. Langeron, P. Cuvillon, C. Ibanez-Esteve, F. Lenfant, B. Riou, and Y. Le Manach, "Prediction of difficult tracheal intubation: Time for a paradigm change," *Anesthesiology*, vol. 117, no. 6, pp. 1223–1233, 2012.

[20] D. Z. Ferson, W. H. Rosenblatt, M. J. Johansen, I. Osborn, and A. Ovassapian, "Use of the intubating lma-fastrach in 254 patients with difficult-to-manage airways," *Anesthesiology*, vol. 95, no. 5, pp. 1175–1181, 2001.

[21] I. A. Du Rand, J. Blaikley, R. Booton et al., "British Thoracic Society guideline for diagnostic flexible bronchoscopy in adults," *Thorax*, vol. 68, no. 1, pp. i1–i44, 2013.

[22] F. S. Xue, C. W. Li, K. P. Liu et al., "Circulatory responses to fiberoptic intubation in anesthetized children: A comparison of oral and nasal routes," *Anesthesia & Analgesia*, vol. 104, no. 2, pp. 283–288, 2007.

[23] R. N. Kaddoum, Z. Ahmed, A. A. D'Augsutine, and M. M. Zestos, "Guidelines for elective pediatric fiberoptic intubation," *Journal of Visualized Experiments*, no. 47, 2011.

[24] N. Pirlich and R. R. Noppens, "Local airway anaesthesia for awake fibreoptic intubation," *Trends in Anaesthesia and Critical Care*, vol. 10, pp. 22–28, 2016.

[25] J. L. Benumof, "Management of the difficult adult airway: With special emphasis on awake tracheal intubation," *Anesthesiology*, vol. 75, no. 6, pp. 1087–1110, 1991.

[26] G. Frova, A. Guarino, F. Petrini, G. Merli, M. Sorbello, and S. Baroncini, "Gruppo di Studio SIAARTI "Vie Aeree Difficili". Recommendations for airway control and difficult airway management in paediatric patients," *Minerva Anestesiol*, vol. 72, no. 9, pp. 723-48, 2006.

[27] M. Karišik, D. Janjević, and M. Sorbello, "Fiberoptic bronchoscopy versus video laryngoscopy in pediatric airway management," *Acta clinica Croatica*, vol. 55, pp. 51–54, 2016.

[28] K. K. Kuroiwa, M. Nishizawa, N. Kondo, H. Nakazawa, and T. Hirabayashi, "Remifentanil for sedation and analgesia during awake division of tongue flap in children: a report of two cases," *JA Clinical Reports*, vol. 3, no. 1, 2017.

53

Epidural Analgesia with Ropivacaine during Labour in a Patient with a SCN5A Gene Mutation

A. L. M. J. van der Knijff-van Dortmont,[1] **M. Dirckx,**[1] **J. J. Duvekot,**[2]
J. W. Roos-Hesselink,[3] **A. Gonzalez Candel,**[1] **C. D. van der Marel,**[1] **G. P. Scoones,**[1]
V. F. R. Adriaens,[1] **and I. J. J. Dons-Sinke**[1]

[1]*Department of Anesthesiology, Erasmus University Medical Centre, Rotterdam, Netherlands*
[2]*Department of Obstetrics and Gynaecology, Erasmus University Medical Centre, Rotterdam, Netherlands*
[3]*Department of Cardiology, Erasmus University Medical Centre, Rotterdam, Netherlands*

Correspondence should be addressed to A. L. M. J. van der Knijff-van Dortmont; a.vandortmont@erasmusmc.nl

Academic Editor: Richard Riley

SCN5A gene mutations can lead to ion channel defects which can cause cardiac conduction disturbances. In the presence of specific ECG characteristics, this mutation is called Brugada syndrome. Many drugs are associated with adverse events, making anesthesia in patients with SCN5A gene mutations or Brugada syndrome challenging. In this case report, we describe a pregnant patient with this mutation who received epidural analgesia using low dose ropivacaine and sufentanil during labour.

1. Introduction

There are several known SCN5A gene mutations, leading to ion channel defects causing either decreased sodium or calcium influx or increased potassium efflux from the cardiomyocyte [1]. Patients may suffer syncope or sudden cardiac death secondary to polymorphic ventricular tachycardia or ventricular fibrillation. However, the majority of patients remain completely asymptomatic. A small percentage of patients with this gene mutation suffer from Brugada syndrome (BrS). This is a rare, autosomal dominant, arrhythmogenic disorder characterized by the presence of a typical electrocardiographic (ECG) pattern (right bundle branch block and persistent ST-segment elevation in the right precordial leads) and it is associated with a risk of sudden cardiac death [2]. The only effective prevention of sudden cardiac death in patients with heart rhythm disturbances is an implantable cardioverter defibrillator (ICD) [3].

Many drugs have been associated with arrhythmogenic events in BrS patients. Because of the unknown phenotype in patients with a SCN5A gene mutation, avoidance of arrhythmogenic medication is advised [3]. Bupivacaine is one of the drugs that should be avoided (evidence class II a) [4]. Spinal anesthesia using bupivacaine has been used in pregnant [5] and male patients without provoking arrhythmias [6, 7]. A pregnant, SCN5A-positive patient had an uneventful epidural during labour and delivery using a 10 mL bolus of bupivacaine 0,125% followed by an epidural infusion of bupivacaine 0,125% plus 2 μg fentanyl at 10 mL/hour, without any recorded ECG changes during labour [8].

In this case report, we describe the use of low dose ropivacaine for epidural analgesia during labour and delivery in a patient with a SCN5A mutation.

2. Case Report

A 31-year-old patient, carrier of SCN5A mutation, with no history of syncope or aborted sudden cardiac arrest, presented at the preoperative assessment clinic of our anesthetic department at 27 weeks of gestation. She used no medication. Past medical history included surgical correction of an atrial ventricular septum defect at the age of 8. Cardiac ultrasound showed mild left sided atrioventricular valve regurgitation and a good left ventricular function. An ECG showed a first

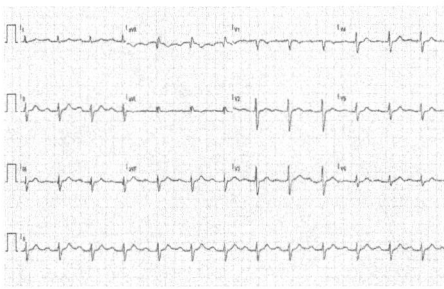

FIGURE 1: Patient's ECG, showing a first degree heart block with an intraventricular conduction delay. PR interval: 302 ms, QRS duration: 144 ms, and ventricular rate: 76 beats per minute.

degree heart block with an intraventricular conduction delay; see Figure 1. Because of these findings, she was included in a clinical research project relating to the association of cardiac septum defects, conduction disturbances, and SCN5A mutations. Her genotype showed a splice-site mutation c.4719C>T in exon 27 of the SCN5A gene. This rare mutation, which was only once found in another patient in Netherlands, is the most likely cause of her cardiac conduction disturbances. The father of our patient who also has cardiac conduction disturbances was found to have the same gene mutation.

The obstetric history included one spontaneous abortion and one instrumental vaginal delivery of a healthy male neonate complicated by a retained placenta requiring manual removal under uncomplicated general anesthesia. With regard to the SCN5A mutation and local anesthetics at her first labour, epidural analgesia was considered a relative contraindication due to the possibility of arrhythmias and she was offered patient-controlled analgesia using remifentanil.

Having experienced her previous delivery as being very traumatic, she specifically requested epidural analgesia during labour in her current pregnancy. After a multidisciplinary discussion with our cardiologists, gynaecologists, and anesthesiologists, it was agreed to induce labour at 38 weeks of gestation with early titrated epidural analgesia under continuous rhythm monitoring. Ropivacaine 0.1% with sufentanil 1 μg/mL was considered the safest anesthetic medication. The patient was fully informed about the risks and possible adverse events.

At 38 weeks of pregnancy, she was admitted at the department of obstetrics. Monitoring consisted of continuous ECG, saturation, and noninvasive blood pressure monitoring and the presence of a resident cardiologist.

The epidural space was located at 5 cm using 18-gauge Tuohy needle at the L3-4 intervertebral space. An epidural catheter was inserted and a test dose of 2.5 mL ropivacaine 0.1% with sufentanil 1 μg/mL was administered resulting in no changes in ECG, heart rate, blood pressure, or sensory block.

Ten minutes later, a loading dose of 8 mL of the same mixture was given through the epidural catheter. After 20 minutes, a bilateral sensory block (to ice) to the T10 dermatome level was achieved. Patient-controlled epidural

analgesia (PCEA) was started using an infusion of ropivacaine 0.1% with sufentanil 1 μg/mL 5 mL/h with a patient-controlled bolus dose of 5 mL with a lockout interval of 30 minutes.

Labour was induced by amniotomy and an intravenous oxytocin infusion in increasing dosage, and the first stage progressed uneventfully.

At 9 cm dilatation, the patient experienced increasing pain which was managed by injection of 5 mL of lidocaine 1% through the epidural catheter, because of the pharmacologic profile of the fast onset and intensive blockade.

A healthy male neonate was spontaneously delivered 6.5 hours after starting the epidural. No hypotension or cardiac arrhythmias were recorded during this period, neither was a change in her heart block noted by the resident cardiologist.

The patient was continuously monitored for 24 hours postpartum on the obstetric high care unit; during this period no arrhythmias occurred.

3. Discussion

To our knowledge, this is the first case report in literature using epidural ropivacaine during labour in a patient with this gene mutation. For the diagnosis of BrS, the presence of a typical ECG pattern is mandatory. Our patient did not have this specific ECG pattern, although her ECG showed conduction disturbances. Because of her gene mutation and ECG abnormalities, she was advised to avoid the same medications as BrS patients.

A retrospective analysis of 104 pregnant Brugada patients with a total of 219 deliveries evaluated pregnancy outcomes. Three women, with an ICD inserted prior to pregnancy, had arrhythmia episodes recorded during pregnancy. Four other patients with aborted sudden cardiac death before pregnancy had no events during pregnancy. Of the 24 patients with syncope prior to pregnancy, only six experienced recurrent syncope during pregnancy [9]. However, a case report describes a patient, 12-week pregnant, presenting with a polymorphic ventricular tachycardia that failed to respond to routinely used drug therapy and defibrillation, as the first manifestation of BrS [10].

There are case reports describing the use of epidural bupivacaine infusions in male patients with BrS resulting in a Brugada-type ECG pattern [11], PVCs and ventricular fibrillation [12], and ventricular tachycardia and electrical storm in an undiagnosed Brugada patient with a SCN5A mutation [13]. There are however also cases with known BrS who had uneventful epidural analgesia [14, 15].

In contrast to spinal anesthesia, epidural analgesia requires a much higher volume of local anesthetic, therefore necessitating the use of the lowest effective concentration. Continuous epidural infusion with either ropivacaine or bupivacaine provides good labour pain relief, but use of ropivacaine resulted in higher plasma concentration in comparison to bupivacaine [16]. However, for a number of reasons, ropivacaine was considered the local anesthetic of choice. In our daily practice, we are used to the combination of ropivacaine 0.1% and sufentanil 1 μg/mL, for our labour epidurals using PCEA. This mixture is prepared by our pharmacy, which reduces the risk of errors in medication. Bupivacaine seems to be more toxic than equivalent doses of ropivacaine with regard to the cardiovascular system. The PR interval, QRS duration, and QT interval (corrected for heart rate) are increased more when bupivacaine is given intravenously compared to intravenous ropivacaine, despite the mean plasma concentration of bupivacaine being lower than that of ropivacaine [17]. The cardiovascular changes, such as increased heart rate, decrease in stroke volume, and ejection fraction, are the same in both drugs. And finally, ropivacaine is presumably safer because it dissociates from the cardiac sodium channel more rapidly than bupivacaine does and thus produces a less pronounced inhibition of the cardiac sodium channel current [18].

In BrS patients, it is important that even the smallest ECG changes should be noticed and in case of changes epidural infusion must be discontinued [11]. For the perioperative monitoring, multilead ECG, preferably with ST trend analysis of the right cardiac leads, is advised [4, 19]. In this case, we did not perform but it is advisable in next cases.

As there is no clear advice in the literature on the duration of postoperative ECG monitoring in BrS patients, we continued ECG monitoring until 24 hours after removal of the epidural catheter. This decision was based on the fact that terminal half-life of ropivacaine after a 48-hour continuous epidural infusion is 7,4 hours [20]. Furthermore, Vernooy et al. [13] described the fact that the ventricular arrhythmias and the typical Brugada-like ECG disappear within 24 hours after discontinuing bupivacaine epidural infusion.

Good communication and cooperation between obstetricians, cardiologists, and anesthesiologists is mandatory. Furthermore, the patient should be informed of and involved in all decisions. One should avoid prolonged use of an epidural infusion and keep the concentration of the local anesthetic as low as possible, since the risk of provoking arrhythmia is related to the dose and duration of the medication used. There is always a risk of ventricular tachycardia or fibrillation, with potential disastrous consequences for mother and the unborn baby; a defibrillator should be on the ward to start advanced life support when necessary. Furthermore, a plan should be made for the management of hypotension and ventricular arrhythmias since the standard treatment is different from that in the ACLS plan. It is worth having isoprenaline available on the labour ward [4, 10].

With all precautions, we think that the use of ropivacaine for epidural analgesia during labour in patients considered as having SCN5A gene mutation with this phenotype is justified, although more experience and research are needed.

Competing Interests

The authors declare that they have no competing interests.

References

[1] A. Khan, S. Mittal, and M. V. Sherrid, "Current review of Brugada syndrome: from epidemiology to treatment," *Anadolu Kardiyoloji Dergisi*, vol. 9, no. 2, pp. 12–16, 2009.

[2] R. Brugada, O. Campuzano, G. Sarquella-Brugada, J. Brugada, and P. Brugada, "Brugada syndrome," *Methodist DeBakey Cardiovascular Journal*, vol. 10, no. 1, pp. 25–28, 2014.

[3] Y. Mizusawa and AA. Wilde, "Brugada syndrome," *Circulation: Arrhythmia and Electrophysiology*, vol. 5, pp. 606–616, 2012.

[4] P. G. Postema, C. Wolpert, A. S. Amin et al., "Drugs and Brugada syndrome patients: review of the literature, recommendations, and an up-to-date website," *Heart Rhythm*, vol. 6, no. 9, pp. 1335–1341, 2009.

[5] J. Bramall, A. Combeer, J. Springett, and R. Wendler, "Caesarean section for twin pregnancy in a parturient with Brugada syndrome," *International Journal of Obstetric Anesthesia*, vol. 20, no. 2, pp. 181–184, 2011.

[6] J. S. Kim, S. Y. Park, S. K. Min et al., "Anaesthesia in patients with Brugada syndrome," *Acta Anaesthesiologica Scandinavica*, vol. 48, no. 8, pp. 1058–1061, 2004.

[7] S. E. T. Alves and M. J. Bezerra, "Spinal anaesthesia in Brugada syndrome: a case report. Posterpresentation," in *Proceedings of the 29th Annual ESRA Congress*, p. E100, Porto, Portugal, September 2010.

[8] B. Kloesel, M. J. Ackerman, J. Sprung, B. J. Narr, and T. N. Weingarten, "Anesthetic management of patients with Brugada syndrome: a case series and literature review," *Canadian Journal of Anesthesia*, vol. 58, no. 9, pp. 824–836, 2011.

[9] M. Rodríguez-Mañero, R. Casado-Arroyo, A. Sarkozy et al., "The clinical significance of pregnancy in Brugada syndrome," *Revista Española de Cardiología (English Edition)*, vol. 67, no. 3, pp. 176–180, 2014.

[10] M. B. Sharif-Kazemi, Z. Emkanjoo, A. Tavoosi et al., "Electrical storm in Brugada syndrome during pregnancy," *Pacing and Clinical Electrophysiology*, vol. 34, no. 2, pp. e18–e21, 2011.

[11] N. Phillips, M. Priestley, A. R. Denniss, and J. B. Uther, "Brugada-type electrocardiographic pattern induced by epidural bupivacaine," *Anesthesia and Analgesia*, vol. 97, no. 1, pp. 264–267, 2003.

[12] Y. Kaneda, N. Fujita, K. Ueda et al., "Surgically treated primary lung cancer associated with Brugada syndrome: report of a case," *Surgery Today*, vol. 31, no. 9, pp. 817–819, 2001.

[13] K. Vernooy, S. Sicouri, R. Dumaine et al., "Genetic and biophysical basis for bupivacaine-induced ST segment elevation and VT/VF. Anesthesia unmasked Brugada syndrome," *Heart Rhythm*, vol. 3, no. 9, pp. 1074–1078, 2006.

[14] C. J. Edge, D. J. Blackman, K. Gupta, and M. Sainsbury, "General anaesthesia in a patient with Brugada syndrome," *British Journal of Anaesthesia*, vol. 89, no. 5, pp. 788–791, 2002.

[15] A. Ripley, J. Castro, and J. Gadsden, "Local anesthetics, neuraxial anesthesia, and the Brugada syndrome," *Journal of Clinical Anesthesia*, vol. 25, no. 1, pp. 78–79, 2013.

[16] L. Irestedt, A. Ekblom, C. Olofsson, A.-C. Dahlström, and B.-M. Emanuelsson, "Pharmacokinetics and clinical effect during continuous epidural infusion with ropivacaine 2.5 mg/ml or bupivacaine 2.5 mg/ml for labour pain relief," *Acta Anaesthesiologica Scandinavica*, vol. 42, no. 8, pp. 890–896, 1998.

[17] D. B. Scott, A. Lee, D. Fagan, G. M. R. Bowler, P. Bloomfield, and R. Lundh, "Acute toxicity of ropivacaine compared with that of bupivacaine," *Anesthesia & Analgesia*, vol. 69, no. 5, pp. 563–569, 1989.

[18] P. Arlock, "Actions of three local anaesthetics: lidocaine, bupivacaine and ropivacaine on guinea pig papillary muscle sodium channels (V_{max})," *Pharmacology Toxicology*, vol. 63, no. 2, pp. 96–104, 1988.

54

Previously Undiagnosed Spinal and Bulbar Muscular Atrophy as a Cause of Airway Obstruction after Robot-Assisted Laparoscopic Prostatectomy

Miyuki Niki,[1] Taihei Tachikawa,[2] Yuka Sano,[1] Hiroki Miyawaki,[1] Aisa Matoi,[3] Yukari Okano,[1] Nobutaka Kariya,[1] Tsuneo Tatara,[1] and Munetaka Hirose[1]

[1]*Department of Anesthesiology and Pain Medicine, Hyogo College of Medicine, Nishinomiya, Hyogo, Japan*
[2]*Department of Anesthesia, Meiwa Hospital, Nishinomiya, Hyogo, Japan*
[3]*Intensive Care Unit, Hyogo College of Medicine Hospital, Nishinomiya, Hyogo, Japan*

Correspondence should be addressed to Munetaka Hirose; mhirose@hyo-med.ac.jp

Academic Editor: Anjan Trikha

Background. Preoperative vocal cord paralysis is a risk factor for postoperative respiratory distress following extubation after general anesthesia. We present an unusual case where a geriatric patient developed airway obstruction after robot-assisted laparoscopic prostatectomy. *Case Presentation*. A 67-year-old male, who had suffered from left vocal cord paralysis of unknown etiology, was scheduled for robot-assisted laparoscopic prostatectomy (RALP). General anesthesia was performed without any problems. The patient, however, developed airway obstruction one hour after extubation and was reintubated following commencement of mechanical ventilation for one day. At the age of 70 years, the patient received an emergency tracheostomy due to bilateral vocal cord paralysis and then was diagnosed with spinal and bulbar muscular atrophy (SBMA). Although no muscle weakness of either upper or lower extremities was observed, rocuronium showed hypersensitivity during total laryngectomy under general anesthesia. *Conclusions*. Vocal cord paralysis combined with postoperative laryngeal edema, the cause of which was presumed to be SBMA, likely caused airway obstruction after RALP. As neuromuscular symptoms progress gradually in patients with SBMA, muscle relaxants should be used carefully, even if patients with SBMA present no immobility of their extremities.

1. Background

A 6-degree head-down tilt position during surgery induces fluid shift from the lower to the upper body, along with cardiopulmonary baroreceptor reflex responses including bradycardia, an increase in urinary excretion of sodium, and thermoregulatory changes [1, 2]. In addition to these physiological responses, a steep 25–40-degree head-down tilt position during robot-assisted laparoscopic prostatectomy (RALP) may cause postoperative laryngeal edema [3]. Severe laryngeal edema requiring reintubation after RALP, however, occurs rarely and the reason why it occurs only rarely is uncertain [4].

On the other hand, spinal and bulbar muscular atrophy (SBMA), also known as Kennedy's disease or Kennedy-Alter-Sung disease, is a rare neurodegenerative disorder of lower motor neurons with an X-linked recessive inheritance pattern and occurs virtually only in adult males [5–7]. There are several potential anesthetic risk factors, including laryngospasm, hyperkalemia with use of depolarizing muscle relaxants, increased sensitivity to nondepolarizing muscle relaxants, and postoperative respiratory failure or aspiration [7].

We report a case of a male patient who was reintubated due to airway obstruction after undergoing general anesthesia for RALP. He was subsequently diagnosed with SBM three years later. The patient provided written permission for the authors to publish this report.

2. Case Presentation

A 67-year-old male, ASA physical status II, diagnosed with prostatic adenocarcinoma was scheduled for RALP under general anesthesia. He had suffered from left vocal cord paralysis of unknown etiology since the age of 50 years. He had also been diagnosed with adenomatous goiter at the age of 56.

After assessment by the anesthesiologists, it was decided that despite the steep head-down tilt position the patient would tolerate general anesthesia, using a tracheal tube with a smaller diameter. General anesthesia was induced with 100 mg of propofol, 50 μg of fentanyl, and 50 mg of rocuronium intravenously and was maintained with 600 μg of fentanyl, intravenous continuous infusion of remifentanil ($0.1–0.4\,\mu g \cdot kg^{-1} \cdot min^{-1}$), sevoflurane (end-tidal: 1.0–1.5%), and rocuronium. Intravenous rocuronium was injected intermittently following the simulated effect-site concentration of rocuronium during surgery.

Following induction, the patient was intubated under direct laryngoscopy with a cuffed tracheal tube, ID 6.5 mm, after observing that there were no laryngeal or pharyngeal abnormalities besides the left vocal cord paralysis via a fiber-optic bronchofiberscope. There were no intraoperative problems with surgery or anesthesia.

After surgery concluded, intravenous 120 mg sugammadex (2 mg/ideal body weight) was administered for reversal of rocuronium. The patient was extubated without any problems with the Aldrete score of 10 and transferred to our intensive care unit (ICU) for routine observation after RALP. Surgical time was 6 h and 31 min and anesthetic time was 8 h 36 min. Total amount of crystalloid infused was 2950 mL, intraoperative urine output was 740 mL, and intraoperative blood loss was 300 mL.

In the intensive care unit, the patient developed dyspnea with paradoxical respiration about one hour after extubation. Fiber-optic bronchofiberscope examination revealed airway obstruction due to laryngeal edema with vocal cord paralysis. Midazolam was injected intravenously, and the patient was reintubated with an uncuffed tracheal tube, ID 5.0 mm, after we were unable to pass an ID 5.5 mm uncuffed tracheal tube through the edematous larynx. The patient was positioned in head-up tilt, and intravenous methylprednisolone was administered following commencement of mechanical ventilation. The patient was successfully extubated 12 h after reintubation and reported no dyspnea thereafter. He was discharged from ICU 3 days after the operation.

At the age of 68, the patient underwent left thyroidectomy due to adenomatous goiter. Intravenous 70 mg of propofol and 100 μg of fentanyl were administered for induction of general anesthesia, and 50 mg of rocuronium was used to facilitate tracheal intubation with a 6.5 mm ID endotracheal tube. Surgery proceeded and general anesthesia was maintained with sevoflurane (end-tidal: 1.0–1.5%), 100 μg of fentanyl, intravenous continuous infusion of remifentanil ($0.1–0.3\,\mu g \cdot kg^{-1} \cdot min^{-1}$), and 100 mg of rocuronium. There were no intraoperative problems. At the end of the procedure, reversal of muscle relaxant was achieved using 120 mg of sugammadex. Video-laryngoscopy confirmed that there was no laryngeal edema present. The tracheal tube was removed without any problems. Total surgical time was 1 h 11 min, and anesthetic time was 2 h 8 min.

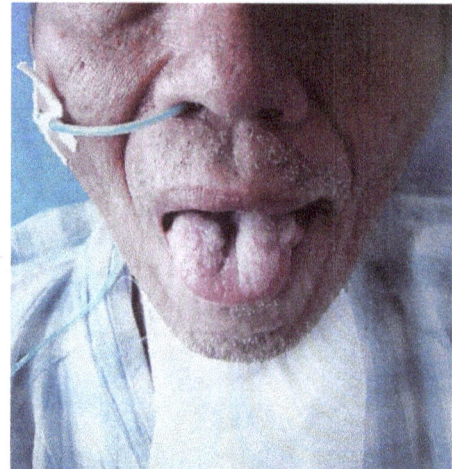

FIGURE 1: Atrophy and fasciculation of the tongue at the time of diagnosis of spinal and bulbar muscular atrophy (SBMA).

At the age of 69 years, the patient underwent uneventful inguinal hernia repair under spinal anesthesia, using 3.2 ml of 0.5% bupivacaine. The highest level of spinal block achieved was Th8.

At the age of 70 years, the patient suffered from dysphagia and dyspnea suddenly with the development of pyrexia within one month. An emergency tracheostomy was performed under local anesthesia after bilateral vocal cord paralysis was identified. Clinical examination revealed bulbar paralysis with atrophy and fasciculation of the patient's tongue (Figure 1).

Although the patient had no muscle weakness of either upper or lower extremities, deep tendon reflexes were suppressed. After genetic testing revealed an expanded CAG repeat, the number of which was 45 times, in the androgen receptor (AR) gene, he was diagnosed with SBMA. The patient did not have gynecomastia, testicular atrophy, glucose intolerance, or hyperlipidemia, Brugada syndrome, or a high level of plasma creatine kinase; these findings occasionally accompany SBMA.

Total laryngectomy was scheduled after he was diagnosed as having SBMA. His tracheostomy tube was replaced to an armoured tracheal tube under general anesthesia using 6.0% end-tidal concentration of desflurane and 50 μg of fentanyl. Train-of-four ratio (TOFR), which was measured by stimulating the left ulnar nerve using TOF-Watch (Organon, Dublin, Ireland), was 1.0 before rocuronium injection. Two min after the injection of 30 mg of rocuronium (0.6 mg/ideal body weight), TOFR reached 0. General anesthesia was maintained with desflurane (end-tidal: 4.0–4.5%), 100 μg of fentanyl, and intravenous continuous infusion of remifentanil ($0.1–0.3\,\mu g \cdot kg^{-1} \cdot min^{-1}$). Recovery of the first twitch height (T1) of TOFR was delayed at 100 min after rocuronium injection. T2 and T4 were obtained at 150 min and 180 min, respectively. Although 110 mg of sugammadex (2 mg/ideal body weight) was administered at the end of surgery, TOFR remained at 0.5. After we administered the same dose of sugammadex additionally, TOFR recovered to 0.67. We extubated a tracheostomy tube, and his Aldrete score was 10 at the end of anesthesia. The duration of surgery was 2 h 21 min, and the duration of anesthesia was 3 h 39 min. There were no problems in the ICU, and the patient was discharged from ICU the next day of surgery.

3. Discussion

SMBA is characterized by progressive weakness in the lower and upper extremities, bulbar weakness, laryngospasm, gynecomastia, and tremor and occurs only in adult males [5–7]. Some clinical features of SMBA resemble the early stages of amyotrophic lateral sclerosis. SMBA is caused by the enlargement of a CAG repeat in the AR gene on the X chromosome, which encodes glutamine tract in ARs. The number of CAG repeats over 38 is diagnostically useful and is often associated with androgen insensitivity [8]. Its estimated prevalence is 1-2 per 100,000 [9]. Suggested pathophysiological mechanisms of neurodegeneration involve formation of nuclear inclusions by the polyglutamine-expanded AR (polyQ AR) and/or release of toxic soluble form of oligomerized polyQ AR and alterations of the ubiquitin-proteasome system and of autophagy pathways [10] Neuronal and muscular dysfunction may be a consequence of loss of normal functions of AR and/or gain of functions of toxic form of polyQ ARs which accumulate in motor neurons [10].

Given that SMBA is a motor neuron disease with bulbar dysfunction, many anesthesiologists may be concerned about the use of neuromuscular blocking drugs and their reversal agents. Interestingly, however, there have been no reported complications following the use of these agents so far [7, 11]. In this case, neither rocuronium nor sugammadex, used during the first and second instances of general anesthesia, was associated with any complications when the patient was 67 and 68 years old. In the third instance of general anesthesia at the age of 70 after the patient was diagnosed with SBMA, however, rocuronium showed hypersensitivity because of the prolonged neuromuscular blocking effect of rocuronium with insufficient recovery of TOFR after the administration of sugammadex [12]. Although he had no muscle weakness at the extremities, dysfunction of motor neurons might cause this hypersensitivity to nondepolarizing muscle relaxant. If a patient shows immobilization at the extremities, anesthesiologists need to take their anesthetic management into consideration that depolarizing muscle relaxant could induce hyperkalemia, as immobilization upregulates immature types of nicotinic acetylcholine receptors at the skeletal muscle [13]. As neuromuscular symptoms progress gradually in patients with SBMA, muscle relaxants should be used carefully, even if patients with SBMA present no immobility of their extremities.

Niesen et al. examined the anesthetic records of six patients with SBMA who underwent general anesthesia and identified one 66-year-old patient who developed severe postoperative glottic edema after surgery for a tibial fracture [7]. Although this patient had proximal muscle weakness and bulbar dysfunction preoperatively, the cause of glottic edema was unclear.

Androgens inhibit activation of complement by enhancing C1-esterase inhibitor [14]. In hereditary angioneurotic edema, activation of the classical complement pathway, caused by the deficiency of C1-esterase inhibitor, induces laryngeal edema, and androgens have been used for treatment in this disease [15].

As such, it is speculated that, in our present case, activation of the classical complement pathway due to androgen insensitivity in SBMA likely augmented his laryngeal edema after the steep head-down tilt position was employed during RALP. Before this procedure, he had existing left vocal cord paralysis, which may have been caused by the loss of lower motor neurons supplying the laryngeal muscles. In view of this, it is our opinion that vocal cord paralysis secondary to SBMA, combined with postoperative laryngeal edema, likely caused airway obstruction after RALP.

4. Conclusion

In this patient, preoperative vocal cord paralysis combined with laryngeal edema, which was facilitated by a steep head-down tilt position during surgery, caused airway obstruction after extubation. SBMA was diagnosed three years later and is presumed to be the cause of the patient's bulbar symptomatology. As motor dysfunction progresses slowly in SBMA patients, anesthetic management needs to be carefully tailored, paying particular condition to the clinical presentation.

References

[1] M. Hirose, Y. Hara, J. Iwasa, and M. Matsusaki, "Thermoregulatory response in female patients during lower abdominal surgery in the head-down tilt position," *Acta Anaesthesiologica Scandinavica*, vol. 40, no. 4, pp. 475–479, 1996.

[2] M. Hirose, S. Hashimoto, and Y. Tanaka, "Effect of the Head-down Tilt Position During Lower Abdominal Surgery on Endocrine and Renal Function Response," *Anesthesia & Analgesia*, vol. 76, no. 1, pp. 40–44, 1993.

[3] J. Saito, S. Noguchi, A. Matsumoto et al., "Impact of robot-assisted laparoscopic prostatectomy on the management of general anesthesia: efficacy of blood withdrawal during a steep Trendelenburg position," *Journal of Anesthesia*, vol. 29, no. 4, pp. 487–491, 2015.

[4] S. V. N. Phong and L. K. D. Koh, "Anaesthesia for robotic-assisted radical prostatectomy: Considerations for laparoscopy in the Trendelenburg position," *Anaesthesia and Intensive Care*, vol. 35, no. 2, pp. 281–285, 2007.

[5] W. R. Kennedy, M. Alter, and J. H. Sung, "Progressive proximal spinal and bulbar muscular atrophy of late onset: a sex-linked recessive trait," *Neurology*, vol. 18, no. 7, pp. 671–680, 1968.

[6] P. Fratta, N. Nirmalananthan, L. Masset et al., "Correlation of clinical and molecular features in spinal bulbar muscular atrophy," *Neurology*, vol. 82, no. 23, pp. 2077–2084, 2014.

[7] A. D. Niesen, J. Sprung, Y. S. Prakash, J. C. Watson, and T. N. Weingarten, "Case series: anesthetic management of patients

with spinal and bulbar muscular atrophy (Kennedy's disease)," *Canadian Journal of Anesthesia*, vol. 56, no. 2, pp. 136–141, 2009.

[8] A. R. L. Spada, E. M. Wilson, D. B. Lubahn, A. E. Harding, and K. H. Fischbeck, "Androgen receptor gene mutations in X-linked spinal and bulbar muscular atrophy," *Nature*, vol. 352, no. 6330, pp. 77–79, 1991.

[9] P. Weydt, A. Sagnelli, A. Rosenbohm et al., "Clinical Trials in Spinal and Bulbar Muscular Atrophy—Past, Present, and Future," *Journal of Molecular Neuroscience*, vol. 58, no. 3, pp. 379–387, 2016.

[10] L. K. Beitel, C. Alvarado, S. Mokhtar, M. Paliouras, and M. Trifiro, "Mechanisms mediating spinal and bulbar muscular atrophy: Investigations into polyglutamine-expanded androgen receptor function and dysfunction," *Frontiers in Neurology*, vol. 4, p. 53, 2013.

[11] R. Takeuchi, H. Hoshijima, K. Doi, and H. Nagasaka, "The use of sugammadex in a patient with Kennedy's disease under general anesthesia," *Saudi Journal of Anaesthesia*, vol. 8, no. 3, pp. 418–420, 2014.

[12] Y. Sugi, K. Nitahara, T. Shiroshita, and K. Higa, "Restoration of train-of-four ratio with neostigmine after insufficient recovery with sugammadex in a patient with myasthenia gravis," *A & A Case Reports*, vol. 1, no. 3, pp. 43–45, 2013.

[13] J. A. J. Martyn, M. Jonsson Fagerlund, and L. I. Eriksson, "Basic principles of neuromuscular transmission," *Anaesthesia*, vol. 64, supplement 1, no. 1, pp. 1–9, 2009.

[14] T. Hidvégi, G. K. Fehér, T. Fehér, E. Koó, and G. Füst, "Inhibition of the complement activation by an adrenal androgen, dehydroepiandrosterone," *Complement*, vol. 1, pp. 201–206, 1984.

[15] B. Visy, G. Füst, L. Varga et al., "Sex hormones in hereditary angioneurotic oedema," *Clinical Endocrinology*, vol. 60, no. 4, pp. 508–515, 2004.

Dexmedetomidine as Part of a Multimodal Analgesic Treatment Regimen for Opioid Induced Hyperalgesia in a Patient with Significant Opioid Tolerance

Richard K. Patch III,[1] Jason S. Eldrige,[2] Susan M. Moeschler,[2] and Matthew J. Pingree[3]

[1]Division of Critical Care Medicine, Department of Anesthesiology & Perioperative Medicine and Division of Pulmonary and Critical Care Medicine, Department of Medicine, Mayo Clinic, Rochester, MN, USA
[2]Division of Pain Medicine, Department of Anesthesiology & Perioperative Medicine, Mayo Clinic, Rochester, MN, USA
[3]Department of Physical Medicine and Rehabilitation, Mayo Clinic, Rochester, MN, USA

Correspondence should be addressed to Richard K. Patch III; patch.richard@mayo.edu

Academic Editor: Alparslan Apan

Acute postoperative pain in patients with opioid tolerance creates a significant management challenge for anesthesiologists and pain medicine physicians. A multimodal approach is key; however other factors can complicate management such as opioid induced hyperalgesia. We present the case of a patient on large amounts of intrathecal opioids for chronic pain syndrome with opioid induced hyperalgesia after an exploratory laparotomy. Dexmedetomidine was utilized successfully as part of a controlled multimodal analgesic plan and should be a consideration for opioid tolerant patients experiencing opioid induced hyperalgesia.

1. Introduction

Chronic pain, as defined by the American Society of Anesthesiologists, is pain not directly related to neoplastic involvement extending in duration beyond the expected temporal boundary of injury [1]. The International Association for the Study of Pain (IASP) further defines chronicity as pain which is present for at least three months duration or longer [2]. According to a recent Institute of Medicine (IOM) report, over 100 million Americans suffer from chronic pain; this is a leading cause of disability and represents more US patients than those with cardiovascular disease [3–5]. Opioids are one option for the treatment of chronic pain, yet their effectiveness as a long-term therapeutic option has not been established [6, 7]. Chronic pain patients on large amounts of opioids represent a management conundrum for anesthesiologists, primary care providers, and pain medicine physicians in the outpatient and perioperative setting [6, 7]. Given the extreme tolerance to opioid medications that may be exhibited in this population, multimodal analgesia is of the utmost importance.

Opioid induced hyperalgesia (OIH) is defined as a state of enhanced nociceptive sensitization due to exposure to opioids [8]. Opioid induced hyperalgesia is not located at the site of injury and is typically diffuse and ill defined. No established diagnostic criteria exist to diagnose OIH. It is suspected when pain is perceived to increase with increasing opioid use [9]. Opioid induced hyperalgesia can occur in the acute setting and one does not need to be receiving chronic opioids for it to occur. The pathophysiology of OIH has yet to be completely elucidated. One possibility is activation of descending pain pathways from the medulla resulting in certain neurons uniquely responding to opioids [9]. Another possibility is alteration of the central glutaminergic system and the excitatory NMDA neurotransmitter [8]. Regardless of the mechanism OIH in patients on chronic opioids complicates their management.

Dexmedetomidine, a highly selective α-2 agonist, may be an increasingly important adjunct to consider within the multimodal approach to postoperative pain management. Dexmedetomidine is a potent anxiolytic, while also providing opioid-sparing analgesic effects [10]. The mechanism of antinociception has not been completely elucidated, but it is believed that it is secondary to α-2 receptor stimulation in the central nervous system and spinal cord. We present a case of a patient with chronic pain on large amounts of intrathecal narcotics who developed OIH after abdominal surgery in which dexmedetomidine was utilized as part of a multimodal analgesic regimen.

2. Case Description

A 55-year-old female presented for a laparotomy with abdominal exploration, small bowel resection, and lysis of adhesions secondary to sclerosing mesenteritis. The patient had a history of chronic pain syndrome. In 1997 she had an intrathecal drug delivery device implanted to treat refractory chronic back pain in the context of four prior lumbar laminectomies and fusion at an outside medical facility. Her chronic abdominal pain began in 2009 after a small bowel obstruction required an exploratory laparotomy, at which time fibrotic strictures were found which required small bowel resection at the ileum. The patient's pain continued and she went on to undergo cholecystectomy in 2010. In 2011 she underwent evaluation by a local gastroenterologist, with upper endoscopy revealing signs of bile reflux gastritis and retained food. Concomitant motility testing revealed gastroparesis and she was ultimately diagnosed with narcotic-related gastroparesis. In an attempt to decrease the amount of opioids she was receiving from her intrathecal device, she had a spinal cord stimulator (SCS) placed as a therapeutic adjunct. Her pain was marginally improved with the stimulator, though this device ultimately failed and stopped working. Despite the SCS failure, the patient elected not to have the stimulator explanted. Throughout this time course, the patient was also treated concurrently with multiple medication regimens including gabapentin, long acting morphine, fluoxetine, and benzodiazepines.

In 2013, due to continued abdominal pain and increasing intrathecal opioid requirements, a repeat CT scan of the abdomen showed enhancement of the terminal ileum and rectosigmoid colon with a new mass-like area of mesenteric inflammation. The diagnosis of sclerosing mesenteritis was considered and she presented to our institution for further evaluation and management.

During preoperative evaluation, the patient stated her abdominal pain was constant, 24 hours a day, seven days a week. Utilizing the Agency for Healthcare Research and Quality's numeric pain intensity scale (NPIS) her pain was always an eight out of ten. Additionally, it was exacerbated with food, alcohol, the cold, and stress. She noted that she went to sleep and awoke with the same level of pain. Her current medication regimen included trazadone 200 mg orally at night and probiotics. The intrathecal drug delivery system (IDDS) included fentanyl (25,000 mcg/mL) and Bupivacaine (15 mg/mL), infusing at continuous infusion doses of 6000 mcg and 8 mg per day, respectively. Additionally, there were 11 pre-set boluses for fentanyl at 1200 mcg each (given over three-minute durations) per day. In summation, the patient was receiving a total daily dose of 19,702 mcg of fentanyl intrathecally when accounting for both continuous

infusion and bolus dosing; this correlates with an oral morphine equivalent (OME) of 591 grams per day. This amount was calculated using a 100 : 1 conversion between intravenous and intrathecal fentanyl, a 100 greater fold potency of fentanyl, and a 3 : 1 conversion between oral and intravenous morphine.

Preoperatively, regional analgesia with an epidural was extensively discussed with the patient; however given her multiple back surgeries and chronic back pain, she declined. As previously mentioned, the patient was treated with gabapentin in the past without any benefit and, as such, she declined preoperative administration. Her operative course was unremarkable. Anesthesia was induced with propofol and succinylcholine, endotracheal intubation was uneventful, and maintenance was provided with isoflurane in air and oxygen. Intraoperative opioids were rotated to hydromorphone totaling 15 mg and additional analgesia consisted of a ketamine infusion of 0.2 mg/kg/hr, acetaminophen 1000 mg IV, ketorolac 15 mg IV, and local infiltration of the wound with 20 cc of liposomal bupivacaine. Antiemetics included droperidol, ondansetron, and dexamethasone while ciprofloxacin was administered for surgical site prophylaxis due to a penicillin allergy. Her hemodynamics were satisfactory throughout the case and she was extubated at the end and transferred to the postanesthetic care unit (PACU) for recovery.

In the PACU the patient's pain was extremely difficult to control. She received escalating boluses of hydromorphone totalling an additional 6 mg and 40 mg of ketamine in addition to an increase in her ketamine infusion to 0.3 mg/kg/hr. The inpatient pain service, who manages both acute and chronic pain, was contacted to assist with management. The patient was hypertensive and tachycardic with a normal temperature, elevated respiratory rate, and oxygen saturations of 98% on 2 L nasal cannula. Examination revealed an unremarkable cardiopulmonary exam with a soft but diffusely tender abdomen to palpation. She noted her pain was progressively becoming worse over the course of her PACU stay and was some of the worst pain she had ever experienced. Her hemoglobin was 10 g/dL down from 11.7 g/dL preoperatively; electrolytes and coagulation profile were all within normal limits. After discussion with the surgical service, no intra-abdominal process was felt to be the etiology and she was diagnosed with an acute pain crisis complicated by OIH. Given the use of high dose intrathecal opioids, substantial ketamine infusion, and current multimodal regimen, we elected to initiate a dexmedetomidine infusion. Per institutional protocol, she was transferred to the progressive care unit (PCU) for monitoring during this infusion.

While in the PCU her pain continued to be difficult to control. She required a dexmedetomidine infusion of 0.8 mcg/kg/hr, ketamine infusion of 0.7 mg/kg/hr with 10 mg IV boluses every 30 minutes as needed, lidocaine patches around her incision, an additional dose of ketorolac, and scheduled acetaminophen. A narcotic patient controlled analgesia (PCA) system was not prescribed given signs and symptoms of OIH. Boluses of 1 mg of hydromorphone every 30 minutes as needed were available and she had continued use of her personal therapy manager (PTM) to provide the previously prescribed intrathecal fentanyl boluses. This regimen provided adequate postoperative analgesia. Additionally, the patient was found to be hemodynamically stable throughout her admission without any overt signs of pain-sedation mismatch.

Over the course of next 48 hrs the dexmedetomidine and ketamine infusions were weaned while the interval of IV boluses of hydromorphone and ketamine was progressively increased to every four hours. On postoperative day three she was transferred to the floor and transitioned from intravenous opioids to oral hydromorphone. At the request of the patient, oral medications were chosen rather than making adjustments to the IDDS. Throughout her hospitalization she experienced no opioid related adverse events such has constipation or sedation. She was discharged on hospital day seven with a prescription of hydromorphone 4 mg orally as needed every 6 hrs and plans to follow-up with her primary pain physician. At her three-month follow-up, her chronic abdominal pain was noted to be better and her intrathecal fentanyl usage had been reduced to 11,000 mcg per day. Furthermore, she was to be evaluated by a pain rehabilitation center at home to address her ongoing pain syndrome.

3. Discussion

Chronic pain continues to be one of the most common presenting complaints in the primary care setting. Opioids are an option for nonmalignant pain though chronic use remains controversial, with a general paucity of evidence for long-term benefit [6]. As a result of chronic use, however, patients often develop clinically significant opioid tolerance and opioid induced hyperalgesia. Dexmedetomidine may offer distinct clinical advantages in this patient population, due to opioid-sparing effects as well as anxiolysis. Interestingly, previously published work by Belgrade and Hall also suggests that dexmedetomidine may help physiologically reset opioid sensitivity in otherwise tolerant individuals and in patients suffering from OIH [11]. The precise mechanism of antinociception has not been fully elucidated, but it is α-2 receptor stimulation in the central nervous system and spinal cord is thought to play a vital role [10].

Perioperatively, data for the use of dexmedetomidine as part of a multimodal analgesic regimen is becoming well established. A meta-analysis in 2012 of close to 1800 patients, of which 339 received dexmedetomidine, revealed that systemic α-2 agonists decreased postoperative opioid consumption and pain intensity [12]. Additional trials have shown that the addition of dexmedetomidine to a sufentanil infusion achieved better analgesic effect and greater patient satisfaction in patients undergoing abdominal hysterectomy for 72 hours postoperatively [13]. Intraoperative infusions of dexmedetomidine have also shown that postoperative pain scores and Ramsay Sedation Scale scores were lower and morphine consumption was lower during the first 24 hrs after surgery [14]. When dexmedetomidine was added to propofol and remifentanil in patients undergoing an abdominal colectomy, they had lower visual analog pain scores and consumed less morphine compared to the addition of saline to propofol and remifentanil [15]. Moreover, pain scores were lower at

rest for the first 48 hrs after laparoscopic colorectal surgery; however this group had no difference in morphine utilization [16]. An additional meta-analysis in 2013 examined randomized controlled trials of postoperative pain control utilizing dexmedetomidine compared to placebo at one, two, four, 24, and 48 hours postoperatively [17]. Nine of the trials examined postoperative pain scores revealing that patients receiving dexmedetomidine had lower pain scores at all time points. It is noteworthy that while the mean difference in pain scores remained statistically significant, the means decreased from −1.59 at one hour to −0.41 at 48 hours. Patients receiving dexmedetomidine also had lower morphine consumption at one, two, four, 24, and 48 hours postoperatively [17]. Fourteen of the trials showed significantly higher intraoperative bradycardia in dexmedetomidine treated patients with a relative risk (RR) of 2.66 and a number needed to harm (NNH) of 6.25. The dexmedetomidine group also had higher rates of postoperative bradycardia; however this result failed to show any significance [17].

Less well established is the role of dexmedetomidine for treatment of OIH. In a small retrospective case series 11 patients with OIH and intractable pain were given a dexmedetomidine infusion. Seven of the eleven patients had substantial reductions in their baseline opioid requirements [11]. Patients undergoing laparoscopically assisted vaginal hysterectomy with remifentanil-induced hyperalgesia from an infusion of 0.3 μg/kg/min were randomized to a dexmedetomidine infusion or saline. The group that did not receive dexmedetomidine had a decreased mechanical hyperalgesia threshold, increased pain intensity at one, six, 12, and 24 hrs [18]. Additionally, the morphine consumption was significantly higher leading the authors to conclude that dexmedetomidine reduced the hyperalgesic effect of remifentanil and may have a role in OIH. In a case series of recurrent vasoocclusive episodes in three adolescents with sickle-cell disease who exhibited features consistent with OIH, dexmedetomidine was shown to decrease opioid consumption and pain scores [19].

Ketamine has also been a long established adjuvant both for intraoperative and for postoperative analgesia, specifically in opioid tolerant patients [20]. It played a key role in the management of our patient's postoperative pain as it allowed us to reduce opioids that could exacerbate OIH, while still providing primary analgesic effects itself. Ketamine exerts its analgesic properties by antagonism of the n-methyl-d-aspartate (NMDA) receptor thus reducing presynaptic release of glutamate [21]. This mechanism also allows reduction of central sensitization and the windup phenomena in chronic pain. Low dose ketamine infusions are also a useful adjunct in opioid tolerant patients experiencing acute pain. In opioid dependent patients undergoing spine surgery, ketamine infusions reduced opioid requirements in the first 48 hrs after surgery [22]. The combination of ketamine and dexmedetomidine for acute pain in a patient with chronic regional pain syndrome type I (CRPS-1) was reported to provide a synergistic effect without sequela [23].

Interestingly, our patient received wound infiltration by the surgical team instead of application of a more specific regional anesthetic technique. While neuraxial blocks were discussed and considered (epidural versus paravertebral block/catheter), there was legitimate clinical concern for aberrant anatomy and/or disrupting the indwelling intrathecal system due to a known history of several prior back surgeries and the absence of precise outside medical records to clarify IDDS implantation technique. Other peripheral blocks, such as transversus abdominus plane (TAP) block, could have been placed but the expectation was that such a block would not help the significant visceral pain component expected after exploratory laparotomy. Additionally, it should be noted that there is randomized clinical trial data suggesting that surgical wound infiltration is as effective at pain control as epidural or TAP block interventions [24, 25].

We recognize that other preoperative strategies, such as weaning intrathecal opioids, could have been employed as a viable therapeutic path to attenuate concerns of opioid tolerance and OIH. However, in our case, there were at least two relevant barriers to this clinical consideration. First, the patient was being managed by an out-of-state pain physician who had very different ideas on appropriate medical management of the patient's pain. Intrathecal doses of such magnitude, which exceed reasonable limits suggested by national guidelines such as the Polyanalgesic Consensus Conference (PACC), imply a general unwillingness by both patient and provider to vastly restrict opioid dosing (as would be required) [26]. Additionally, even if an overt willingness to wean had been encountered, both distance and time presented significant barriers. Distance and location otherwise complicated the sort of long-term longitudinal care and follow-up that would be required to wean such high intrathecal doses. The length of time required to significantly wean such high doses may also have presented a moral dilemma; though the surgery was not emergent, the lysis of adhesions for progressive sclerosing mesenteritis presented a clear palliative medical need that could not be easily ignored [22].

Perioperative lidocaine infusion is another adjunct used for postoperative pain that could have been utilized in our patient. However, a systemic review concluded that currently the evidence is low to moderate that the intervention will reduce pain in early postoperative phase, one to four hours, and there is no evidence that that it will reduce pain at 48 hours [27]. Additionally, data on lidocaine infusions in patients with intrathecal drug delivery devices is limited and, given the significant amount of intrathecal opioids the patient was receiving, their effect on her postoperative pain and OIH would likely have been minimal.

4. Conclusion

In conclusion, we present the case of OIH in a patient with an intrathecal drug delivery device receiving an oral morphine equivalent of 591 gms of intrathecal fentanyl that required an aggressive multimodal postoperative analgesic regimen after exploratory laparotomy. Dexmedetomidine was utilized as part of that regimen with safe and effective results. Our patient was monitored in a PCU setting and there were no hemodynamic sequela. We propose that dexmedetomidine is a useful adjunct for the management of OIH, particularly in

a patient who is significantly opioid tolerant with high opioid requirements.

References

[1] American Society of Anesthesiologists Task Force on Chronic Pain Management and the American Society of Regional Anesthesia and Pain Medicine, "Practice Guidelines for Chronic Pain Manageme," *Anesthesiology*, vol. 112, no. 4, pp. 810–833, 2010.

[2] Classification of chronic pain. Descriptions of chronic pain syndromes and definitions of pain terms. Prepared by the International Association for the Study of Pain, Subcommittee on Taxonomy," *Pain Suppl*, vol. 3, pp. S1-226, 1986.

[3] Institute of Medicine, *Relieving Pain in America: A Blueprint for Transforming Prevention, Care, Education, and Research,* The National Academies Press, Washington, DC, 2011.

[4] V. L. Roger, A. S. Go, D. M. Lloyd-Jones et al., "Heart Disease and Stroke Statistics—2011 Update," *American Heart Association*, vol. 123, no. 4, pp. e18–e209, 2011.

[5] V. J. Dzau and P. A. Pizzo, "Relieving pain in America: Insights from an institute of medicine committee," *JAMA - Journal of the American Medical Association*, vol. 312, no. 15, pp. 1507-1508, 2014.

[6] D. Dowell, T. M. Haegerich, and R. Chou, "CDC guideline for prescribing opioids for chronic pain—United States, 2016," *Journal of the American Medical Association*, vol. 315, no. 15, pp. 1624–1645, 2016.

[7] R. Chou, J. A. Turner, E. B. Devine et al., "The effectiveness and risks of long-term opioid therapy for chronic pain: a systematic review for a national institutes of health pathways to prevention workshop," *Annals of Internal Medicine*, vol. 162, no. 4, pp. 276–286, 2015.

[8] M. Lee, S. Silverman, H. Hansen, V. Patel, and L. Manchikanti, "A comprehensive review of opioid-induced hyperalgesia," *Pain Physician*, vol. 14, no. 2, pp. 145–161, 2011.

[9] P. Yi and P. Pryzbylkowski, "Opioid Induced Hyperalgesia," *Pain Medicine (United States)*, vol. 16, pp. S32–S36, 2015.

[10] A. K. M. Chan, C. W. Cheung, and Y. K. Chong, "Alpha-2 agonists in acute pain management," *Expert Opinion on Pharmacotherapy*, vol. 11, no. 17, pp. 2849–2868, 2010.

[11] M. Belgrade and S. Hall, "Dexmedetomidine infusion for the management of opioid-induced hyperalgesia," *Pain Medicine*, vol. 11, no. 12, pp. 1819–1826, 2010.

[12] G. Blaudszun, C. Lysakowski, N. Elia, and M. R. Tramèr, "Effect of perioperative systemic $\alpha2$ agonists on postoperative morphine consumption and pain intensity: systematic review and meta-analysis of randomized controlled trials," *Anesthesiology*, vol. 116, no. 6, pp. 1312–1322, 2012.

[13] C. Ren, M. Chi, Y. Zhang et al., "Dexmedetomidine in postoperative analgesia in patients undergoing hysterectomy: A CONSORT-prospective, randomized, controlled trial," *Medicine (United States)*, vol. 94, no. 32, Article ID e1348, 2015.

[14] S. Abu-Halaweh, F. Obeidat, A. R. Absalom et al., "Dexmedetomidine versus morphine infusion following laparoscopic bariatric surgery: effect on supplemental narcotic requirement during the first 24 h," *Surgical Endoscopy and Other Interventional Techniques*, vol. 30, no. 8, pp. 3368–3374, 2016.

[15] D.-J. Ge, B. Qi, G. Tang, and J.-Y. Li, "Intraoperative dexmedeto-midine promotes postoperative analgesia and recovery in patients after abdominal colectomy: A CONSORT-prospective, randomized, controlled clinical trial," *Medicine (United States)*, vol. 94, no. 43, Article ID e1727, 2015.

[16] C. W. Cheung, Q. Qiu, A. C. L. Ying, S. W. Choi, W. L. Law, and M. G. Irwin, "The effects of intra-operative dexmedetomidine on postoperative pain, side-effects and recovery in colorectal surgery," *Anaesthesia*, vol. 69, no. 11, pp. 1214–1221, 2014.

[17] A. Schnabel, C. H. Meyer-Frießem, S. U. Reichl, P. K. Zahn, and E. M. Pogatzki-Zahn, "Is intraoperative dexmedetomidine a new option for postoperative pain treatment? A meta-analysis of randomized controlled trials," *Pain*, vol. 154, no. 7, pp. 1140–1149, 2013.

[18] C. Lee, Y.-D. Kim, and J.-N. Kim, "Antihyperalgesic effects of dexmedetomidine on high-dose remifentanil-induced hyperal-gesia," *Korean Journal of Anesthesiology*, vol. 64, no. 4, pp. 301–307, 2013.

[19] K. A. Sheehy, J. C. Finkel, D. S. Darbari, M. F. Guerrera, and Z. M. N. Quezado, "Dexmedetomidine as an Adjuvant to Anal-gesic Strategy During Vaso-Occlusive Episodes in Adolescents with Sickle-Cell Disease," *Pain Practice*, vol. 15, no. 8, pp. E90–E97, 2015.

[20] J. Jouguelet-Lacoste, L. La Colla, D. Schilling, and J. E. Chelly, "The Use of Intravenous Infusion or Single Dose of Low-Dose Ketamine for Postoperative Analgesia: A Review of the Current Literature," *Pain Medicine (United States)*, vol. 16, no. 2, pp. 383–403, 2015.

[21] N. Garg, N. B. Panda, K. A. Gandhi et al., "Comparison of small dose ketamine and dexmedetomidine infusion for postoper-ative analgesia in spine surgery - A prospective randomized double-blind placebo controlled study," *Journal of Neurosurgical Anesthesiology*, vol. 28, no. 1, pp. 27–31, 2016.

[22] R. W. Loftus, M. P. Yeager, J. A. Clark et al., "Intraoperative ket-amine reduces perioperative opiate consumption in opiate-dependent patients with chronic back pain undergoing back surgery," *Anesthesiology*, vol. 113, no. 3, pp. 639–646, 2010.

[23] B. S. Nama Sharanya, D. R. Meenan, and W. T. Fritz, "The use of sub-anesthetic intravenous ketamine and adjuvant dexmedeto-midine when treating acute pain from CRPS," *Pain Physician*, vol. 13, no. 4, pp. 365–368, 2010.

[24] M. J. Hughes, E. M. Harrison, N. J. Peel et al., "Randomized clin-ical trial of perioperative nerve block and continuous local anaesthetic infiltration via wound catheter versus epidural analgesia in open liver resection (LIVER 2 trial)," *British Journal of Surgery*, vol. 102, no. 13, pp. 1619–1628, 2015.

[25] M. M. Tawfik, Y. M. Mohamed, R. E. Elbadrawi, M. Abdel-khalek, M. M. Mogahed, and H. M. Ezz, "Transversus abdo-minis plane block versus wound infiltration for analgesia after cesarean delivery: A randomized controlled trial," *Anesthesia and Analgesia*, vol. 124, no. 4, pp. 1291–1297, 2017.

[26] T. R. Deer, J. E. Pope, S. M. Hayek et al., "The Polyanalgesic Con-sensus Conference (PACC): Recommendations for Intrathecal Drug Delivery: Guidance for Improving Safety and Mitigating Risks," *Neuromodulation*, vol. 20, no. 2, pp. 155–176, 2017.

[27] P. Kranke, J. Jokinen, N. L. E. Pace et al., "Continuous intra-venous perioperative lidocaine infusion for postoperative pain and recovery," *The Cochrane Database of Systematic Reviews*, vol. 7, article CD009642, 2015.

56

Quadratus Lumborum Block as Sole, Homeostatic-Preserving Anesthetic for a Patient with Multiple System Atrophy Undergoing Open Inguinal Hernia Repair

M. D. Luca La Colla⑩ **and R. M. D. Schroeder**

Department of Anesthesiology, Duke University Medical Center, Durham, NC, USA

Correspondence should be addressed to M. D. Luca La Colla; lacolla.luca@gmail.com

Academic Editor: Ehab Farag

Quadratus Lumborum (QL) block has been successfully used for different abdominal procedures in the past. Multiple system atrophy (MSA) is a progressive neurodegenerative disorder characterized mainly by autonomic instability, motor impairment, and cognitive dysfunction. We report a case of a patient with MSA with a history of multiple episodes of unplanned admissions following outpatient minor surgical procedures under general anesthesia scheduled to undergo open inguinal hernia repair. In our patient, QL block was successfully used for surgical anesthesia and it resulted in hemodynamic stability and an opioid-free perioperative course.

1. Introduction

Quadratus Lumborum (QL) block was first described in 2007 by Blanco [1] and can provide reliable analgesia following different abdominal [2] as well as hip procedures [3, 4] and even amputations [5].

Multiple system atrophy (MSA) is a progressive neurodegenerative disorder characterized mainly by autonomic failure (including autonomic instability) and motor impairment. Anesthesia of any kind in affected patients carries significant risk [6]. Inguinal hernia repair (IHR) is one of the most commonly performed surgical procedures and is routinely performed under general, spinal, or even local anesthesia with sedation. All of these pose significant risk for patients afflicted with MSA.

To the best of our knowledge QL block has never been used as primary anesthetic choice for inguinal hernia repair in adults.

Written informed consent for both anesthesia and publication of patient's data in an anonymous form was obtained and documented in the patient's chart. The 2013 CARE checklist for writing case reports was followed.

2. Description of the Case

A 69-year-old male with a history of MSA and obstructive sleep apnea was scheduled for elective open repair of a symptomatic right inguinal hernia. In particular, he suffered from autonomic dysfunction, severe orthostatic hypotension, and cognitive impairment with several unplanned admissions following outpatient minor orthopedic surgical procedures due to "slowness to wake up" (according to his wife) or delirium requiring restraints after postoperative opioid administration.

Given his history, it was felt that avoiding general anesthesia was advisable. His severe orthostatic hypotension also made subarachnoid block potentially unsuitable considering the risk of hypotension. There was also concern that he would not be able to cooperate with local anesthesia performed by the surgeon without deep sedation. Considering the patient's prior history and comorbidities, a QL block was chosen as the sole anesthetic.

Written informed consent for both anesthesia and publication of the patient's data in an anonymous form was obtained and documented in the patient's chart. The 2013 CARE checklist for writing case reports was followed.

The patient was transferred to the preoperative holding area and ASA standard monitors were applied. He was placed in the supine position slightly tilted to the left to better expose the right flank and received fentanyl 50 mcg for sedation. After sterile preparation and using standard aseptic technique, a high-frequency linear array probe covered by sterile plastic sleeve was placed horizontally on the umbilicus and moved laterally. Both rectus abdominis and the 3 muscle layers of the abdominal wall were identified and traced posteriorly to the point where the deep fascia of the transversus abdominis merges with the thoracolumbar fascia. A 20-G 10-cm nonstimulating echogenic Tuohy needle was advanced in-plane with the probe until appropriate location for a QL type I block according to Blanco and McDonnell [1] was achieved. Needle positioning was confirmed by careful hydrodissection with normal saline and, after negative aspiration, 20 ml of 0.5% ropivacaine was injected and appropriate, posterior spread observed.

After a few minutes the patient was brought to the operating room and loss of pin-prick sensation was documented from T9 to L1 on the right side.

Prior to incision, the surgeon (unfamiliar with this block) decided to perform local infiltration along the incision site (no iliohypogastric and/or ilioinguinal block) with 6 mL of 0.25% bupivacaine. Intraoperative sedation was accomplished with low-dose propofol (10 mcg/kg/min). No additional parenteral opioids or sedative agents were administered. The patient's vital signs were stable and remained within 20% of his preoperative values. Of note, the patient did not require any additional supplementation of local anesthetic and the surgeon was pleasantly surprised.

Postoperative analgesia was supplemented by IV acetaminophen 1 g.

The patient was brought to the PACU awake, oriented, and pain-free, and he was discharged to the floor within 45 minutes. There was no evidence of delirium, agitation, or other issues during the perioperative period, and he was discharged home the following day after receiving 2 scheduled doses of acetaminophen 975 mg and pregabalin 100 mg overnight.

3. Discussion

Multiple System Atrophy is a group of neurodegenerative syndromes characterized by autonomic dysfunction, cerebellar abnormalities, corticospinal degeneration and Parkinson-like symptoms. MSA patients are at risk for hemodynamic instability (due to impairment of baroreceptor activity and sympathetic hypersensitivity), airway problems including laryngeal stridor, central sleep apnea (with increased risk of prolonged ventilation, reintubation and emergency tracheostomy following general anesthesia), and gastric aspiration. These patients are also at risk for delirium and/or agitation making cooperation with regional, neuraxial, and especially local anesthesia potentially problematic. While there are published reports of surgical procedures under single-shot spinal anesthesia [7], the general consensus

among practitioners seems to be that if possible, low-dose spinal or epidural anesthesia should be used and titrated carefully to minimize hemodynamic compromise [6]. Should general anesthesia be necessary, an arterial line should be placed [8].

Previous reports of reliable and widespread coverage with QL block [3, 4] led us to choose this block over the more popular TAP block. QL block has been shown to provide superior analgesia compared to TAP block after low abdominal surgery in children [9]. Scimia et al. [10] published a single case report of the use of an ultrasound-guided transversalis fascia block for a patient undergoing inguinal herniorrhaphy. According to some authors, though, the QL type 1 block (the approach we used in this case) and the transversalis fascia block are essentially the same block because the patterns of spread of the injectate are similar [11]. Therefore, Scimia et al. might have performed a QL-1 block.

In our opinion, the better coverage obtained by the QL-1 block compared to the traditional TAP block is due to more reliable block of the iliohypogastric/ilioinguinal as well as genitofemoral nerves in the posterior pararenal space. Even though prospective comparisons between QL and TAP block in adults are currently ongoing, preliminary data from a study in children show that QL provides superior and longer-lasting analgesia than TAP block [9]. For these reasons it was felt that QL-1 was a better choice than TAP block, general, and even spinal anesthesia and this approach allowed us to avoid arterial line placement for a minor surgical procedure. The QL block provided excellent surgical anesthesia with a single needle pass, caused as minimal if any perturbations in autonomic tone, and posed no risk to our patient's vocal cord function. Finally, it allowed him to remain as awake and oriented as possible, thus minimizing the risk of drug-induced delirium either intra- or postoperatively. The patient and his family, who had been far more concerned about anesthetic than surgical risk, were extremely pleased with the result.

In summary, we report the first use of QL type 1 block which provided excellent and complete surgical anesthesia for open inguinal repair in a patient with MSA, preventing further interventions that would likely have caused hemodynamic compromise or mental status changes. Even though further studies are necessary, this case report suggests that options other than general and spinal anesthesia are available and may be preferable in patients with MSA undergoing abdominal surgical procedures.

Authors' Contributions

Both authors Luca La Colla and Rebecca Schroeder helped with performing the actual anesthetic, writing the case report, and final editing.

References

[1] R. Blanco and J. G. McDonnell, "Optimal point of injection: The quadratus lumborum type I and II blocks," http://www.respond2articles.com/ANA/forums/post/1550.aspx.

[2] V. R. Kadam, "Ultrasound-guided quadratus lumborum block as a postoperative analgesic technique for laparotomy," *Journal of Anaesthesiology Clinical Pharmacology*, vol. 29, no. 4, pp. 550–552, 2013.

[3] L. La Colla, A. Uskova, and B. Ben-David, "Single-shot quadratus lumborum block for postoperative analgesia after minimally invasive hip arthroplasty a new alternative to continuous lumbar plexus block?" *Regional Anesthesia and Pain Medicine*, vol. 42, no. 1, pp. 125-126, 2017.

[4] L. La Colla, B. Ben-David, and R. Merman, "Quadratus Lumborum Block as an Alternative to Lumbar Plexus Block for Hip Surgery: A Report of 2 Cases," *A & A case reports*, vol. 8, no. 1, pp. 4–6, 2017.

[5] H. Ueshima and H. Otake, "Lower limb amputations performed with anterior quadratus lumborum block and sciatic nerve block," *Journal of Clinical Anesthesia*, vol. 37, p. 145, 2017.

[6] S. Agarwal and R. Aggarwal, "Anesthetic considerations in a patient with multiple system atrophy-cerebellar for lower limb surgery," *Saudi Journal of Anaesthesia*, vol. 11, no. 3, pp. 365-366, 2017.

[7] J.-M. Malinovsky, A. Cozian, and O. Rivault, "Spinal anesthesia for transurethral prostatectomy in a patient with multiple system atrophy [2]," *Canadian Journal of Anesthesia*, vol. 50, no. 9, pp. 962-963, 2003.

[8] M.-S. Jang, J. H. Han, S. W. Park, J.-M. Kang, and W. J. Kang, "General anesthesia for a patient with multiple system atrophy," *Korean Journal of Anesthesiology*, vol. 67, pp. S34–S35, 2014.

[9] G. Öksüz, B. Bilal, Y. Gürkan et al., "Quadratus Lumborum Block Versus Transversus Abdominis Plane Block in Children Undergoing Low Abdominal Surgery: A Randomized Controlled Trial," *Regional Anesthesia and Pain Medicine*, vol. 42, no. 5, pp. 674–679, 2017.

[10] P. Scimia, E. Basso Ricci, E. Petrucci, A. U. Behr, F. Marinangeli, and P. Fusco, "Ultrasound-Guided Transversalis Fascia Plane Block," *A & A Case Reports*, p. 1, 2017.

[11] O. Choquet and X. Capdevila, "Quadratus Lumborum 1 and Transversalis Fascia Blocks: Different Names for the Same Posterior Pararenal Space Block," *Regional Anesthesia and Pain Medicine*, vol. 42, no. 4, pp. 547-548, 2017.

57

Preoperative Fasting Guidelines in Children: Should They Be Revised?

Hazem Kafrouni ⓘ and Rami El Ojaimi

Saint George Hospital-University Medical Center, Beirut, Lebanon

Correspondence should be addressed to Hazem Kafrouni; hazemkafrouni@yahoo.com

Academic Editor: Jian-jun Yang

Children presenting with ingestion of foreign bodies need gastroscopy as a primary management modality. A controversy lies regarding guidelines for preoperative fasting among children with low risk of aspiration and intraoperative complications. This case report represents cases of children who ingested foreign bodies and underwent fasting at different times preoperatively. With mounting evidence questioning the benefits of long durations of fasting in decreasing the risk of aspiration and with studies showing that fasting for more than 2 hours after ingestion of clear fluid does not significantly alter gastric pH or volume, these incidental findings raise the question of whether it is safe to keep children NPO, for a shorter duration before the administration of anesthesia. In addition, this report shows that current guidelines are in need of revision.

1. Introduction

General anesthesia has been documented to attenuate protective laryngeal reflexes and to increase the risk of pulmonary aspiration. According to American Society of Anesthesiologists (1999), Association of Paediatric Anaesthetists of Great Britain and Ireland (2003), and European Society of Anaesthesia (2005), the times needed are 2 h of preoperative fasting for clear fluids, 4 h of fasting for breast milk, and 6 h of fasting for solids [1]. Glucose gradually becomes hepatic glycogenolysis during fasting, in which ketogenesis becomes the main source of energy. Ketoacidosis has been distinguished among children who are less than 3 years old who fasted for more than 7 hours; this has affected the levels of ketone bodies and led to hypotension on induction of anesthesia [2]. According to literature, children who were allowed to drink 2h preoperatively, had lower gastric pH than those who fasted for a duration longer than 2 hours. Moreover, these children were reported to be less irritable than others [3, 4].

2. Case Description

Three pediatric patients presented with ingestion of a foreign body and were sent for gastroscopy for retrieval. All three patients had full stomachs and thus rapid sequence intubation with cricoid pressure using xylocaine, propofol, fentanyl, and succinylcholine was performed for induction of general anesthesia, before the procedure.

Case 1. A 5-year-old boy (height: 108 cml weight: 16.5 kg) who had sandwich 4 hours ago was brought to the operating rooms for removal of a coin that he has ingested 3 hours prior to presentation. A gastroscopy was performed under general anesthesia and the foreign body was successfully retrieved. Interestingly, no food residues were observed in the stomach (Figure 1).

Case 2. A 4-year-old girl (Height: 100.5 cm; weight: 15 kg) who had cereal 3 hours prior to presentation underwent a gastroscopy for the removal of a pebble that is the size of 1 euro coin that she has ingested 4 hours prior to presentation. After ingestion, the patient was directly admitted to the emergency room. The foreign body was successfully retrieved and again the patient had no food in her stomach with only gastric secretions.

Case 3. A 3.5-year-old girl (height: 105 cm; weight: 15.5 Kg) had a gastroscopy to remove a metal coin that she has ingested 4 hours prior to the procedure. The mother also reports that

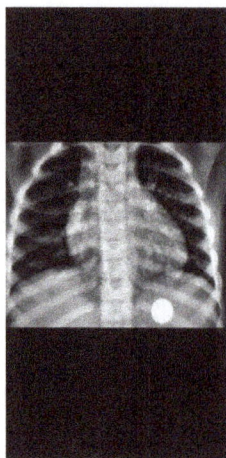

FIGURE 1

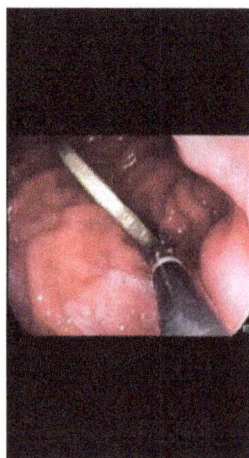

FIGURE 2

the girl had a cup of cereals an hour before ingesting the coin. Again, the girl was found to have only gastric secretions with no food and the coin was successfully retrieved (Figure 2).

3. Discussion

Preoperative fasting in children undergoing anesthesia is recommended to decrease the risk of aspiration of gastric contents. Despite the guidelines, fasting periods are often exceeded in pediatrics [5]. Long periods of fasting in children, however, may lead to symptoms of dehydration or discomfort [6], thus exceeding the fasting time may be more harmful than useful. Current guidelines recommend a fasting time of 2 h for clear fluids, 4 h for breast milk, and 6 h for other milk and solids before induction of deep sedation or general anesthesia [7]. In addition, the rigid approach to fasting has led to orders of nil per os after midnight leading to considerably long fasting time of up to 15 hours [8]. In addition to the discomfort of fasting, a fasting state poses the body under significant metabolic stress decreasing its ability to deal with stress, and with depletion of glycogen stores lean body mass is sacrificed to meet the metabolic demands [6].

Three children were admitted to our hospital for endoscopic removal of a foreign body that they have accidentally ingested. By direct observation of gastric contents in children with a foreign body, we found that the patients had empty stomachs despite not adhering to the fasting guidelines. With mounting evidence questioning the benefits of long durations of fasting in decreasing the risk of aspiration, and with studies showing that fasting for more than 2 hours after ingestion of clear fluid does not significantly alter gastric pH or volume [5]; these incidental findings raise the question of whether it is safe to keep children NPO for a shorter duration before the administration of anesthesia and whether the current guidelines are in need of revision. Our case report presents cases that may reinforce a more liberal approach to preoperative fasting as it reflects a potential exaggeration in fasting time for solids but is indeed not enough to support any changes to the current recommendations. However, further investigation and studies are needed. Since the timing of the fasting was not enough as compared to international guidelines, successful gastroscopy was established, the matter that raised the question. These issues are necessary but, because of the ethical issues that accompany performing random gastroscopies, the evaluation of children who have swallowed a foreign body and necessitate gastroscopy for removal may provide very useful information as to the importance of strict fasting guidelines, if their last PO intake is accounted for before the procedure.

To note that, individual digestion is different according to patients' body nature specificity, and thus a universal law cannot be concluded out of these cases.

Disclosure

In our study, we made sure that ethical issues were minimized as much as possible. Especially that our report addresses pediatric patients who are considered a vulnerable population. However, our study is scientifically valid and contributed to better health outcomes among patients who were fairly selected and any chance of autonomy was avoided.

References

[1] I. Smith, P. Kranke, I. Murat et al., "Perioperative fasting in adults and children: Guidelines from the european society of anaesthesiology," *European Journal of Anaesthesiology*, vol. 28, no. 8, pp. 556–569, 2011.

[2] B. G. Arun and G. Korula, "Preoperative fasting in children: an audit and its implications in a tertiary care hospital," *Journal of Anaesthesiology Clinical Pharmacology*, vol. 29, no. 1, pp. 88–91, 2013.

[3] J. M. Baden, M. Kelley, R. S. Wharton, B. A. Hitt, V. F. Simmon, and R. I. Mazze, "Mutagenicity of halogenated ether anesthetics," *Anesthesiology*, vol. 46, no. 5, pp. 346–350, 1977.

[4] American Society of Anesthesiologists Committee., "Practice Guidelines for Preoperative Fasting and the Use of Pharmacologic Agents to Reduce the Risk of Pulmonary Aspiration: Application to Healthy Patients Undergoing Elective Procedures," *Anesthesiology*, vol. 90, no. 3, pp. 896–905, 1999.

[5] M. Subrahmanyam and M. Venugopal, "Perioperative fasting: A time to relook," *Indian Journal of Anaesthesia*, vol. 54, no. 5, pp. 374-375, 2010.

[6] N. Dennhardt, C. Beck, D. Huber et al., "Optimized preoperative fasting times decrease ketone body concentration and stabilize mean arterial blood pressure during induction of anesthesia in children younger than 36 months: a prospective observational cohort study," *Pediatric Anesthesia*, vol. 26, no. 8, pp. 838–843, 2016.

[7] K. R. Ingebo, N. J. Rayhorn, R. M. Hecht, M. T. Shelton, G. H. Silber, and M. D. Shub, "Sedation in children: Adequacy of two-hour fasting," *Journal of Pediatrics*, vol. 131, no. 1 I, pp. 155–158, 1997.

[8] T. Engelhardt, G. Wilson, L. Horne, M. Weiss, and A. Schmitz, "Are you hungry? Are you thirsty?—fasting times in elective outpatient pediatric patients," *Pediatric Anesthesia*, vol. 21, no. 9, pp. 964–968, 2011.

58

Ropivacaine Plasma Concentrations after 192-Hour High Dose Epidural Ropivacaine Infusion in a Pediatric Patient without Side Effects

Glenn van de Vossenberg ⓘ,[1] **Selina van der Wal,**[1] **Andrea Müller,**[1] **Edward Tan,**[2] **and Kris Vissers** ⓘ[1]

[1]*Department of Anesthesiology, Pain and Palliative Medicine, Radboudumc, Nijmegen, Netherlands*
[2]*Department of Surgery, Radboudumc, Netherlands*

Correspondence should be addressed to Glenn van de Vossenberg; glenn.vandevossenberg@radboudumc.nl

Academic Editor: Anjan Trikha

This case report discusses continuous epidural administration of ropivacaine 0.56 mg kg^{-1} h^{-1} for 8 days in a 7-year-old trauma patient to prevent pain, after performing a lower right and upper left leg guillotine amputation. Venous sampling after 8 days revealed bound and unbound ropivacaine concentrations of 1.1 mg/l and 0.06 mg/l in plasma, respectively. Arterial sampling for bound and unbound ropivacaine was 1.2 mg/l and 0.05 mg/l in plasma, respectively. In this case report, long-term high dose epidural infiltration of ropivacaine did not result in severe side effects or complications. Further studies are needed to explore safety of these concentrations in larger populations of children.

1. Introduction

Since cocaine was introduced in the 19th century by Carl Köller and Sigmund Freud, the use of local anesthetics (LA) has evolved enormously. Local anesthetics can be used to produce local, locoregional, and neuraxial nerve blockade. Binding of LA to various subtypes of sodium channels (Na$_v$) in the nervous system produces nerve blockade. Currently 7 subtypes of Na$_v$ are known in the nervous system. Blocking on these receptors can potentially cause minor side effects such as a metallic taste or tingling, but also severe side effects such as seizures and cardiac arrest. All these symptoms and adverse effects are referred to as local anesthetic systemic toxicity (LAST) [1]. In pediatrics little is known about the absolute maximum dosages for epidural infusion of ropivacaine. Only two studies [2, 3] have been performed in pediatrics assessing the save use of ropivacaine given via continuous epidural infusion for maximum dose of 0.4 mg kg^{-1} h^{-1}. In this case report we present and discuss a case of continuous administration of ropivacaine 0.56 mg kg^{-1} h^{-1} in the epidural space for over 8 days to control severe pain after bilateral amputation and reveal its concentration in venous and arterial plasma after 8 days. Written informed consent was obtained from the patient's parent for publication of this report.

2. Clinical Presentation

A previously healthy 7-year-old male presented to a community hospital with severe lower extremity trauma due to accident with a truck. The patient was instantly brought to the OR and the surgeon performed a lower right leg and an upper left leg guillotine amputation. During surgery the patient received one litre of crystalloids, two units of packed cells, and one unit plasma and remained hemodynamically stable with low noradrenaline dosage. For postoperative analgesia a n. ischiadicus and a n. popliteal catheter were placed during surgery in the left and right lower extremity, respectively. Since much postoperative pain was expected ropivacaine infusion of 0.2 mg kg^{-1} h^{-1} was started over each catheters (0.4 mg kg^{-1} h^{-1} in total), postoperatively. Intravenous infusion of esketamin 0,2 mg kg^{-1} h^{-1} and morphine 20 mcg kg^{-1} h^{-1} was started additionally. Initially peripheral catheters were preferred since less hemodynamic consequences were expected. Postoperative analgesia was generally sufficient scoring NRS 0 at rest and NRS 2 during movement. However, after one week his pain management was not sufficient anymore, most probably due to peripheral catheter manipulation after several debridements and stump closure on OR. Therefore, the peripheral catheters were removed and since the patient was hemodynamically stable and had no fever anymore a tunneled epidural catheter (L4-L5) was placed and ropivacaine 0.4 mg kg^{-1} h $^{-1}$ infusion was started epidurally. This resulted in adequate pain management during rest and additional morphine was stopped since it caused itching. However, during wound treatment the next day the patient experienced again nonacceptable pain. A bolus of esketamin did not reduce pain to acceptable levels. Moreover, infusion of esketamin is controversial since it may induce liver enzyme disorder and it was stopped [4]. One day after epidural placement a bolus of 10 ml ropivacaine 0.375% with 5 mcg of sufentanil resulted in adequate pain relief, and we increased continuous epidural infusion to 0,48 mg kg^{-1} h $^{-1}$ of ropivacaine. Initially a bilateral sensory block was present at T12/L1 without a motor block. We observed the patient in a medium care unit with continuously pulse oximetry, 3-lead ECG (no qualitative 12-lead ECG analysis) and blood pressure monitoring. Furthermore, our nurses are trained to recognize symptoms of LAST and the patient was monitored on a daily basis by the acute pain service. Since we did not observe symptoms of LAST whatsoever, no side effects of epidural bupivacaine 0.5 mg kg^{-1} h $^{-1}$ were described in literature [5], the department of pediatric anesthesiology approved these high concentrations, and adequate pain relief was obtained and these high dosages were accepted. After taking into account the weight loss due to amputation we were actually infusing at 0.56 mg kg^{-1} h $^{-1}$.

Since few studies are performed to assess intravenous ropivacaine concentration after subsequent epidural infusion for days in pediatrics, we obtained venous and arterial samples after 8 days of epidural ropivacaine infusion and continued epidural infusion. Venous sampling resulted in 1.1 mg/l and 0.06 mg/l bound and unbound ropivacaine concentration, respectively. Arterial sampling resulted in 1.2 mg/l and 0.05 mg/l bound and unbound ropivacaine concentration, respectively. To our knowledge there were no other laboratory tests which we could perform to monitor for ropivacaine toxicity, other than more frequent testing which we did not find ethical to do in a child.

After 11 days, our patient was transferred, with the epidural in situ, to another hospital closer to his hometown. In follow-up, we learned that the epidural catheter was luxated during transport and thus removed. At this moment, the pain was tolerated well. No long-term side effects such as paresthesia were observed.

3. Discussion

As far as we know, this case report is the first report on administering 0.56 mg kg^{-1} h $^{-1}$ ropivacaine epidurally for 8 consecutive days in a pediatric case with severe trauma and hence pain. Therefore, we sampled venous and arterial concentrations of ropivacaine after 8 days. The unbound and bound

ropivacaine concentrations fractions showed an equal distribution in the arterial and venous compartment. However, Knudsen et al. [6] showed a 2-fold and 4-fold higher arterial than venous ropivacaine concentration after IV-infusion for bound and unbound fraction, respectively. Different concentrations of local anesthetics in the venous and arterial compartment were observed in other studies after extravascular administration as well and they show that an equilibrium was reached after 2h of extravascular administration [7, 8]. This effect is known as the so-called flip-flop effect and is caused by slow distribution of local anesthetics and is also identified in epidural infusion. This helps us understand why we found an equal distribution of plasma ropivacaine concentrations in the venous and arterial compartment in our patient.

Furthermore, Knudsen et al. showed first adverse effects for unbound ropivacaine at 0.15 mg/l in adults; the concentrations measured in our case were well below this concentration. The question what concentrations of ropivacaine are necessary to cause LAST symptoms in pediatrics cannot be directly answered with this comparison because of the different pharmacology between children and adults such as bigger volume of distribution in children (not important in this case since steady-state was attained) and a higher susceptibility for LA in peripheral blocks [9]. However, the higher concentrations measured in this case report are not causing LAST symptoms in this patient. Evidence is available that toxic concentration for bupivacaine is reached at 3.7 mg l^{-1} in children [10]. Unfortunately no study revealed thus far the toxic concentration of ropivacaine for children.

Concentrations we measured in this case report are in line with other studies by Bösenberg et al. [2] and Berde et al. [3]. Since they only assessed infusion for 24-72h, we showed what concentration of ropivacaine after 192h is not accumulating. This was also shown by Berde et al., who showed stable and decreased concentrations of unbound ropivacaine throughout epidural infusion. Because we only report one case one should be prudent with generalization, especially since we only sampled at day 8.

Gustorff et al. [11] described a case report where they performed ropivacaine continuous epidural infusion at 1.14 mg kg^{-1} h $^{-1}$ with an optional bolus of 1.36 mg kg^{-1}. After 70 hours they measured a total concentration of 1.54 ml l^{-1} in plasma. Unfortunately they did not mention the bound and unbound concentration, so it is difficult to compare our measurement with their data other than stating that their total concentration was higher than we found. This can be easily explained by the fact that they were infusing at higher rates and in addition had a bolus function.

Based on this case report we cannot advise to allow higher concentrations of epidural ropivacaine as advised in current literature in infants than 0.4 mg kg^{-1} h $^{-1}$, since we only took one measurement and thus cannot describe the typical pharmacological profile of 0.56 mg kg^{-1} h $^{-1}$. Further studies are needed to explore safety of these concentrations in larger populations of children. However, we can conclude that we did not observe any side effect nor symptoms of LAST. Moreover, the unbound ropivacaine plasma concentrations we measured did not reach toxic levels if compared to current literature. So we advise clinicians to consider titrate ropivacaine infiltration to higher concentrations when pain treatment is difficult to manage. Of course, it is mandatory to monitor regularly for symptoms of LAST when higher concentrations of ropivacaine are infused epidurally. Moreover, clinical symptoms are most important to observe since it is known that large variability exists in serum free/total local anesthetic concentration and sensitivity to local anesthetics [7]. Unfortunately, only few laboratories offer the possibility of assessing the concentration of ropivacaine in plasma, so clinicians must take into account the fact that it might take some time (weeks) before ropivacaine concentrations are measured.

Authors' Contributions

Glenn van de Vossenberg was responsible for care taking of patient, interpretation of data, and drafting and writing the case report. Selina van de Wal was responsible for care taking of patient, drafting, and revising. Andrea Muller and Edward Tan were responsible for care taking of patient and revising. Kris Vissers performed revision.

References

[1] J. F. Butterworth, "Models and mechanisms of local anesthetic cardiac toxicity: A review," *Regional Anesthesia and Pain Medicine*, vol. 35, no. 2, pp. 167–176, 2010.

[2] A. T. Bösenberg, J. Thomas, L. Cronje et al., "Pharmacokinetics and efficacy of ropivacaine for continuous epidural infusion in neonates and infants," *Pediatric Anesthesia*, vol. 15, no. 9, pp. 739–749, 2005.

[3] C. B. Berde, M. Yaster, O. Meretoja et al., "Stable plasma concentrations of unbound ropivacaine during postoperative epidural infusion for 24-72 hours in children," *European Journal of Anaesthesiology*, vol. 25, no. 5, pp. 410–417, 2008.

[4] I. M. Noppers, M. Niesters, L. P. H. J. Aarts et al., "Drug-induced liver injury following a repeated course of ketamine treatment for chronic pain in CRPS type 1 patients: a report of 3 cases," *PAIN*, vol. 152, no. 9, pp. 2173–2178, 2011.

[5] C. B. Berde, "Convulsions Associated With Pediatric Regional Anesthesia," *Anesthesia & Analgesia*, vol. 75, no. 2, pp. 164–166, 1992.

[6] K. Knudsen, M. B. Suurküla, S. Blomberg, J. Sjövall, and N. Edvardsson, "Central nervous and cardiovascular effects of I.V. infusions of ropivacaine, bupivacaine and placebo in volunteers," *British Journal of Anaesthesia*, vol. 78, no. 5, pp. 507–514, 1997.

[7] P. Dureau, B. Charbit, N. Nicolas, D. Benhamou, and J.-X. Mazoit, "Effect of intralipid® on the dose of ropivacaine or levo-bupivacaine tolerated by volunteers," *Anesthesiology*, vol. 125, no. 3, pp. 474–483, 2016.

[8] L. E. Mather and M. J. Cousins, "Local Anaesthetics and their Current Clinical Use," *Drugs*, vol. 18, no. 3, pp. 185–205, 1979.

[9] M. Jöhr, "Regional anaesthesia in neonates, infants and children," *European Journal of Anaesthesiology*, vol. 32, no. 5, pp. 289–297, 2015.

[10] J. J. McCloskey, S. E. Haun, and J. K. Deshpande, "Bupivacaine toxicity secondary to continuous caudal epidural infusion in children," *Anesthesia & Analgesia*, vol. 75, no. 2, pp. 287–290, 1992.

[11] B. Gustorff, P. Lierz, P. Felleiter, T. H. Knocke, K. Hoerauf, and H. G. Kress, "Ropivacaine and bupivacaine for long-term epidural infusion in a small child," *British Journal of Anaesthesia*, vol. 83, no. 4, pp. 673-674, 1999.

59

Ultrasound-Guided Subclavian Vein Cannulation in Neonate via Supraclavicular Approach

Onur Balaban and Tayfun Aydın

Department of Anesthesiology & Pain Medicine, Dumlupinar University Hospital, Merkez, Kutahya, Turkey

Correspondence should be addressed to Onur Balaban; obalabandr@gmail.com

Academic Editor: Kuang-I Cheng

Central venous cannulation of infants may be challenging. Ultrasonography is recommended and has been found superior to classic landmark technique in pediatric central venous cannulation. The cannulation of the subclavian vein using supraclavicular approach under real-time ultrasound guidance is a novel technique. It may have advantages over ultrasound-guided jugular vein cannulation in specific patients. We report a case of 3200-gram 20-day-old anencephalic neonate who had a diffuse generalized edema. The neonate was cannulated successfully via subclavian vein using supraclavicular approach under ultrasound guidance.

1. Introduction

Central venous cannulation in infants weighing less than 10 kilograms or younger than 1 year may be difficult even with ultrasound (US) guidance. Younger age decreases success rate and increases complication rate of central venous cannulation. Ultrasonography is recommended and has been found superior to classic landmark technique, especially for pediatric patients [1, 2]. The Agency for Healthcare Research and Quality reported that the use of US guidance for the placement of central venous catheters is one of the highest patient safety practices with the strongest evidence [3]. The use of US during catheterization in pediatric patients is also recommended by the National Institute of Clinical Excellence (NICE) [4]. In pediatric patients, ultrasound-guided central venous catheter placement decreases complications and decreases placement attempts compared with the landmark technique [5].

There are many approaches and techniques using ultrasound guidance during cannulation. The cannulation of the subclavian vein (SCV) using supraclavicular approach under real-time US guidance is a novel technique. It may have advantages over ultrasound-guided jugular vein cannulation in specific patients. We report a case of US-guided subclavian vein cannulation in a neonate who had a short neck and diffuse edema, using supraclavicular approach.

2. Case

Informed consent was obtained from the family of the patient for the case report. A 3200-gram, 20-day-old neonate was intubated after delivery and being followed in the neonatal intensive care unit. Multiple peripheral vascular access attempts were unsuccessful. The neck was short and there was a generalized edema involving the neck. As there was not enough space for needle insertion and manipulation at the neck for jugular cannulation, we decided to place a subclavian vein catheter under US guidance using supraclavicular approach. An experienced anesthetist about US-guided jugular and subclavian vein cannulation in adults and infants performed the cannulation. Before the procedure, 5 milligrams per kilogram intramuscular ketamine was administered. The neonate was placed in supine position with the head turned to the opposite of needle insertion site (Figure 1). A sheet was placed under the infant's shoulder for an optimum position to facilitate US scanning and cannulation. The anesthetist stood at the right side of the infant and performed the cannulation. A nurse pulled the right arm of the infant along the body during the procedure. The skin was prepared for aseptic condition and a 10-megahertz frequency linear transducer was placed in a sterile cover. Sterile gel was used as coupling agent. The jugular vein and carotid artery were visualized transversally at the tracheal cartilage

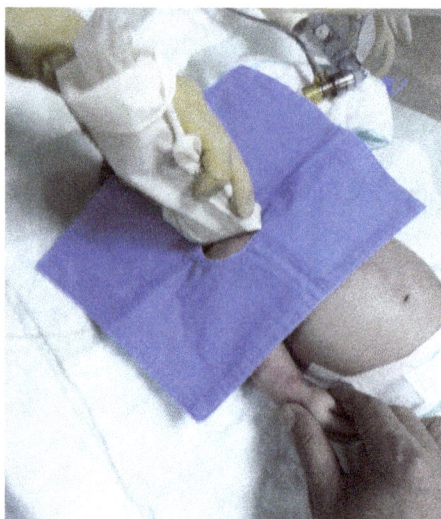

FIGURE 1: The position of the patient and ultrasound transducer during cannulation.

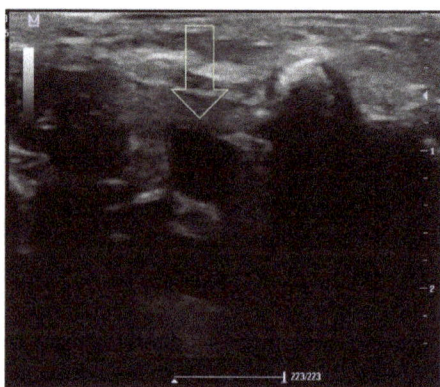

FIGURE 2: The ultrasound image of the subclavian vein. Yellow arrow is showing the subclavian vein.

level. Then the transducer was moved laterally and rotated slightly, following the jugular vein, until SCV was visualized. A transverse cross-sectional image of SCV was visualized at supraclavicular region. Also, subclavian artery was visualized posterior to the vein (Figure 2). There was no enough space for alignment and tilting maneuvers of the transducer due to anatomical difficulties of the patient and pleura could not be visualized. Vascular flux was verified by color Doppler before the puncture to identify subclavian artery and the SCV. Using out-of-plane technique and visualizing the transverse cross-sectional view of SCV, the needle was inserted into the vein visualizing the tip under real-time US guidance. An open-end needle was inserted without an attached syringe, to avoid collapse of the vein when negative pressure is applied by syringe. When the tip of the needle was seen in the vein and blood reflux was observed, the guide wire was inserted through the needle into the vein. Then, a 22-gauge catheter (Certofix Mono Paed S 110, Braun, Melsungen, Germany) was introduced over the guide wire. The procedure was completed at first attempt, without any complication such as hematoma,

arterial puncture, or pneumothorax. The place of catheter in SCV was verified by US scan and a chest X-ray.

3. Discussion

Ultrasound guidance technique is becoming gold standard for central venous cannulation. The success rate is increased and the complications related to central venous catheter (CVC) placement are decreased [6]. Failure rates for CVC placement in children range from 5% to 19% with reported complication rates from 2.5% to 22% [5]. US-guided CVC placement decreases complications and increases the success rate at first attempt compared to the landmark technique in pediatric patients [5]. A meta-analysis by Hind et al. reported that the use of 2-dimensional US guidance was associated with increased success of cannulation of internal jugular vein and SCV [1]. Another meta-analysis of 26 randomized controlled trials showed that patients receiving CVC can obtain significant benefit from US [7].

There are many techniques and approaches for central venous cannulation. Internal jugular, subclavian, and femoral vein are commonly used sites [1]. The femoral vein is the most common attempted site during pediatric resuscitation in emergency departments [2]. Femoral vein cannulation is associated with a low complication rate during insertion in hypovolemic patients or patients with low cardiac output, compared to the internal jugular and subclavian catheters [8]. Disadvantages of femoral cannulation are a higher incidence of thromboembolic and infectious complications [2]. Although the most popular site has been the femoral vein, recently, the internal jugular vein (IJV) has been favored when ultrasound is used [6]. During cannulation, IJV may collapse under probe or needle pressure. High puncture of the IJV often is exposed to difficulties like tunnelization difficulty because of the neck shortness, whereas low puncture of the IJV hampers the insertion of the metallic guide that gets stopped against the medial wall [9]. Subclavian vein cannulation does not present these difficulties because of its anterior wall fixation on clavicle. This brings protection against venous collapse and enables lateral insertion of needle, allowing an axial insertion of the metallic guide [9]. SCV is less affected by collapse and easily accessed to tunnel and fixed to a patient's shoulder [10]. Infraclavicular placement of the CVC is not recommended for a long period of time, because of the risk of catheter rupture caused by the costoclavicular pinch [9]. Supraclavicular cannulation of SCV may be more suitable for long-term cannulation.

Reports on pediatric SCV cannulation have been rare. A supraclavicular approach was suggested by Yoffa and known since 1965 but was rarely used [11]. Physicians have been hesitant to use this technique in blind puncture, because of the pleural and vascular closeness of insertion site. In a retrospective analysis, the authors used subclavian approach as first choice and cannulated 148 pediatric patients [12]. They concluded that subclavian central venous cannulation is a safe procedure with minimal complications in pediatric patients. Pirotte and Veyckemans described a novel US-guided approach for SCV cannulation in infants and children [13]. The principle of this technique is to place the US probe at the supraclavicular level to obtain a longitudinal view of the SCV. This approach offers a longitudinal view of intrathoracic segment of the SCV reaching (via the innominate vein on left side) the IJV at the level of the Pirogoff confluent. The authors reported a high success rate and no major complications. The limitation of this approach is that the US shadow of the clavicle may not allow following the entire course of the needle. Guilbert et al. placed CVCs to the SCV of 40 children and neonates under US guidance [10]. They scanned the internal jugular vein from thyroid cartilage level to the supraclavicular region until the brachiocephalic vein and the SCV could be viewed in long axis. Viewing the brachiocephalic vein and the SCV in long axis, they performed needle in-plane puncture under ultrasound guidance. Rhondali et al. used a supraclavicular technique for SCV cannulation in 37 infants [9]. They placed the US probe at the supraclavicular level to obtain a longitudinal view of the SCV and gain access to the vein by in-plane needle puncture. Park et al. reported a case series of SCV cannulation in 11 pediatric patients weighing 1.1 kg to 15 kg [6]. They visualized the vein using infraclavicular approach and performed the puncture using needle in-plane technique. Kulkarni et al. reported cannulation of subclavian vein by a supraclavicular approach under ultrasound guidance in a series of 150 children and they routinely used this method in pediatric cardiac surgery patients [14]. Nardi et al. used an in-plane technique and a longitudinal axis visualization of subclavian vein in a prospective observational study for pediatric patients [15]. Ultrasound-guided subclavian vein cannulation was found feasible in low birth weight even weighing less than 1,500 g [16].

All of these studies confirm that US helps to find the location of the vascular structures, demonstrates preexisting intravascular clots, and defines anatomically inaccessible vessels. As a different approach from these studies, we preferred needle out-of-plane technique visualizing a transverse cross-sectional view of the subclavian vein. The patient's neck anatomy and diffuse generalized edema did not allow a perfect longitudinal view of the SCV. This approach provided the optimal ultrasonographic vision of the vein at the supraclavicular region.

In conclusion, needle out-of-plane technique with visualization of transverse cross-sectional view of subclavian vein is a successful alternative for supraclavicular subclavian vein cannulation in specific patients. Our case supports recent previous studies that are showing positive results for ultrasound-guided supraclavicular puncture of the subclavian vein in pediatric patients.

References

[1] D. Hind, N. Calvert, R. McWilliams et al., "Ultrasonic locating devices for central venous cannulation: meta-analysis," *British Medical Journal*, vol. 327, no. 7411, pp. 361–364, 2003.

[2] K. Al Sofyani, G. Julia, B. Abdulaziz, C. Yves, and R. Sylvain, "Ultrasound guidance for central vascular access in the neonatal and pediatric intensive care unit," *Saudi Journal of Anaesthesia*, vol. 6, no. 2, pp. 120–124, 2012.

[3] P. G. Shekelle, R. M. Wachter, P. J. Pronovost et al., "Making health care safer II: an updated critical analysis of the evidence for patient safety practices," *Evidence Report/Technology Assessment*, no. 211, pp. 1–945, 2013.

[4] National Institute for Clinical Excellence. Guidance on the Use of Ultrasound Location Devices for Placing Central Venous Catheters. Technology Appraisal Guidance No 49, September 2002 https://www.nice.org.uk/.

[5] C. D. Froehlich, M. R. Rigby, E. S. Rosenberg et al., "Ultrasound-guided central venous catheter placement decreases complications and decreases placement attempts compared with the landmark technique in patients in a pediatric intensive care unit," *Critical Care Medicine*, vol. 37, no. 3, pp. 1090–1096, 2009.

[6] S. I. Park, Y. H. Kim, S. Y. So, M. J. Kim, H. J. Kim, and J. K. Kim, "Ultrasound-guided subclavian catheterization in pediatric patients with a linear probe: a case series," *Korean Journal of Anesthesiology*, vol. 64, no. 6, pp. 541–544, 2013.

[7] S.-Y. Wu, Q. Ling, L.-H. Cao, J. Wang, M.-X. Xu, and W.-A. Zeng, "Real-time two-dimensional ultrasound guidance for central venous cannulation: a meta-analysis," *Anesthesiology*, vol. 118, no. 2, pp. 361–375, 2013.

[8] P. Skippen and N. Kissoon, "Ultrasound guidance for central vascular access in the pediatric emergency department," *Pediatric Emergency Care*, vol. 23, no. 3, pp. 203–207, 2007.

[9] O. Rhondali, R. Attof, S. Combet, D. Chassard, and M. De Queiroz Siqueira, "Ultrasound-guided subclavian vein cannulation in infants: supraclavicular approach," *Paediatric Anaesthesia*, vol. 21, no. 11, pp. 1136–1141, 2011.

[10] A.-S. Guilbert, L. Xavier, C. Ammouche et al., "Supraclavicular ultrasound-guided catheterization of the subclavian vein in pediatric and neonatal ICUs: a feasibility study," *Pediatric Critical Care Medicine*, vol. 14, no. 4, pp. 351–355, 2013.

[11] M. B. Yoffa, "Supraclavicular subclavian veni-puncture and catheterization," *The Lancet*, vol. 2, pp. 614–617, 1965.

[12] A. Çitak, M. Karaböcüoğlu, R. Üçsel, and N. Uzel, "Central venous catheters in pediatric patients—subclavian venous approach as the first choice," *Pediatrics International*, vol. 44, no. 1, pp. 83–86, 2002.

[13] T. Pirotte and F. Veyckemans, "Ultrasound-guided subclavian vein cannulation in infants and children: a novel approach," *British Journal of Anaesthesia*, vol. 98, no. 4, pp. 509–514, 2007.

[14] V. Kulkarni, K. P. Mulavisala, R. K. Mudunuri, and J. R. Byalal, "Ultrasound-guided supraclavicular approach to the subclavian vein in infants and children," *British Journal of Anaesthesia*, vol. 108, no. 1, article 162, 2012.

[15] N. Nardi, E. Wodey, B. Laviolle et al., "Effectiveness and complications of ultrasound-guided subclavian vein cannulation in children and neonates," *Anaesthesia Critical Care and Pain Medicine*, vol. 35, no. 3, pp. 209–213, 2016.

[16] U. Lausten-Thomsen, Z. Merchaoui, C. Dubois et al., "Ultrasound-guided subclavian vein cannulation in low birth weight neonates," *Pediatric Critical Care Medicine*, vol. 18, no. 2, pp. 172–175, 2017.

60

Bronchoesophageal Fistula Stenting Using High-Frequency Jet Ventilation and Underwater Seal Gastrostomy Tube Drainage

Nitish Fokeerah, Xinwei Liu, Yonggang Hao, and Lihua Peng

Department of Anesthesiology, The First Affiliated Hospital of Chongqing Medical University, No. 1, Youyi Road, Yuanjiagang, Yuzhong District, Chongqing 400016, China

Correspondence should be addressed to Xinwei Liu; 1594390020@qq.com

Academic Editor: Anjan Trikha

Managing a patient scheduled for bronchoesophageal fistula repair is challenging for the anesthetist. If appropriate ventilation strategy is not employed, serious complications such as hypoxemia, gastric distension, and pulmonary aspiration can occur. We present the case of a 62-year-old man with a bronchoesophageal fistula in the left main stem bronchus requiring the insertion of a Y-shaped tracheobronchial stent through a rigid bronchoscope, under general anesthesia. We successfully managed this intervention and herein report this case to demonstrate the effectiveness of underwater seal gastrostomy tube drainage used in conjunction with high-frequency jet ventilation during bronchoesophageal fistula stenting.

1. Introduction

Bronchoesophageal fistula (BEF) is a pathological communication between the bronchial tree and the esophagus. BEF usually result from aerodigestive malignancies, blunt or penetrating chest trauma, chronic granulomatous infections, or ingestion of foreign bodies and corrosive substances, or it can be congenital [1, 2]. BEF is a life-threatening condition which if left untreated will ultimately lead to overwhelming sepsis and death [1]. Therefore, timely diagnosis and treatment are of paramount importance. Isolating the bronchus from the esophagus remains the basis of management of this pathology. This can be achieved through the insertion of a tracheobronchial stent (TBS). However, this intervention has various complex anesthetic implications. Nevertheless, we successfully managed the stenting of an acquired BEF using high-frequency jet ventilation (HFJV) and gastric drainage system, whereby the patient's gastrostomy tube was connected to an underwater seal bottle.

2. Case Report

A 62-year-old man (weight 60 kg, height 170 cm, and BMI: 20.8 kg/m^2), chronic smoker and working as a stone breaker for the past 40 years, complained of cough and hemoptysis since 15 years and progressive shortness of breath for last one year. His symptoms got exacerbated and he was admitted to our hospital. Both fiberoptic bronchoscopy (Figure 1) and computed tomography scan of the chest (Figure 2) showed the presence of a 7 mm by 8 mm BEF in the left main stem bronchus, 3.2 cm distal to the carina. The etiology was chronic tracheobronchitis secondary to chronic nontuberculous mycobacterium (NTM) infection caused by *Mycobacterium fortuitum*. Besides the BEF, the patient also had underlying pneumonia, pneumoconiosis, and mild chronic obstructive pulmonary disease.

The patient was scheduled for the insertion of a Y-shaped covered self-expandable metal stent (CSEMS) (Micro-Tech Y-stent, Nanjing, China) through a rigid bronchoscope, under general anesthesia. Three weeks prior to the scheduled surgery, oral feeding was discontinued for both solids and liquids and a percutaneous endoscopic gastrojejunostomy was performed for enteral feeding. The patient also received total parenteral nutrition, intravenous fluids, antibiotics, and oxygen by face mask. Moreover, a thorough discussion between the interventionist and anesthetist was undertaken regarding the surgical procedure and its anesthetic implications.

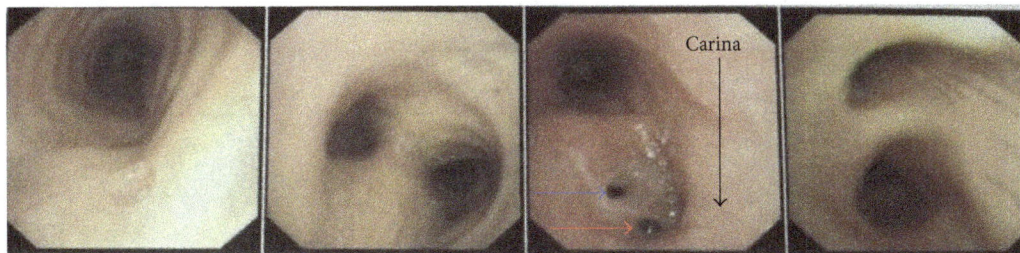

FIGURE 1: Bronchoscopy showing the presence of a bronchoesophageal fistula (blue arrow) and an ulcer (red arrow) in the left main bronchus.

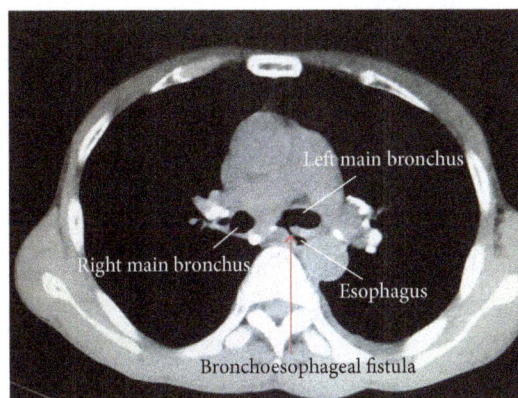

FIGURE 2: Computed tomography of the chest depicting the presence of a bronchoesophageal fistula between the left main bronchus and the esophagus.

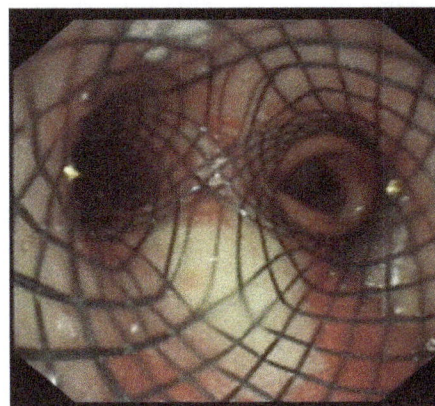

FIGURE 4: Correct position of the Y-shaped tracheobronchial stent, sealing the left bronchoesophageal fistula.

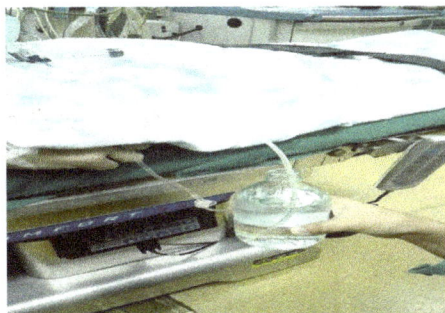

FIGURE 3: Patient lying on the operating table with his gastrostomy tube connected to an underwater seal bottle.

In the operation room, Ringer's lactate drip was started. Standard monitoring included pulse oximetry, electrocardiography, temperature, and invasive blood pressure monitoring via a left radial artery catheter. The gastrostomy tube was suctioned and connected to an underwater seal bottle containing a 10 cm column of water (Figure 3). Topical anesthesia was achieved by atomization of the nasopharynx and oropharynx with 4 mL of lidocaine 2%. The patient was preoxygenated with 100% oxygen at 5 L/min via a tight-fitting face mask for 3 minutes. Thereafter, injection penehyclidine 0.5 mg, hydrocortisone 100 mg, and omeprazole 40 mg were administered, followed by induction with propofol 100 mg

and sufentanil 10 mcg. The patient was gently ventilated manually to ascertain the ability to ventilate before giving the muscle relaxant. Simultaneously, we could observe few gas bubbles in the underwater seal bottle, but ventilation was not substantially compromised, thus indicating the efficacy of the gastric drainage system. Succinylcholine 40 mg was injected and eventually the trachea was intubated with the rigid bronchoscope. Additional lidocaine was applied to the tracheobronchial tree in a "spray-as-you-go" manner via the bronchoscope. Then, the HFJV machine (KR-IV [A], Nanchang GENE Medical Devices, Jiangxi, China) was connected to the ventilating port of the bronchoscope. Ventilation parameters included frequency 100/min, driving pressure 25 psi, I : E ratio 1 : 2, and FiO_2 0.7. Anesthesia was maintained with an infusion of propofol 40–60 mcg/kg/min and remifentanil 0.15–0.2 mcg/kg/min. The case proceeded uneventfully, with serial blood gas analysis performed (Table 1) to assess ventilation. No hypoxemia took place and patient remained hemodynamically stable throughout the procedure. However, transitory hypercapnia occurred (Table 1). This case was managed without the use of long acting muscle relaxant, as the patient did not have airway reflexes such as coughing and laryngospasm, patient remained apneic, and the condition for bronchoscopy was good during the intervention.

Once the stent (size: 18 × 30 mm – L 14 × 30 mm – R 14 × 10 mm) was deployed and its correct position confirmed (Figure 4), the bronchoscope was removed and HFJV stopped.

TABLE 1: Serial arterial blood gas analyses.

	Enter OR	Preinduction	15 minutes after HFJV	Stent inserted	HFJV stopped	Entered PACU	Left PACU
PaO$_2$ (mmHg)	75	278	244	105	149	387	110
PaCO$_2$ (mmHg)	38	38	62	76	82	51	42
pH	7.40	7.48	7.32	7.25	7.20	7.34	7.37
SpO$_2$ (%)	97	100	99	97	99	100	99

OR, operation room; HFJV, high frequency jet ventilation; PACU, postanesthesia care unit; PaO$_2$, partial pressure of oxygen in blood; PaCO$_2$, partial pressure of carbon dioxide in blood; SpO$_2$, peripheral capillary oxygen saturation.

An "i-gel" laryngeal mask airway (LMA) was inserted and conventional ventilation started. The patient was shifted to postanesthesia care unit, where emergence from anesthesia and recovery were quick and uneventful. On postoperative day 2, bronchoscopy showed correct position of the stent and patient was allowed to start oral feeding. Four days after the intervention, the patient was clinically stable and discharged from the hospital. One month later, the patient attended the outpatient department; he was asymptomatic and bronchoscopy showed that the CSEMS was in the correct position, sealing the BEF. The whole procedure including anesthesia induction and emergence took 55 minutes to be accomplished. Surgical time was 30 minutes.

3. Discussion

Anesthesia for patients with BEF requiring tracheobronchial stent insertion is challenging for the anesthetist. The challenges include a shared airway, underlying pulmonary pathologies, and coexisting advanced enterorespiratory malignancies. Furthermore, the use of intermittent positive pressure ventilation (IPPV) causes leakage of air through the BEF leading to two main complications. Firstly, distention of the stomach and probable gastric regurgitation leading to pulmonary soiling. Secondly, ventilation of the fistula accounts for inadequate lung ventilation, hypoxemia, atelectasis, and carbon dioxide (CO$_2$) retention. This case report highlights the various anesthetic considerations for the successful management of BEF.

HFJV has been very effective in this case. In contrast to conventional ventilation, HFJV delivers very small tidal volume (V_T) at high frequency, at a lower airway pressure [3, 4], thus decreasing gas outflow through the fistula. Typically, V_T delivered by HFJV is less than the anatomical dead space. Moreover, there is minimal diaphragmatic excursion [3], which provides a motionless surgical field. However, HFJV may cause inadequate CO$_2$ elimination and hypercapnia. In this case, the maximum PaCO$_2$ level was 82 mmHg, duration of hypercapnia was about 15 minutes, and no hypoxemia took place. Hence, this permissive hypercapnia did not require temporary interruption of the HFJV to provide controlled ventilation. Cheng et al. [5] reported that transient hypercapnia (PaCO$_2$ < 100 mmHg) does not prolong the recovery time, nor is it associated with serious complications. Another effective method to assess ventilation during interventional

bronchoscopy is transcutaneous capnography (Ptc$_{CO2}$). In addition, Gupta et al. [6] reported that using heliox (mixture of 80% helium and 20% oxygen) improves CO$_2$ elimination during HFJV.

Furthermore, we used an underwater seal drainage system, whereby the patient's gastrostomy tube was connected to an underwater seal bottle containing a 10 cm column of water. This strategy increases the resistance to gas flow from the airway to the esophagus. Therefore, gas will leak through the fistula only if the airway pressure exceeds the underwater seal pressure (10 cm H$_2$O). There are several benefits of this technique. Firstly, it accounts for better pulmonary ventilation by minimizing gas outflow through the fistula. Secondly, any gas leak to the stomach will be drained through the gastrostomy tube, not increasing the hydrostatic pressure of the stomach, hence no gastric regurgitation. To the best of our knowledge, a gastric underwater seal has not been used in the management of BEF in adults. This technique has been used in the management of congenital tracheoesophageal fistula (TEF) in infants. Donn et al. [7] successfully ventilated two newborns with congenital TEF, using HFJV in conjunction with gastric underwater seal. Likewise, Sosis and Amoroso [8] effectively ventilated an infant with congenital TEF using positive pressure ventilation, with the newborn's gastrostomy tube connected to an underwater seal. This methodology has also been demonstrated to alleviate gastric distension caused by aerophagia by using underwater seal nasogastric tube drainage [9].

There are alternative means of providing effective ventilation for the management of enterorespiratory fistulas. For instance, manual jet ventilation (MJV) can be used. MJV offers more efficient ventilation and CO$_2$ elimination compared to HFJV, due to adequate expiratory time and better chest and lung recoil during expiration [10]. Dolan and Moore [11] ventilated the lungs by passing the jet catheter of the HFJV distal to the fistula, thus minimizing gas leakage. Other options include endobronchial intubation, Univent endobronchial blocker, and double lumen tube to the unaffected bronchus [12, 13]. More complex fistulas have been managed successfully with bilateral endobronchial intubation [14], extracorporeal membrane oxygenation [15], and cardiopulmonary bypass [16]. Some authors reported sealing the fistula prior to the intervention, using a modified esophageal balloon [17], or a Sengstaken–Blakemore tube [18]. Garg et al. [19] reported two cases in children where they sealed the TEF using Fogarty and Foley catheter. In our case, if the surgeon would not have used rigid bronchoscope, we could have used an LMA, avoid muscle relaxant, maintain the patient's spontaneous breathing, and under FOB guidance place the jet catheter of a MJV into the right bronchus to provide intermittent ventilation if required. The jet catheter must be withdrawn upwards into the trachea at the time of stent deployment.

The anesthetic goal for stenting a BEF is to use drugs which are quick in onset, short acting, and readily eliminated. Muscle relaxant is needed to provide optimal relaxation for insertion of the rigid bronchoscope and manipulation of the airway, in order to prevent coughing, laryngospasm, and chest rigidity. We used succinylcholine and performed a rapid sequence induction (RSI). However, succinylcholine is short acting and eventually a top-up dose of another muscle relaxant may be necessary if the patient shows signs of discomfort, starts spontaneous respiration which is hindering with the surgery, or develops airway reflexes. Ideally, rocuronium is the muscle relaxant of choice for this type of intervention. We may use 1.2 mg/kg of rocuronium and perform a RSI. At the end of the surgery, we can promptly antagonize the rocuronium with sugammadex. However, sugammadex is not available in our hospital. Regarding anesthesia maintenance, Wang et al. [20] described that propofol and remifentanil TCI in association with HFJV for bronchoscopy procedures provide multiple benefits. Total intravenous anesthesia (TIVA) is ideal, since the airway remains essentially open to the atmosphere and use of inhaled anesthetics will lead to pollution of the operation room. Furthermore, in the authors' case, atomization of the airway with lidocaine suppressed the cough reflex, prevented laryngospasm, and reduced the need for systemic opioids and sedatives, hence favoring early recovery.

After the placement of the stent, we should advocate the early return of spontaneous respiration, early extubation, and weaning from the ventilator. Therefore, after the intervention, insertion of an LMA is preferred to an endotracheal tube. Endotracheal intubation requires a deeper depth of anesthesia, which will prolong the recovery, and it may also cause coughing and laryngospasm which may cause displacement of the newly placed stent.

Besides all these aspects, a key determining factor is constant and effective communication and cooperation between the interventionist and anesthetist, which plays a pivotal role in the success of this surgery.

In conclusion, anesthetic management for BEF stenting is challenging. However, we successfully managed the surgery using HFJV in conjunction with an underwater seal gastrostomy tube drainage system. The latter has played a crucial role in the success of our case and is a novel strategy for BEF management in adults. Nevertheless, we will consider enhancing our management, in view of optimizing our anesthetic plan for similar eventual interventions. Various other ways to manage a case of BEF have been reported in medical literature. Anyhow, whatever method is chosen, a planned and multidisciplinary approach to successfully tackle this complex issue of bronchoesophageal fistula will be required.

Disclosure

Nitish Fokeerah is the first author.

Competing Interests

The authors declare that there is no conflict of interests regarding the publication of this paper.

Acknowledgments

Source of funding is Anesthesiology Department of the First Affiliated Hospital of Chongqing Medical University.

References

[1] A. N. Rodriguez and J. P. Diaz-Jimenez, "Malignant respiratory-digestive fistulas," *Current Opinion in Pulmonary Medicine*, vol. 16, no. 4, pp. 329–333, 2010.

[2] J. Singh, V. A. Olcese, T. A. D'Amico, and M. M. Wahidi, "Adult tracheoesophageal fistula: a multidisciplinary approach," *Clinical Pulmonary Medicine*, vol. 15, no. 3, pp. 145–152, 2008.

[3] J. Pawlowski, "Anesthetic considerations for interventional pulmonary procedures," *Current Opinion in Anaesthesiology*, vol. 26, no. 1, pp. 6–12, 2013.

[4] V. Pathak, I. Welsby, K. Mahmood, M. Wahidi, N. MacIntyre, and S. Shofer, "Ventilation and anesthetic approaches for rigid bronchoscopy," *Annals of the American Thoracic Society*, vol. 11, no. 4, pp. 628–634, 2014.

[5] Q. Cheng, J. Zhang, H. Wang, R. Zhang, Y. Yue, and L. Li, "Effect of acute hypercapnia on outcomes and predictive risk factors for complications among patients receiving bronchoscopic interventions under general anesthesia," *PLoS ONE*, vol. 10, no. 7, Article ID 0130771, 2015.

[6] V. K. Gupta, E. N. Grayck, and I. M. Cheifetz, "Heliox administration during high-frequency jet ventilation augments carbon dioxide clearance," *Respiratory Care*, vol. 49, no. 9, pp. 1038–1044, 2004.

[7] S. M. Donn, L. K. Zak, M. E. A. Bozynski, A. G. Coran, and K. T. Oldham, "Use of high-frequency jet ventilation in the management of congenital tracheoesophageal fistula associated with respiratory distress syndrome," *Journal of Pediatric Surgery*, vol. 25, no. 12, pp. 1219–1221, 1990.

[8] M. Sosis and M. Amoroso, "Respiratory insufficiency after gastrostomy prior to tracheoesophageal fistula repair," *Anesthesia and Analgesia*, vol. 64, no. 7, pp. 748–750, 1985.

[9] A. W. Solomon, J. C. Bramall, and J. Ball, "Underwater-seal nasogastric tube drainage to relieve gastric distension caused by air swallowing," *Anaesthesia*, vol. 66, no. 2, pp. 124–126, 2011.

[10] E. Evans, P. Biro, and N. Bedforth, "Jet ventilation," *Continuing Education in Anaesthesia, Critical Care & Pain*, vol. 7, no. 1, pp. 2–5, 2007.

[11] A. M. Dolan and M. F. Moore, "Anaesthesia for tracheobronchial stent insertion using an laryngeal mask airway and high-frequency jet ventilation," *Case Reports in Medicine*, vol. 2013, Article ID 950437, 5 pages, 2013.

[12] C. S. Chan, "Anaesthetic management during repair of tracheo-oesophageal fistula," *Anaesthesia*, vol. 39, no. 2, pp. 158–160, 1984.

[13] C. R. Grebenik, "Anaesthetic management of malignant tracheo-oesophageal fistula," *British Journal of Anaesthesia*, vol. 63, no. 4, pp. 492–496, 1989.

[14] J. M. Ford and J. A. Shields, "Selective bilateral bronchial intubation for large, acquired tracheoesophageal fistula," *AANA Journal*, vol. 80, no. 1, pp. 49–53, 2012.

[15] N. F. Collins, L. Ellard, E. Licari, E. Beasley, S. Seevanayagam, and L. Doolan, "Veno-venous extracorporeal membrane oxygenation and apnoeic oxygenation for tracheo-oesophageal fistula repair in a previously pneumonectomised patient," *Anaesthesia and Intensive Care*, vol. 42, no. 6, pp. 789–792, 2014.

[16] N. B. Slamon, J. H. Hertzog, S. H. Penfil, R. C. Raphaely, C. Pizarro, and C. D. Derby, "An unusual case of button battery-induced traumatic tracheoesophageal fistula," *Pediatric Emergency Care*, vol. 24, no. 5, pp. 313–316, 2008.

[17] T. Inada, M. Umemoto, T. Ohshima, O. Sawada, and Y.-S. Nakamuradagger, "Anesthesia for insertion of a Dumon stent in a patient with a large tracheo-esophageal fistula," *Canadian Journal of Anaesthesia*, vol. 46, no. 4, pp. 372–375, 1999.

[18] J. Nakada, S. Nagai, M. Nishira, R. Hosoda, T. Matsura, and Y. Inagaki, "Sealing of a tracheoesophageal fistula using a sengstaken-blakemore tube for mechanical ventilation during general anesthesia," *Anesthesia & Analgesia*, vol. 106, no. 4, pp. 1218–1219, 2008.

[19] R. Garg, R. Pandey, P. Khanna, and D. Narang, "Airway management of undiagnosed tracheoesophageal fistula detected accidentally intraoperatively," *Paediatric Anaesthesia*, vol. 20, no. 10, pp. 970–972, 2010.

[20] H. B. Wang, C. X. Yang, B. Zhang, Y. Xia, H. Z. Liu, and H. Liang, "Efficacy of target-controlled infusion of propofol and remifentanil with high frequency jet ventilation in fibre-optic bronchoscopy," *Singapore Medical Journal*, vol. 54, no. 12, pp. 689–694, 2013.

61

Case Report of Subanesthetic Intravenous Ketamine Infusion for the Treatment of Neuropathic Pain and Depression with Suicidal Features in a Pediatric Patient

Garret Weber ⓘ, JuHan Yao, Shemeica Binns, and Shinae Namkoong

Department of Anesthesiology, New York Medical College, Valhalla, NY, USA

Correspondence should be addressed to Garret Weber; garret.weber@wmchealth.org

Academic Editor: Kuang-I Cheng

Chronic neuropathic pain and depression are often comorbid. Ketamine has been used to treat refractory pain. There is emerging evidence for use in depression. We present a case of a pediatric patient who was successfully treated with subanesthetic intravenous ketamine infusion for chronic neuropathic pain and suicidality.

1. Introduction

Neuropathic pain is often difficult to treat despite multimodal analgesia. Similarly, refractory depression has limited treatment options available. Intravenous ketamine infusion has been increasingly used for the treatment of neuropathic pain. Several recent trials have also shown that intravenous ketamine infusion has a rapid antidepressant effect [1, 2]. There are especially limited research and evidence on the efficacy of the dual treatment of major depression and neuropathic pain in the pediatric population. We present a case of an adolescent with severe depression, suicidality, and neuropathic leg pain who failed multiple antidepressant and analgesic modalities who was successfully treated with subanesthetic intravenous ketamine infusion. To our knowledge this is the first reported case with dual use of intravenous ketamine infusion to treat neuropathic pain and suicidal depression in the pediatric patient.

The patient's healthcare proxy (mother) provided written consent for publication as the patient is a minor.

2. Case Description

A 14-year-old female presented to an outpatient psychiatrist with severe depression and suicidal ideation. She was admitted to the pediatric psychiatric unit for evaluation and treatment.

Her medical history was significant for anxiety, depression with multiple suicide attempts, postconcussive syndrome, chronic migraines, and previous diagnosis of complex regional pain syndrome of the lower extremities. While being admitted for depression and suicidality, she also complained of exacerbation of her bilateral leg pain, which significantly limited her mobility and worsened her mood.

She was admitted two months prior for bilateral generalized neuropathic leg pain which limited her mobility. A lumbar magnetic resonance image (MRI) was unremarkable. She tried multiple classes of pain medications including acetaminophen, nonsteroidal anti-inflammatory agents, tricyclic antidepressants, gabapentinoids, antiepileptics, and opioids. Additional interventions included acupuncture, physical therapy, occupational therapy, guided imagery therapy, and epidural steroid injection.

Upon readmission for suicidality, the pain management team was consulted. On her psychiatric evaluation, patient had a depressed, flat affect endorsing suicidality. The patient reported despair regarding her chronic pain as well as flashbacks to a previous concussion after a fall several years prior with subsequent development of her neuropathic type pain. She had also reported several instances of self-injurious behaviors including cutting and two suicide attempts with a shoelace and pillowcase. She was placed on continuous observation. The patient's chronic outpatient psychiatric medications include fluoxetine and aripiprazole. While she was an inpatient, the patient was also trialed on bupropion but was discontinued due to increased agitation and irritability. She also reported severe burning bilateral leg pain. In addition, she described her pain in terms of "shooting", reporting painful paresthesias, dysesthesias, and hyperalgesia as well as a "numbness" characterization to her bilateral leg pain, which followed a neuropathic pattern.

Her lumbar spine was mildly tender to palpation, but her neurological exam was otherwise intact. While her characterization of pain was neuropathic in nature, she did not meet the criteria for complex regional pain syndrome. There were no allodynic features, vasomotor, pseudomotor, or tropic changes on exam. Despite her prescribed regimen of pregabalin, ibuprofen, acetaminophen, lidocaine 5% patch, tizanidine, and subsequently oxycodone as needed, her pain continued. She had also been tried previously on morphine with also minimal efficacy. The patient also underwent a ten-day trial of duloxetine with minimal improvement and reported worsening severe depressive symptoms, suicidal ideations, and neuropathic pain. It was then recommended to start an intravenous ketamine infusion which was theorized to have a more rapid clinical onset and effect.

Patient was transferred to the pediatric intensive care unit for intravenous ketamine infusion and monitoring. Prior to starting intravenous ketamine infusion, her leg pain was rated 7/10 on the numerical rating scale (NRS, 0-10 with 10 being the worst pain) of burning quality. There was no weakness or changes in sensation, though there was limited mobility secondary to pain. Intravenous ketamine infusion was started at 7 micrograms/kilogram/minute (mcg/kg/min). The ketamine infusion was used 24 hours per day for the entire duration of the treatment with ketamine infusion. The total dose was titrated based on the specific mcg/kg/min. The patient's weight (72 kg) was used for the dosing calculation.

The patient remained hemodynamically stable with no dysphoria or hallucinations. On day one of intravenous ketamine infusion, the patient had significant improvement of her depressive symptoms, as noted by psychiatry and pain management teams, and the maximum NRS throughout the day was 6/10. On day two, she reported less pain in her legs with a maximum NRS of 5/10, and significant improvement in her mood with no further suicidal ideations. On day three, intravenous ketamine infusion was increased to 8 micrograms/kilogram/minute; however physical exam revealed nystagmus and visual changes and was decreased to 7 micrograms/kilogram/minute. Patient's pain maximum NRS score remained at 5/10. On day four, maximum NRS score reduced to 4/10 and self-reported 70% pain relief since initiation of intravenous ketamine infusion. She also had functional improvement in her legs and was able to ambulate freely. On day five, dosage was titrated down to 4 micrograms/kilogram/minute with maximum NRS score of 0/10 and sustained improvement in mood. Intravenous ketamine infusion was further reduced to 2 micrograms/kilogram/minute and discontinued that same day. She was able to tolerate physical therapy and maintain analgesia. Psychiatric reassessment determined her to be no longer at suicide risk, and she was discharged with no

immediate sequelae and was placed on chronic aripiprazole, topiramate, and lithium by her outpatient psychiatrist.

The patient had five months of symptom relief after her first intravenous ketamine infusion. She was readmitted five months later with repeated suicide attempts, depression, and worsening bilateral upper and lower extremity neuropathic pain, though with decreased baseline NRS. Due to her dramatic improvement and sustained relief with intravenous ketamine infusion during her last admission, as well as the lack of other successful treatment options, she was again admitted to the pediatric intensive care unit for five days of intravenous ketamine infusion with resolution of her neuropathic pain and suicidal/depressive symptoms allowing for discharge home without any immediate sequelae.

3. Discussion

To our knowledge this is the first reported successful pediatric use of intravenous ketamine infusion for the dual treatment of depression with suicidality and chronic neuropathic pain. There is one recent report on the use of ketamine for chronic pain and depression in an adult, but none in the pediatric population [1].

In this case the diagnosis of neuropathic pain was made based on clinical descriptors and history. As noted in a recent review, by Gilron et al., there is no absolute pathognomonic sign or symptom of neuropathic pain [3]. Consequently the patient's diagnosis was made based on her descriptors and symptoms in setting of persistent pain that seemed to reflect a neuropathic pain pattern rather than a nociceptive, nonneuropathic painful condition. The authors of this case acknowledge that there are screening tools used for diagnosis of neuropathic pain and quantitative objective sensory testing. These were not used in our patient, especially in light of her ongoing psychiatric, severe, comorbid symptoms.

Neuropathic pain is nerve pain secondary to peripheral or central nervous injury or dysfunction. It often presents as spontaneous burning or lancinating pain. Other symptoms include allodynia, hyperesthesia, hyperalgesia, and the symptoms are typically persistent even after the primary insult has resolved. The current management for the treatment of neuropathic pain is limited due to minimal evidence of efficacy. Traditional first-line agents include gabapentinoids, tricyclic antidepressants, or serotonin-norepinephrine reuptake inhibitors (SNRIs) [4].

Opioids have had mixed efficacy for neuropathic pain. The evidence supporting use for chronic noncancer pain in children and adolescents is low and limited at best [5]. Furthermore, opioids are considered second/third-line therapy because of their questionable long-term efficacy as well as the risks of opioid related adverse effects which commonly include sedation, gastrointestinal effects including constipation and nausea/vomiting. Additionally respiratory depression can occur. Also, opioid misuse and addiction potential is a serious consideration [3]. Given our patient's comorbid advanced psychiatric state, chronic opioid therapy and further titration were not deemed to be a safe and viable option.

Combination therapy is often required due to noneffi-cacy of monotherapy. Additional nonpharmacological treat-ment includes cognitive behavioral therapy, physical therapy, biofeedback, and transcutaneous electrical nerve stimulation (TENS) [6]. Despite a multimodal treatment approach, neu-ropathic pain can be refractory, and multiple novel targets for neuropathic pain are being studied [7].

The mechanism of neuropathic pain differs for peripheral and central pain. Peripheral sensitization occurs due to an injury to axons of a peripheral nerve. This insult leads to spontaneous activation, abnormal excitability, and increased sensitivity to chemical, mechanical, and thermal stimuli [8]. When this occurs in the spinothalamic tract, central sensitization occurs with increased spontaneous activity and increased responses to all afferent impulses. This increase in synaptic efficiency and reduced inhibition lead to a greater response to nociceptive stimuli [8, 9]. Central sensitization has been proposed as an explanation for persistent neuro-pathic pain [10]. There is also the "windup" phenomenon in which repetitive nociceptive stimuli are potentiated in the spinal cord causing increased cortical perception of pain [11].

Ketamine is an N-methyl-D-aspartate (NDMA) recep-tor antagonist. The NMDA receptors are mechanistically involved with central sensitization [8–10]. Ketamine's inhi-bition of the NMDA receptors helps decrease peripheral and central sensitization, promoting analgesia. In addition, NMDA receptors are involved in the development of opioid tolerance. Ketamine's antagonistic action on NMDA recep-tors may prevent opioid tolerance in chronic pain patients. Additional mechanisms of ketamine as an analgesic include its effect on substance P. Ketamine has been shown to directly inhibit substance P receptors, which is also increased in painful hyperalgesic states [12].

The mechanistic role of ketamine in the treatment of depression, however, is less well defined. First-line treat-ment for depression is a combination of psychotherapy with an antidepressant, generally a selective serotonin reuptake inhibitor (SSRI) based on efficacy and side effect profile [13]. Additional classes of medications such as serotonin-norepinephrine reuptake inhibitors, atypical antidepressants, tricyclic antidepressants, or monoamine oxidase inhibitors are often used to treat depression refractory to first-line agents. Electrical convulsive therapy (ECT) is another treat-ment modality for severe depression refractory to pharmaco-logic agents. While ECT provides a rapid response and thus has utility in the acute setting, it requires general anesthesia and has complications including somatic injury and dental trauma, as well as confusion and amnesia [14].

As an alternative, ketamine has emerged for treatment of major depressive disorder with or without suicidality. Several trials demonstrated a large reduction in the severity of depression within 24 hours of intravenous ketamine infusion with lasting antidepressant efficacy [2]. A systematic litera-ture review also demonstrated reduction in suicidal ideation for treatment resistant depression with the use of ketamine [15]. An additional benefit is the rapid antidepressant effect compared with most first-line antidepressant medications.

The antidepressant mechanism of ketamine is unclear at this point but may involve ketamine's NMDA antagonism. In fact, citalopram and fluoxetine, both SSRIs, have been shown to have functional effects of NMDA receptor blockade [16]. Ketamine, by inhibiting NMDA receptors, leads to increased production of brain-derived neurotrophic factor (BDNF) and mammalian target of rapamycin complex 1 (mTORC1), both of which are associated with synaptogenesis and have been shown to be decreased in patients with major depression [16].

One limitation of using ketamine is the higher level monitoring. Due to state regulations, at our institution, patients receiving an intravenous ketamine infusion require an intensive care unit or step down unit for the first 24 hours; it is therefore a resource burden [17]. Furthermore, the long-term cognitive effects and optimal subanesthetic dosing and duration for the dual treatment of neuropathic pain and depression need to be elucidated. Additionally, the described subanesthetic intravenous ketamine infusion is an off-label use in pediatric neuropathic pain and depression.

In summary, we have shown successfully in our trial that subanesthetic intravenous ketamine infusion has the potential for emerging use in the pediatric population for neuropathic pain and depression given its rapid-onset antide-pressant and analgesic effects as well as favorable safety profile at subanesthetic dosing.

Authors' Contributions

Garret Weber, JuHan Yao, Shemeica Binns, and Shinae Namkoong carried out conception and design, acquisition, analysis, and interpretation of data, and drafting. They reviewed the paper and gave final approval.

References

[1] D. Bigman, S. Kunaparaju, and B. Bobrin, "Use of ketamine for acute suicidal ideation in a patient with chronic pain on prescribed cannabinoids," *BMJ Case Reports*, vol. 2017, 2017.

[2] B. Romeo, W. Choucha, P. Fossati, and J.-Y. Rotge, "Meta-analysis of short- and mid-term efficacy of ketamine in unipolar and bipolar depression," *Psychiatry Research*, vol. 230, no. 2, pp. 682–688, 2015.

[3] I. Gilron, R. Baron, and T. Jensen, "Neuropathic pain: Principles of diagnosis and treatment," *Mayo Clinic Proceedings*, vol. 90, no. 4, pp. 532–545, 2015.

[4] A. B. O'Connor and R. H. Dworkin, "Treatment of neuropathic pain: an overview of recent guidelines," *American Journal of Medicine*, vol. 122, supplement 10, pp. S22–S32, 2009.

[5] T. E. Cooper, E. Fisher, A. L. Gray et al., "Opioids for chronic non-cancer pain in children and adolescents," *Cochrane Database of Systematic Reviews*, vol. 26, no. 7, Article ID CD012538, pp. 1–23, 2017.

[6] V. Guastella, G. Mick, and B. Laurent, "Non pharmacologic treatment of neuropathic pain," *La Presse Médicale*, vol. 37, no. 2, pp. 354–357, 2008.

[7] D. Bouhassira and N. Attal, "Emerging therapies for neuro-pathic pain: new molecules or new indications for old treat-ments?" *Pain*, pp. 576–582, 2018.

[8] O. Elsewaisy, B. Slon, and J. Monagle, "Analgesic effect of subanesthetic intravenous ketamine in refractory neuropathic pain: a case report," *Pain Medicine*, vol. 11, no. 6, pp. 946–950, 2010.

[9] D. Bridges, S. W. N. Thompson, and A. S. C. Rice, "Mechanisms of neuropathic pain," *British Journal of Anaesthesia*, vol. 87, no. 1, pp. 12–26, 2001.

[10] A. Truini and G. Cruccu, "Pathophysiological mechanisms of neuropathic pain," *Neurological Sciences*, vol. 27, no. 2, pp. s179–s182, 2006.

[11] P. K. Eide, "Wind-up and the NMDA receptor complex from a clinical perspective," *European Journal of Pain*, vol. 4, no. 1, pp. 5–15, 2000.

[12] G. J. Iacobucci, O. Visnjevac, L. Pourafkari, and N. D. Nader, "Ketamine: An update on cellular and subcellular mechanisms with implications for clinical practice," *Pain Physician*, vol. 20, no. 2, pp. E285–E301, 2017.

[13] S. C. Marcus and M. Olfson, "National trends in the treatment for depression from 1998 to 2007," *Archives of General Psychiatry*, vol. 67, no. 12, pp. 1265–1273, 2010.

[14] C. H. Kellner, M. Fink, R. Knapp et al., "Relief of expressed suicidal intent by ECT: A consortium for research in ECT study," *The American Journal of Psychiatry*, vol. 162, no. 5, pp. 977–982, 2005.

[15] L. Reinstatler and N. A. Youssef, "Ketamine as a potential treatment for suicidal ideation: a systematic review of the literature," *Drugs in R&D*, vol. 15, no. 1, pp. 37–43, 2015.

[16] S. E. Strasburger, P. M. Bhimani, J. H. Kaabe et al., "What is the mechanism of Ketamine's rapid-onset antidepressant effect? A concise overview of the surprisingly large number of possibilities," *Journal of Clinical Pharmacy and Therapeutics*, vol. 42, no. 2, pp. 147–154, 2017.

[17] B. Zittel, "IV Drug Administration of Ketamine for the Treatment of Intractable Pain," Edited by Department NYSE, 2011. http://www.op.nysed.gov/prof/nurse/nurse-iv-ketamine.htm.

62

Management of a Parturient with Mast Cell Activation Syndrome: An Anesthesiologist's Experience

Sangeeta Kumaraswami ⓘ and Gabriel Farkas

Department of Anesthesiology, New York Medical College at Westchester Medical Center, Valhalla, NY, USA

Correspondence should be addressed to Sangeeta Kumaraswami; sangeeta.kumaraswami@wmchealth.org

Academic Editor: Ehab Farag

Mast cell activation syndrome (MCAS) is a disorder in which patients experience symptoms and signs attributable to inappropriate mast cell activation and mediator release. Multiorgan involvement in patients can result in significant morbidity and possible mortality. Limited literature exists regarding anesthetic management of patients with MCAS. We report a case of vaginal delivery with neuraxial labor analgesia in a parturient with this condition and highlight the importance of multidisciplinary planning for uneventful outcomes. Stress can trigger life-threatening symptoms, and counseling is important to allay patients' fears. Optimum medical control, adequate premedication, avoidance of triggers, and preparedness to treat serious mediator effects are key. We review MCAS and discuss anesthetic considerations for patients with this mast cell disorder.

1. Introduction

Mast cell activation syndrome (MCAS) is a condition in which patients experience recurrent and episodic symptoms of mast cell degranulation. Patients with this disorder appear to represent a growing proportion of the mast cell disorder patient population [1, 2]. There is paucity of literature on this subject relevant to an anesthesiologist. Our pregnant patient had symptomatology suggestive of a mast cell mediated disorder with significant suffering and disability. Written consent was taken from her for publication of this case report.

2. Case

A 24-year-old female G3P2 was admitted for induction of labor at 39 weeks' gestation. Her pregnancy had been uneventful except for a diagnosis of gestational hypertension (diet controlled). During a scheduled obstetric visit at 39 weeks, she met criteria for preeclampsia with resulting hospitalization. She had history of 2 prior vaginal deliveries with neuraxial analgesia, both following induction of labor for preeclampsia.

Her medical history was significant for iron deficiency anemia (received iron infusions for treatment), hypothyroidism (controlled with levothyroxine), celiac disease, and a recent diagnosis of MCAS. A few months after the birth of her second child 2 years ago, she began experiencing potentially life-threatening reactions. These reactions typically followed a pattern of abdominal discomfort and diarrhea followed by extremity and facial swelling, hives, and throat itching. Triggers included certain foods, drugs, and physical or emotional stress. The patient reported frequent emergency room (ER) visits for this condition. Self-administration of epinephrine autoinjector and diphenhydramine resulted in relief of symptoms during most episodes. Occasional treatment with corticosteroids was necessary without need for overt resuscitative measures related to fluid replacement or airway management. A treatment regimen for MCAS was started and avoidance of known triggers including nonsteroidal anti-inflammatory drugs (NSAIDs) and histamine-rich foods was advised. Her surgical history included a bone marrow biopsy, esophagogastroduodenoscopy, and colonoscopy with no complications. Her physical examination was significant for obesity (body mass index 33) and an unremarkable back and airway examination.

TABLE 1: Classification of disorders associated with mast cell activation[*].

PRIMARY	SECONDARY	IDIOPATHIC
(i) Clonal mast cell disorders (e.g., mastocytosis) (ii) Monoclonal mast cell activation syndrome	(i) Allergic disorders (e.g., asthma, rhinitis) (ii) Mast cell activation associated with inflammatory or neoplastic disorders (iii) Physical urticaria (iv) Chronic autoimmune urticaria	(i) Urticaria (ii) Angioedema (iii) Anaphylaxis (iv) Mast cell activation syndrome(MCAS)[†]

[*][†]The term MCAS has been used interchangeably in the literature to denote both the umbrella term and idiopathic MCAS [4, 17].

During routine obstetric visits, she repeatedly requested elective cesarean delivery with general anesthesia due to concern for allergic reactions during labor. Our obstetric team saw no contraindication to a vaginal delivery and after intense counseling including discussion with an anesthesiologist she agreed to a trial of labor with early neuraxial analgesia. A multidisciplinary approach involving an obstetrician, anesthesiologist, hematologist, allergist, neonatologist, nursing personnel, and dietician was used to formulate a plan for delivery. A premedication regimen prior to delivery, with availability of an anaphylaxis treatment kit and resuscitation equipment at bedside, was planned. In addition to the existing daily regimen of cetirizine, famotidine, and montelukast, she was informed to start prednisone 60 mg daily about 48 hours prior to estimated date of delivery. Low-histamine and gluten-free diet precautions were to be followed during her hospital stay.

Following induction of labor with a Foley transcervical balloon and vaginal misoprostol, she requested epidural analgesia. Doses of 125 mg methylprednisolone and 50 mg diphenhydramine were given intravenously as premedication, and the procedure was accomplished with good pain relief. After approximately 4 hours, she complained of increasing pain secondary to uterine contractions. Examination of her lumbar area revealed a dislodged epidural catheter due to unclear reasons. The epidural procedure was repeated after again administering a prophylactic dose of 50 mg diphenhydramine, and catheter placement was done uneventfully. Alcohol based chlorhexidine was used uneventfully for skin antisepsis both times. She received 0.2% ropivacaine infusion through the epidural catheter with adequate pain relief. Oxytocin was used for augmentation of labor with delivery of a healthy neonate without complications. Her postpartum hospital stay was complicated by an unusual episode of abdominal discomfort and itchy throat, after exposure to odor from a citrus fruit (histamine-rich food), consumed by the other patient in her shared room. She was immediately given 50 mg diphenhydramine with resolution of symptoms and shifted to a single occupancy room. Our patient was discharged home on the third day following delivery without any other complications.

3. Discussion

Mast cells are an important part of our body's immune system, originating from the bone marrow and participating in inflammatory processes with production of mediators [3]. A certain level of mast cell activation is physiological

and necessary for maintenance of homeostasis [4]. Mast cell activation syndromes is an umbrella term used to describe disorders in which recurrent and inappropriate mast cell activation and release of mediators occurs, causing symptoms associated with multiple organ systems.

The term was introduced to propose a global unifying classification of all mast cell activation disorders, with division into primary (proliferation of abnormal mast cells), secondary (normal mast cells activated in response to a microenvironmental trigger), and idiopathic (no evidence of primary or secondary cause) as shown in Table 1 [1, 5].

3.1. Presentation and Diagnosis. Typical symptoms and signs are listed in Table 2 [6].

Proposed diagnostic criteria for MCAS are listed in Table 3 [1].

Mast cells can be activated through both IgE and non-IgE dependent mechanisms with release of mediators such as histamine, tryptase, leukotrienes, and prostaglandins. Activation typically occurs in response to triggers, although none may be identified [7]. Clinical manifestations occur secondary to tissue responses to these mediators.

Our patient had episodic symptoms throughout her pregnancy with no disorder identified that could account for them. A bone marrow biopsy done had shown no evidence of mast cell disease, despite some abnormalities in megakaryocyte clustering and reticulum fibrosis. An elevated serum tryptase was found during an ER visit, with normal serum tryptase and blood histamine level in between episodes. With known primary and secondary causes ruled out, a potential diagnosis of idiopathic MCAS was made based on diagnostic criteria. A thorough workup was deferred until after delivery. Patients are often known to undergo extensive medical evaluation to determine an etiology, with a goal to find a yet-to-be identified endogenous or environmental stimulus or mast cell defect.

3.2. Treatment. Avoidance of exposure to identifiable triggers and antimediator therapy, including medications that prevent mast cell degranulation, form the basis of treatment. Multidrug therapy, such as H-1 and H-2 receptor antagonists, mast cell stabilizers, and leukotriene receptor antagonists are used in varying combinations to achieve control. Epinephrine autoinjector and antihistamine drugs are typically used by patients for breakthrough degranulation, with more aggressive treatment done in a hospital setting if necessary. Recently, omalizumab has been shown to prevent

TABLE 2: Common symptoms and signs of MCAS.

Dermatologic	Flushing, pruritus, hives
Cardiovascular	Near syncope or syncope, palpitations, chest pain, dysrhythmias, hypotension, hypertension
Pulmonary	Cough, wheezing
Eyes, ear, nose, throat	Post nasal drip, inflammation (conjunctivitis, rhinitis, sinusitis, pharyngitis, laryngitis), throat itching and swelling
Neurologic	Headache, seizures, tremors
Psychiatric	Cognitive dysfunction, memory difficulties, anxiety, depression, psychoses
Gastrointestinal	Nausea, vomiting, reflux, constipation, diarrhea, abdominal pain, malabsorption
Musculoskeletal	Bone or muscle pain, arthritis, myositis
Immunologic	Types I, II, III, and IV hypersensitivity reaction

TABLE 3: Proposed diagnostic criteria for MCAS.

(1) Episodic symptoms of mast cell mediator release involving ≥2 organ systems

(2) Appropriate response to antimediator therapy

(3) Documented increase in validated systemic markers of mast cell activation during episode (e.g., serum tryptase or urinary markers such as histamine metabolites, prostaglandin D2 or its metabolite, and leukotriene E4)

(4) Primary and secondary causes ruled out

symptoms and reduce adverse events. Cytoreductive and immunomodulating therapies are tried in some cases.

3.3. Anesthetic Considerations. Little is known about the perioperative management of patients with MCAS. The main anesthetic concern is avoidance of mast cell mediator release. In addition to workup for evaluation of comorbidities, a multidisciplinary plan for perioperative management with involvement of the patient is necessary to lessen concerns. Medications taken for MCAS should be continued up to the day of surgery. A premedication regimen of H-1 and H-2 receptor antagonists and corticosteroids are recommended before invasive procedures including those requiring anesthesia, the goal being reduction and blockade of mediators that can cause life-threatening reactions such as anaphylaxis [8]. Benzodiazepines are valuable in reducing anxiety, a known trigger.

Deviation from routine anesthetic techniques is not necessarily warranted although central and peripheral neuraxial techniques reduce risk of multiple drug administration [9]. Adequate premedication, avoidance of triggers, and emergency preparedness are key. A list of possible perioperative triggers is shown in Table 4 [10]. Judicious use and increased vigilance are mandatory if such triggers cannot be avoided.

Data on adverse drug reactions and mast cell disease is scarce. Knowledge of drugs that can cause histamine release is key, with avoidance suggested based on theoretical assumptions. Drugs which are suspected to have caused previous reactions should be avoided [9].

Preprocedural skin testing is not recommended unless a previously documented hypersensitivity reaction exists [11]. Patients may experience reactions to medications they have tolerated previously. With limited knowledge of causative mechanisms, vigilance is key. Usage of perioperative drugs in this context is described in Table 5 [8, 10–14].

Serious perioperative reactions caused by mast cell mediators can be anaphylactic or anaphylactoid. Occurrence of such reactions is likely to be higher as compared to the general population. Clinical features mainly involve the skin and cardiovascular and respiratory systems. Management should focus on withdrawing the offending agent, interrupting the effects of the mediators already released, and preventing more mediator release. Symptomatic and supportive treatment include oxygen, H-1 and H-2 antagonists, corticosteroids, bronchodilators, epinephrine, fluids, and airway resuscitation [10]. Measurement of serum mediators (e.g., tryptase) during the episode, with identification and testing of all exposures, should be done to determine etiology, although results are often negative or insufficiently reliable.

3.4. MCAS and Pregnancy. Data from studies on pregnancy and delivery in patients with mast cell disorders is reassuring [10, 15]. Mast cells exhibit a beneficial function in pregnancy by contributing to implantation, placentation, and fetal growth. Excessive release of mediators can be associated with preterm delivery. Although the use of systemic treatment should be limited or even avoided in pregnancy, optimum management is recommended for maternal and fetal wellbeing. With appropriate medical control, there is no contraindication to pregnancy [16]. Vaginal delivery with early neuraxial analgesia is permissible, in the absence of an obstetric indication for cesarean section. Similar perioperative considerations apply for either mode of delivery. Practitioners should be aware of possible sedation in the newborn when H-1 antagonists are used directly before delivery.

4. Conclusion

MCAS is an area of ongoing research. Our patient had an uneventful pregnancy, labor, and delivery despite the increased morbidity from MCAS. At 3 months' postpartum, she continued to report frequent allergic reactions and currently follows up with a mast cell disorders specialist. With this review, we attempt to add to the limited anesthesia literature regarding MCAS. Knowledge of this condition

TABLE 4: Perioperative triggers and treatments.

Type	Stressor	Treatment
Psychological	Anxiety, emotional stress	Pharmacologic, quiet environment
Mechanical	Pressure (tourniquet and BP cuff), friction (tape) surgery (GI tract a rich source of mast cells)	Minimize operative time, optimal positioning,
	Pain	Multimodal analgesia
Pharmacologic	Histamine releasing drugs	Avoid
Temperature	Hypothermia, hyperthermia, change in temperature	Heat maintenance devices, warm environment, warm intravenous and irrigation fluids
Infection	Bacterial, viral, fungal	As necessary
Foods, odors	Histamine-rich foods, odors (food, perfumes)	Avoid, single occupancy room

BP: blood pressure and GI: gastrointestinal.

TABLE 5: Perioperative drugs and mast cell disease[a].

Class	Drug	Usage in mast cell disorders
Hypnotic/sedative agents	Propofol[b], dexmedetomidine, etomidate, ketamine[b]	Acceptable
	Methohexital, thiopental	Thiopental causes histamine release
Inhalational anesthetics	Halogenated (isoflurane, sevoflurane, desflurane), nitrous oxide	Acceptable
Benzodiazepines[b]	Midazolam, diazepam	Acceptable
Opioids[c]	Morphine, meperidine, codeine	Causes histamine release
	Hydromorphone, fentanyl, sufentanil, alfentanil, remifentanil, buprenorphine	Acceptable
Nonopioid analgesics	Acetaminophen	Acceptable
	NSAIDs (ketorolac, nefopam)	Causes overproduction of leukotrienes (a mast cell mediator)
Neuromuscular blocking agents	Depolarizing NMBA (succinylcholine)	Acceptable
	Nondepolarizing aminosteroids[c] (rocuronium, vecuronium[b] pancuronium)	Acceptable
	Nondepolarizing benzylisoquinolines (atracurium, mivacurium, cisatracurium)	Atracurium and mivacurium cause histamine release
Reversal of neuromuscular blockade	Neostigmine, sugammadex	Acceptable
Local anesthetics[c]	Amides and esters	Acceptable
Antiseptics[c]	Alcohol, chlorhexidine, povidone-iodine	Acceptable
Intravenous fluids	Crystalloids, colloids, albumin, gelatin, hydroxyethyl starch[c]	Acceptable
Common labor and delivery drugs	Oxytocin, prostaglandins, methylergonovine, tocolytic agent (terbutaline)	Acceptable, though role of prostaglandins in causing or worsening reactions is unclear
Antibiotics[c]	Penicillins, cephalosporins, sulfonamides, vancomycin, polymyxin B, clindamycin, fluoroquinolones	Vancomycin and polymyxin B can cause histamine release
Miscellaneous	Adenosine, atropine, glycopyrrolate, ondansetron, beta-blockers, ACEI, protamine, aprotinin (fibrin glue), blood transfusion, dyes, contrast media, and latex[c]	Acceptable; adenosine and protamine can cause histamine release; beta-blockers can attenuate the effect of epinephrine in anaphylaxis; ACEI can augment an anaphylactic reaction

NSAIDs: nonsteroidal anti-inflammatory drugs; NMBA: neuromuscular blocking agents; ACEI: angiotensin converting enzyme inhibitors. [a]Drugs associated with histamine release should be avoided if another equally effective drug can be used; alternatively, they must be administered slowly. [b]Drugs reported to cause in vitro histamine release from human mast cells. [c]Drugs and products associated with high incidence of hypersensitivity reactions in the general population do not need to be avoided unless a previously documented sensitivity exists.

with appropriate planning and preparation will help ensure optimal outcomes.

References

[1] C. Akin, P. Valent, and D. D. Metcalfe, "Mast cell activation syndrome: proposed diagnostic criteria," *The Journal of Allergy and Clinical Immunology*, vol. 126, no. 6, pp. 1099–1104, 2010.

[2] L. B. Afrin, J. Butterfield, M. Raithel, and G. Molderings, "Often seen, rarely recognized: mast cell activation disease: a guide to diagnosis and therapeutic options," *Annals of Medicine*, vol. 48, no. 3, pp. 190–201, 2016.

[3] M. Krystel-Whittemore, K. N. Dileepan, and J. G. Wood, "Mast cell: a multi-functional master cell," *Frontiers in Immunology*, vol. 6, article 620, 2016.

[4] P. Valent, C. Akin, M. Arock et al., "Definitions, criteria and global classification of mast cell disorders with special reference to mast cell activation syndromes: a consensus proposal," *International Archives of Allergy and Immunology*, vol. 157, no. 3, pp. 215–225, 2012.

[5] C. Akin, "Mast cell activation disorders," *The Journal of Allergy and Clinical Immunology: In Practice*, vol. 2, no. 3, pp. 252–257.e1, 2014.

[6] L. Afrin, "Presentation, diagnosis, and management of mast cell activation syndrome," in *Mast Cells: Phenotypic Features, Biological Functions, and Role in Immunity*, D. Murray, Ed., pp. 155–231, Nova Science Publishers, Hauppauge, NY, USA, 2013.

[7] S. Valap, P. Millns, and S. Bulchandani, "Management of a parturient with mast cell activation syndrome," *International Journal of Obstetric Anesthesia*, vol. 22, no. 1, pp. 83-84, 2013.

[8] P. Bonadonna, M. Pagani, W. Aberer et al., "Drug hypersensitivity in clonal mast cell disorders: ENDA/EAACI position paper," *Allergy: European Journal of Allergy and Clinical Immunology*, vol. 70, no. 7, pp. 755–763, 2015.

[9] G. Lerno, G. Slaats, E. Coenen, L. Herregods, and G. Rolly, "Anaesthetic management of systemic mastocytosis," *British Journal of Anaesthesia*, vol. 65, no. 2, pp. 254–257, 1990.

[10] P. Dewachter, M. C. Castells, D. L. Hepner, and C. Mouton-Faivre, "Perioperative management of patients with mastocytosis," *Anesthesiology*, vol. 120, no. 3, pp. 753–759, 2014.

[11] E. W. Richter, K. L. Hsu, and V. Moll, "Successful management of a patient with possible mast cell activation syndrome undergoing pulmonary embolectomy: a case report," *A & A case reports*, vol. 8, no. 9, pp. 232–234, 2017.

[12] M. A. W. Hermans, N. J. T. Arends, R. Gerth van Wijk et al., "Management around invasive procedures in mastocytosis: An update," *Annals of Allergy, Asthma & Immunology*, vol. 119, no. 4, pp. 304–309, 2017.

[13] C. Unterbuchner, M. Hierl, T. Seyfried, and T. Metterlein, "Anaesthesia and orphan disease: rapid sequence induction in systemic mastocytosis," *European Journal of Anaesthesiology*, vol. 34, no. 3, pp. 176–178, 2017.

[14] G. Marone, C. Stellato, P. Mastronardi, and B. Mazzarella, "Mechanisms of activation of human mast cells and basophils by general anesthetic drugs," *Annales Françaises d'Anesthésie et de Réanimation*, vol. 12, no. 2, pp. 116–125, 1993.

[15] K. Ciach, M. Niedoszytko, A. Abacjew-Chmylko et al., "Pregnancy and delivery in patients with mastocytosis treated at the polish center of the European Competence Network on Mastocytosis (ECNM)," *PLoS ONE*, vol. 11, no. 1, Article ID e0146924, 2016.

[16] K. Woidacki, A. C. Zenclussen, and F. Siebenhaar, "Mast cell-mediated and associated disorders in pregnancy: a risky game with an uncertain outcome?" *Frontiers in Immunology*, vol. 5, 231 pages, 2014.

[17] C. Akin, "Mast cell activation syndromes," *The Journal of Allergy and Clinical Immunology*, vol. 140, no. 2, pp. 349–355, 2017.

63

An Undiagnosed Paraganglioma in a 58-Year-Old Female Who Underwent Tumor Resection

**William C. Fox,[1] Matthew Read,[2] Richard E. Moon,[3]
Eugene W. Moretti,[3] and Brian J. Colin[3]**

[1]Department of Anesthesiology, Duke University Medical Center, Box 3823, Durham, NC 27710, USA
[2]Critical Care Medicine, Department of Anesthesiology, Duke University Medical Center, Box 3823, Durham, NC 27710, USA
[3]General, Vascular, Transplant Division, Department of Anesthesiology, Duke University Medical Center,
 Box 3823 Durham, NC 27710, USA

Correspondence should be addressed to William C. Fox; william.c.fox@dm.duke.edu

Academic Editor: Maurizio Marandola

Paragangliomas and pheochromocytomas are rare neuroendocrine tumors that can have high morbidity and mortality if undiagnosed. Here we report a case of an undiagnosed paraganglioma in a 58-year-old female who underwent tumor resection. The patient became severely hypertensive intraoperatively with paroxysmal swings in blood pressure and then later became acutely hypotensive after tumor removal. She was managed in the surgical intensive care unit (SICU) postoperatively and discharged from the hospital without acute complications. We briefly discuss the epidemiology, clinical presentation, perioperative management, and possible complications of these tumors to assist healthcare providers if one were to encounter them.

1. Introduction

Catecholamine-secreting tumors, also known as paragangliomas and pheochromocytomas, are rare neuroendocrine tumors that can have high morbidity and mortality if undiagnosed. Here we present a rare but interesting case of a resection of an undiagnosed paraganglioma in a 58-year-old African-American female. Her past medical history included hypertension, hyperlipidemia, obstructive sleep apnea on CPAP, asthma and COPD, morbid obesity, history of myocardial infarction in her 30s, and report of uncharacterized congestive heart failure and cerebrovascular accident in her early 50s with residual left-sided deficit. She presented for robotic-assisted laparoscopy for resection of an incidentally found right retroperitoneal mass. Two prior CT-guided fine needle aspiration biopsies of the mass were attempted but insufficient for diagnosis. Contrast-enhanced abdomen/pelvis CT revealed a 3.8 × 3.3 cm soft tissue mass at the right renal hilum abutting the inferior aspect of the right renal vein and right aspect of the inferior vena cava (Figure 1). Her home medications included aspirin, amlodipine-benazepril, furosemide, hydralazine, nebivolol,

and spironolactone, as well as gabapentin, ibuprofen, and hydrocodone-acetaminophen for analgesia, and an albuterol inhaler and montelukast for asthma/COPD. Epidemiology, clinical presentation, perioperative management, and possible complications of these tumors are discussed.

2. Case Report

On the morning of surgery, the patient was hemodynamically stable. She received 2 mg IV midazolam preoperatively then underwent induction of general anesthesia with 100 mg IV lidocaine, 250 mcg IV fentanyl, 150 mg IV propofol, and 140 mg IV succinylcholine followed by 40 mg IV rocuronium after endotracheal tube placement. Shortly after incision and insufflation, she became hypertensive. Serial arterial BP readings were close to 250/140 mmHg with HR 60–70 bpm. Despite deepening the anesthetic gas and administering adequate doses of IV opioids and muscle relaxant, the patient's blood pressure did not improve. A total of 65 mg IV labetalol and 20 mg IV hydralazine were administered over the course of an hour. There was intermittent improvement in blood

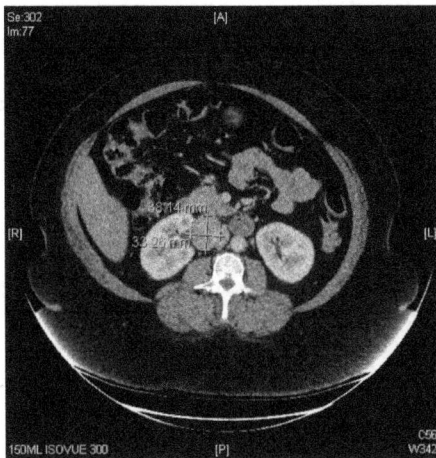

FIGURE 1: CT abdomen/pelvis with contrast.

pressure to as low as 113/80 mmHg that lasted for a few minutes before soon returning to 250/140 mmHg. This cycle repeated during the redosing of antihypertensive agents but adequate control of blood pressure could not be obtained.

A clevidipine bolus (0.5 mg) was administered, followed by infusion at 1 mg/hr. Blood pressure remained close to 160/80 mmHg during the infusion but the patient became acutely tachycardic with HR 130 bpm, so the infusion was paused, resulting in an increase in BP to 257/163 mmHg. An esmolol bolus (100 mg) was administered, followed by an infusion which was started at 50 mcg/kg/min and clevidipine restarted once heart rate was controlled. Doses were escalated to 75 mcg/kg/min and 3 mg/hr, respectively, with BP ranging between 120/80 and 200/120 mmHg. Heart rate decreased to 90–100 bpm.

The procedure was converted from laparoscopic to open given the difficulty of resection due to the tumor's anatomy and patient instability. Her vital signs briefly appeared to "normalize" with BP 120/80 mmHg and HR 90 bpm before tumor removal so both clevidipine and esmolol infusions were discontinued. However, within several minutes of tumor removal, the patient became acutely hypotensive with systolic BP 60 mmHg and HR 80–90 bpm. A total of 400 mcg IV phenylephrine boluses were administered but the BP dropped to as low as 58/40 mmHg. Next, a total of 300 mcg of IV epinephrine was administered over several doses and the patient showed an improvement in blood pressure to 77/48 mmHg. At that time, the pathologist communicated that the tumor was a paraganglioma/pheochromocytoma. Norepinephrine and vasopressin infusions were started at 0.1 mcg/kg/min and 0.04 units/min, respectively. The patient was also given 100 mg IV hydrocortisone. Intraoperative transesophageal echocardiography (TEE) showed a hyperdynamic left ventricle with near collapse during systole and no wall motion abnormalities. The patient had received a total of 4300 ml of crystalloid and 1000 ml of colloid resuscitation intraoperatively prior to TEE.

She was taken to the SICU intubated on both pressors with ongoing fluid resuscitation. 3700 ml of crystalloid was

administered postoperatively. The ICU team extubated and weaned her off pressors by postop day 1. CT brain without contrast did not show any acute intracranial abnormalities and cardiac enzymes were normal. She was discharged from the ward on postop day 4.

3. Discussion

Paragangliomas are rare neuroendocrine tumors that arise from the extra-adrenal autonomic paraganglia. These are small organs consisting mainly of neuroendocrine cells that are derived from the embryonic neural crest and have the ability to secrete catecholamines [1]. Paragangliomas are closely related to pheochromocytomas, which are sometimes referred to as intra-adrenal paragangliomas. The combined estimated annual incidence is approximately 0.8 per 100,000 person years [2]. Most are sporadic, but approximately one-third to one-half are associated with an inherited syndrome. The four genetic syndromes that are associated are multiple endocrine neoplasia 2A and 2B, neurofibromatosis type 1, von Hippel Lindau, and Carney-Stratakis syndrome. The male-to-female ratio is approximately equal among patients with hereditary paraganglioma, while sporadic tumors are more common in women than men (71 versus 29 percent) [3]. Most paragangliomas are diagnosed between third and fifth decade of life.

Paragangliomas can derive from parasympathetic or sympathetic paraganglia with similar frequencies. The majority of sympathetic paragangliomas arise outside of the skull base and neck anywhere along the sympathetic chain. About 75 percent arise in the abdomen, most often at the junction of the inferior vena cava and left renal vein. About 10 percent arise in the thorax. They excrete excess amounts of catecholamine (86 percent in one series) [4], usually almost always norepinephrine.

Manifestations of catecholamine-secreting tumors include hypertension, often paroxysmal, and are associated with episodic headache, sweating, and palpitations. Less commonly there may be orthostatic hypotension, weight loss, hyperglycemia, polyuria, polydipsia, visual blurring, papilledema, or constipation. The patient in this case mentioned postoperatively that she had previous episodes of periodic facial flushing, palpitations, and intermittent chest pain. Given her history of myocardial infarction and cerebrovascular accident, these may have been attributed to her paraganglioma. Also, it is difficult to rule out an adrenal or extra-adrenal tumor based on her CT images. Hence, this should have alerted her physicians of a possible paraganglioma. Although she had two unsuccessful fine needle biopsies, preoperative labs including plasma and urinary metanephrines and catecholamines may have suggested a possible catecholamine-secreting tumor.

Undiagnosed pheochromocytoma has a high perioperative mortality risk, as great as 80 percent perioperatively according to one report [5] and 27 percent in a different series [6]. However, it is hypothesized that, with advancement in perioperative care and optimal management of these tumors as discussed below, the mortality is lower compared to 30 years ago. Patients can become hypertensive during induction, positioning, or tumor resection. Chronic catecholamine excess causes hypovolemia and patients can become severely hypotensive, as in this case, if adequate volume resuscitation is not performed. It is prudent to evaluate for adverse events following hypertensive and hypotensive episodes. Serial neurological evaluations, electrocardiograms, and cardiac enzymes should be considered as part of management. Plasma catecholamine concentrations should return to normal after about a week from tumor resection.

Complications of surgery are primarily due to severe preoperative hypertension, high secretion tumors, or repeat intervention for recurrence. In one study, adverse perioperative events occurred in 32 percent of cases [7]. The most common adverse event was sustained hypertension in 25 percent of the patients. There were no perioperative deaths, myocardial infarctions, or cerebrovascular events. Despite premedication of most patients with phenoxybenzamine and a beta-blocker, varying degrees of intraoperative hemodynamic lability occurred.

In preparation for surgery, preoperative medical therapy should focus on controlling blood pressure and volume resuscitation. An alpha-blocker, preferably phenoxybenzamine is started 10–14 days prior to procedure. Beta blockade may be necessary for control over arrhythmias or tachycardia. It should never be started prior to alpha blockade because blockade of vasodilatory peripheral beta-adrenergic receptors with unopposed alpha-adrenergic receptor stimulation can lead to hypertensive crisis.

Hypertensive crisis may occur intraoperatively despite optimum medical therapy due to various stimuli. A retrospective study at a single institution of 73 patients undergoing resection for pheochromocytoma found higher preoperative plasma norepinephrine concentration, larger tumor size (>4 cm), and more pronounced postural blood pressure fall after alpha blockade (>10 mmHg) correlated with intraoperative hypertensive events [8].

Treatment for hypertensive crisis has included intravenous sodium nitroprusside, phentolamine, or nicardipine infusions. Cardiac arrhythmias can be managed with IV lidocaine bolus or esmolol infusion (extreme caution is necessary when administering a beta blockade without concurrent or preexisting alpha blockade). Magnesium sulfate has also been shown to inhibit catecholamine release. It is a calcium channel antagonist of vascular smooth muscle, which acts to decrease intracellular calcium. One major effect of decreased intracellular calcium would be inactivation of calmodulin-dependent myosin light chain kinase activity and decreased contraction, causing smooth muscle relaxation [9]. Magnesium sulfate appears to be predominantly an arterial vasodilator, reducing peripheral resistance but with minimal effects on venous return or pulmonary capillary wedge pressure. A total of 10–20 grams of magnesium sulfate may be required perioperatively to achieve blood pressure control. One series was successful in preventing catecholamine surge by keeping the plasma magnesium concentration between 2.5 and 3 mmol/L (6.1–7.3 mg/dL), requiring a magnesium infusion of 1-2 grams per hour [10].

Medications that produce histamine release such as morphine and medications that inhibit catecholamine reuptake or cause indirect increase of catecholamines, such as droperidol, ketamine, ephedrine, and metoclopramide, should all be avoided.

In summary, this case illustrates the importance of obtaining a detailed clinical history and evaluation if there is a high suspicion for paraganglioma/pheochromocytoma. Although not all patients with hypertension and an incidentally found adrenal or extra-adrenal tumor on imaging may have a catecholamine-secreting tumor, plasma and urinary metanephrines and catecholamines may assist in the diagnosis of one, especially if there is a history of hypertensive crisis, paroxysmal swings in blood pressure, history of myocardial infarction or cerebrovascular accident, or any other manifestation of catecholamine-secreting tumors. Optimal medical management such as starting patients on alpha-adrenergic antagonists weeks prior to any elective procedure and discussing with the patient perioperative complications and risks are essential. From intraoperative TEE findings, we found that postresection hypotension is almost always associated with hypovolemia from chronic catecholamine secretion and should be treated by aggressive fluid resuscitation. Serial neurological and cardiac evaluations should be considered as part of management in a patient with severe intraoperative hypertension or hypotension.

References

[1] D. Lin, S. E. Carty, and W. F. Young, "Paragangliomas: epidemiology, clinical presentation, diagnosis, and histology," *Uptodate.com*, 2016, http://www.uptodate.com/contents/paragangliomas-epidemiology-clinical-presentation-diagnosis-and-histology.

[2] C. M. Beard, S. G. Sheps, L. T. Kurland, J. A. Carney, and J. T. Lie, "Occurrence of pheochromocytoma in Rochester, Minnesota, 1950 through 1979," *Mayo Clinic Proceedings*, vol. 58, no. 12, pp. 802–804, 1983.

[3] C. C. Boedeker, H. P. H. Neumann, W. Maier, B. Bausch, J. Schipper, and G. J. Ridder, "Malignant head and neck paragangliomas in SDHB mutation carriers," *Otolaryngology—Head and Neck Surgery*, vol. 137, no. 1, pp. 126–129, 2007.

[4] D. Erickson, Y. C. Kudva, M. J. Ebersold et al., "Benign paragangliomas: clinical presentation and treatment outcomes in 236 patients," *The Journal of Clinical Endocrinology & Metabolism*, vol. 86, no. 11, pp. 5210–5216, 2001.

[5] O. F. M. Sellevold, J. Raeder, and R. Stenseth, "Undiagnosed Phaeochromocytoma in the Perioperative Period: Case Reports," *Acta Anaesthesiologica Scandinavica*, vol. 29, no. 5, pp. 474–479, 1985.

[6] M. J. Sutton, S. Sheps, and J. Lie, "Prevalence of clinically unsuspected pheochromocytoma. review of a 50-year autopsy series," *Mayo Clinic Proceedings*, vol. 56, no. 6, pp. 354–360, 1981.

[7] M. A. Kinney, M. E. Warner, J. A. vanHeerden et al., "Perianesthetic risks and outcomes of pheochromocytoma and paraganglioma resection," *Anesthesia & Analgesia*, vol. 91, no. 5, pp. 1118–1123, 2000.

[8] H. Bruynzeel, R. A. Feelders, T. H. N. Groenland et al., "Risk factors for hemodynamic instability during surgery for pheochromocytoma," *The Journal of Clinical Endocrinology & Metabolism*, vol. 95, no. 2, pp. 678–685, 2010.

[9] B. M. Altura, B. T. Altura, and A. Carella, "Mg2+-Ca2+ interaction in contractility of vascular smooth muscle: Mg2+ versus organic calcium channel blockers on myogenic tone and agonist-induced responsiveness of blood vessels," *Canadian Journal of Physiology and Pharmacology*, vol. 65, no. 4, pp. 729–745, 1987.

[10] M. F. James and L. Cronjé, "Pheochromocytoma crisis: The use of magnesium sulfate," *Anesthesia & Analgesia*, vol. 99, no. 3, pp. 680–686, 2004.

Permissions

All chapters in this book were first published in CRA, by Hindawi Publishing Corporation; hereby published with permission under the Creative Commons Attribution License or equivalent. Every chapter published in this book has been scrutinized by our experts. Their significance has been extensively debated. The topics covered herein carry significant findings which will fuel the growth of the discipline. They may even be implemented as practical applications or may be referred to as a beginning point for another development.

The contributors of this book come from diverse backgrounds, making this book a truly international effort. This book will bring forth new frontiers with its revolutionizing research information and detailed analysis of the nascent developments around the world.

We would like to thank all the contributing authors for lending their expertise to make the book truly unique. They have played a crucial role in the development of this book. Without their invaluable contributions this book wouldn't have been possible. They have made vital efforts to compile up to date information on the varied aspects of this subject to make this book a valuable addition to the collection of many professionals and students.

This book was conceptualized with the vision of imparting up-to-date information and advanced data in this field. To ensure the same, a matchless editorial board was set up. Every individual on the board went through rigorous rounds of assessment to prove their worth. After which they invested a large part of their time researching and compiling the most relevant data for our readers.

The editorial board has been involved in producing this book since its inception. They have spent rigorous hours researching and exploring the diverse topics which have resulted in the successful publishing of this book. They have passed on their knowledge of decades through this book. To expedite this challenging task, the publisher supported the team at every step. A small team of assistant editors was also appointed to further simplify the editing procedure and attain best results for the readers.

Apart from the editorial board, the designing team has also invested a significant amount of their time in understanding the subject and creating the most relevant covers. They scrutinized every image to scout for the most suitable representation of the subject and create an appropriate cover for the book.

The publishing team has been an ardent support to the editorial, designing and production team. Their endless efforts to recruit the best for this project, has resulted in the accomplishment of this book. They are a veteran in the field of academics and their pool of knowledge is as vast as their experience in printing. Their expertise and guidance has proved useful at every step. Their uncompromising quality standards have made this book an exceptional effort. Their encouragement from time to time has been an inspiration for everyone.

The publisher and the editorial board hope that this book will prove to be a valuable piece of knowledge for researchers, students, practitioners and scholars across the globe.

List of Contributors

Youmna E. DiStefano and Michael D. Lazar
Department of Anesthesiology, New York Medical College, Valhalla, NY 10595, USA

Frank Schuster, Stephan Johannsen, Marc Lazarus and Norbert Roewer
Department of Anaesthesia and Critical Care, University of Wuerzburg, 97080 Wuerzburg, Germany

Carsten Wessig
Department of Neurology, University of Wuerzburg, 97080 Wuerzburg, Germany

Christoph Schimmer, Ivan Aleksic and Rainer Leyh
Department of Cardiothoracic and Thoracic Vascular Surgery, University of Wuerzburg, 97080 Wuerzburg, Germany

Christopher Allen-John Webb and Paul David Weyker
Columbia University College of Physicians and Surgeons, Columbia University Medical Center, New York, NY 10032, USA

Brigid Colleen Flynn
Columbia University College of Physicians and Surgeons, Columbia University Medical Center, New York, NY 10032, USA
Division of Critical Care, Department of Anesthesiology, Columbia University Medical Center, 622 West 168th Street PH 5-505, New York, NY 10032, USA

Michihiro Sakai
Department of Anesthesiology, Fujisawa Shonandai Hospital, 2345 Takakura, Fujisawa, Kanagawa 252-0802, Japan

Noriko Murakami, Hiroshi Iwama and Akira Nomura
Department of Anesthesiology, Kimitsu Chuo Hospital, 1010 Sakurai, Kisarazu, Chiba 292-8535, Japan

Yuji Kitamura and Shin Sato
Department of Anesthesiology, Chiba University School of Medicine, 1-8-1 Inohana, Chuo-ku, Chiba 260-8677, Japan

Nabil A. Shollik, Sami M. Ibrahim and Ahmed Ismael
Anesthesia Department, HMC-Weill Cornell Medical College, Doha, Qatar

Vanni Agnoletti, Emanuele Piraccini and Ruggero Massimo Corso
Anaesthesia and Intensive Care Section, Department of Emergency, G.B. Morgagni-Pierantoni Hospital, viale Forlanini 34, 47100 Forlì, Italy

Tanu Mehta, Geeta P. Parikh and Veena R. Shah
Department of Anaesthesia and Critical Care, Smt. K.M. Mehta and Smt. G. R. Doshi Institute of Kidney Diseases and Research Center, Dr. H. L. Trivedi Institute of Transplantation Sciences, Civil Hospital Campus, Asarwa, Ahmedabad, Gujarat 380016, India

Kenichi Takahoko, Hajime Iwasaki, Tomoki Sasakawa, Akihiro Suzuki, Hideki Matsumoto and Hiroshi Iwasaki
Department of Anesthesiology and Critical Care Medicine, Asahikawa Medical University, Midorigaoka Higashi 2-1-1-1, Asahikawa, Hokkaido 078-8510, Japan

Loreto Lollo and Andreas Grabinsky
Department of Anesthesiology and Pain Medicine, Harborview Medical Center, University of Washington, No. 359724, 325 Ninth Avenue, Seattle, WA 98104, USA

Tanya K. Meyer
Department of Otolaryngology, Harborview Medical Center, University of Washington, 325 Ninth Avenue, Seattle, WA 98104, USA

Harsha Shanthanna
St. Joseph's Hospital, Department of Anesthesiology, McMaster University, Health Sciences Centre 2U1, 1200 Main Street West, Hamilton, ON, Canada L8N 3Z5

Arlene J. Hudson
Department of Anesthesiology, Uniformed Services University of the Health Sciences, 4301 Jones Bridge Road, Bethesda, MD 20814, USA

Kevin B. Guthmiller and Marian N. Hyatt
San Antonio Military Medical Center, 3551 Roger Brooke Drive, San Antonio, TX 78234m, USA

Trabelsi Walid, Belhaj Amor Mondher, Lebbi Mohamed Anis and Ferjani Mustapha
Departement of Anesthesia and Intensive Care Unit, Tunisian Military Hospital, 1002 Tunis, Tunisia

Eiko Hirai
Department of Anesthesia, Seikei-kai Chiba Medical Center, 1-11-12 Minami-cho, Chuo-ku, Chiba-shi, Chiba 260-0842, Japan

Joho Tokumine
Department of Anesthesiology, Kyorin University School of Medicine, 6-20-2 Shinkawa, Mitaka-shi, Tokyo 181-8611, Japan

Alan Kawarai Lefor
Department of Surgery, Jichi Medical University, 3311-1 Yakushiji, Shimotsuke-shi, Tochigi 329-0498, Japan

Shinobu Ogura
Department of Anesthesiology, Hakujikai Memorial General Hospital, 5-11-1 Shikahama, Adachi-ku, Tokyo 123-0864, Japan

Miwako Kawamata
Nippori Clinic, Medical Center East, Tokyo Women's Medical University, Station Port Tower 4th F 2-20-1 Nishinippori, Arakawa-ku, Tokyo 116-0013, Japan

Yuri Uchiyama, Yasuyuki Tokinaga, Yukitoshi Niiyama, Soshi Iwasaki and Michiaki Yamakage
Sapporo Medical University School of Medicine, Sapporo, S1W16, Chuo-ku, Sapporo-shi, Hokkaido 060-8543, Japan

Kartika Balaji Samala
Sapporo Medical University School of Medicine, Sapporo, S1W16, Chuo-ku, Sapporo-shi, Hokkaido 060-8543, Japan
GSL Medical College and Hospital, Rajahmundry, India

Monu Yadav, Sapna A. Nikhar, Dilip Kumar Kulkarni and R. Gopinath
Department of Anaesthesiology and Critical Care, Nizam's Institute of Medical Sciences, Hyderabad 500082, India

Jahan Porhomayon
VA Western New York Healthcare System, Division of Critical Care and Pain Medicine, Department of Anesthesiology, State University of New York at Buffalo, School of Medicine and Biomedical Sciences, VA Medical Center, Room 203C, 3495 Bailey Avenue, Buffalo, NY 14215, USA

Gino Zadeii
University of Iowa, Mason City Cardiology, Mason City, IA 50401, USA

Nader D. Nader
VA Western New York Healthcare System, Division of Cardiothoracic Anesthesia and Pain Medicine, Department of Anesthesiology, State University of New York at Buffalo School of Medicine and Biomedical Sciences, Buffalo, NY 14215, USA

George R. Bancroft
Department of Anesthesiology, State University of New York at Buffalo, School of Medicine and Biomedical Sciences, Buffalo, NY 14215, USA

Alireza Yarahamadi
Director of Mercy North-Iowa Neurology and Sleep Laboratory, University of Iowa, Mason City Neurology, Mason City, IA 50401, USA

Saptarshi Biswas, Marwa Sidani and Sunil Abrol
Department of Surgery, Brookdale University Hospital Medical Center, Brooklyn, NY 11212, USA

Kalpana Tyagaraj, David A. Gutman, Lynn Belliveau and Dennis E. Feierman
Department of Anesthesiology, Maimonides Medical Center, 4802 10th Avenue, Brooklyn, NY 11219, USA

Adnan Sadiq
Department of Cardiology, Maimonides Medical Center, 4802 10th Avenue, Brooklyn, NY 11219, USA

Alok Bhutada
Department of Neonatology, Maimonides Medical Center, 4802 10th Avenue, Brooklyn, NY 11219, USA

Ismail Demirel, Ayse Belin Ozer and Mustafa K. Bayar
Department of Anaesthesiology and Reanimation, Faculty of Medicine, Firat University, 23119 Elazig, Turkey

Salih Burcin Kavak
Department of Obstetrics and Gynecology, Faculty of Medicine, Firat University, 2311 Elazig, Turkey

Betul Kozanhan, Betul Basaran, Leyla Kutlucan and Sadık Ozmen
Department of Anesthesiology and Reanimation, Konya Training and Research Hospital, Meram Yeniyol Street No. 97, Meram, 42090 Konya, Turkey

Christopher Hoffman, Hawa Abubakar, Pramood Kalikiri and Michael Green
Drexel University College of Medicine, Hahnemann University Hospital, Philadelphia, PA 19102, USA

Selçuk Okur, Müge Arıkan, Gülşen Temel and Volkan Temel
Department of Anesthesiology, Karabük State Hospital, Karabük, Turkey

William R. Hartman, Michael Brown and James Hannon
Department of Anesthesiology, Mayo Clinic, Rochester, MN, USA

Aliki Tympa and Aikaterini Melemeni
Department of Anesthesiology, Aretaieion University Hospital, 76 Vas. Sofias A venue, 11528 Athens, Greece

Dimitrios Hassiakos and Nikolaos Salakos
1st Department of Obstetrics and Gynecology, Aretaieion University Hospital, 76 Vas. Sofias Avenue, 11528 Athens, Greece

Acílio Marques, Carla Retroz-Marques, Sara Mota, Raquel Cabral and Matos Campos
Anaesthesiology Department, Coimbra University Hospital Center, Praceta Mota Pinto, 3001-301 Coimbra, Portugal

Asish Subedi and Balkrishna Bhattarai
Department of Anaesthesiology and Critical Care, BP Koirala Institute of Health Sciences, Dharan 56700, Nepal

Jennifer Knautz, Yogen Asher, Mark C. Kendall and Robert Doty Jr.
Department of Anesthesiology, McGaw Medical Center, Feinberg School of Medicine, Northwestern University, Chicago, IL 60611, USA

Mehmet I. Buget, Emine Ozkan and Suleyman Kucukay
Department of Anesthesiology, Istanbul Medical Faculty, Istanbul University, Fatih, 34093 Istanbul, Turkey

Ipek S. Edipoglu
Department of Anesthesiology, Suleymaniye Obstetrics and Pediatrics Training and Research Hospital, Zeytinburnu, 34116 Istanbul, Turkey

SunWoo Bang
Department of Radiology, Kim Chan Hospital, 228 Hyowon-ro, Gwonseon-gu, Suwon 441-822, Republic of Korea

Kyung Ream Han, Seung Ho Kim, Won Ho Jeong, Eun Jin Kim and Chan Kim
Department of Pain Medicine, Kim Chan Hospital, 228 Hyowon-ro, Gwonseon-gu, Suwon 441-822, Republic of Korea

Jin Wook Choi
Department of Cardiovascular Surgery, Kim Chan Hospital, 228 Hyowon-ro, Gwonseon-gu, Suwon 441-822, Republic of Korea

Bassam M. Shoman, Hany O. Ragab, Ammar Mustafa and Rashid Mazhar
Cardiothoracic Anesthesia Department, Heart Hospital, Hamad Medical Corporation, Doha, Qatar

Minal Joshi, Simon Mardakh, Joel Yarmush, H. Kamath and Joseph Schianodicola
Department of Anesthesiology, New York Methodist Hospital, 506 6th street, Brooklyn, NY 11215, USA

Ernesto Mendoza
Department of Surgery, New York Methodist Hospital, 506 6th Street, Brooklyn, NY 11215, USA

Karan Srivastava and Vikas Y. Sacher
Department of Surgery, University of Miami Miller School of Medicine, Miami, FL 33136, USA

John I. Lew
Department of Surgery, University of Miami Miller School of Medicine, Miami, FL 33136, USA
University of Miami Leonard M. Miller School of Medicine and DeWitt Daughtry Family Department of Surgery, Division of Endocrine Surgery, University of Miami and Jackson Memorial Hospitals, 1120 NW14th Street, CRB-Room 410P (M-875), Miami, FL 33136, USA

Craig T. Nelson
Department of Anesthesiology, University of Miami Miller School of Medicine, Miami, FL 33136, USA

Ebirim N. Longinus, Lagiri Benjamin and Buowari Yvonne Omiepirisa
Department of Anaesthesiology, University of Port Harcourt Teaching Hospital, Port Harcourt, 6173 Rivers State, Nigeria

Santosh Kumar Yadav
Department of Oral and Maxillofacial Surgery, Chitwan Medical College, P.O. Box 42, Bharatpur-10, Chitwan, Nepal

Gopendra Deo
Department of Anesthesiology, Chitwan Medical College, P.O. Box 42, Bharatpur-10, Chitwan, Nepal

Marek Brzezinski, Maren Gregersen, Luiz Gustavo Schuch, Ricarda Sawatzki, Joy W. Chen and Brian Cason
VA Medical Center, Anesthesia Services, 4150 Clement Street, San Francisco, CA 94121, USA

Department of Anesthesia and Perioperative Care, University of California, San Francisco, 521 Parnassus Avenue Room C-450, San Francisco, CA 94143-0648, USA

Grant Gauger
VA Medical Center, Neurosurgery Services, 4150 Clement Street, San Francisco, CA 94121, USA
Department of Neurosurgery, University of California, San Francisco, 400 Parnassus Ave., San Francisco, CA 94143, USA

Jasleen Kukreja
VA Medical Center, Surgery Services, 4150 Clement Street, San Francisco, CA 94121, USA
Department of Surgery, University of California, San Francisco, 400 Parnassus Ave., San Francisco, CA 94143, USA

Eric Kamenetsky
McGaw Medical Center of Northwestern University, Chicago, IL 60611, USA

Antoun Nader and Mark C. Kendall
Feinberg School of Medicine, Northwestern University, Chicago, IL 60611, USA

Eric S. Schwenk, Kishor Gandhi and Eugene R. Viscusi
Department of Anesthesiology, Jefferson Medical College, Suite 8490, 111 South 11th Street, Philadelphia, PA 19107, USA

Ahmed Abdelaal Ahmed Mahmoud, Mark Campbell and Margarita Blajeva
Department of Anaesthesia and Intensive Care Medicine, Tallaght University Hospital (Adelaide and Meath Incorporating National Children's Hospital), Ireland

Dimitrios K. Manatakis, Nikolaos Stamos, Christos Agalianos and Demetrios Davides
1st Surgical Department, Athens Naval and Veterans Hospital, 70 Dinokratous Street, 11521 Athens, Greece

Michail Athanasios Karvelis and Michael Gkiaourakis
Department of Anesthesiology, Athens Naval and Veterans Hospital, 70 Dinokratous Street, 11521 Athens, Greece

Patrick Schober, Stephan A. Loer and Lothar A. Schwarte
Department of Anesthesiology, VU University Medical Center, De Boelelaan 1117, 1007 MB Amsterdam, Netherlands

K. Hakki Karagozoglu
Academic Centre for Dentistry Amsterdam (ACTA) and Department of Oral and Maxillofacial Surgery/Oral Pathology, VU University Medical Center, De Boelelaan 1117, 1007 MB Amsterdam, Netherlands

Jason K. Panchamia, David A. Olsen and Adam W. Amundson
Department of Anesthesiology and Perioperative Medicine, Mayo Clinic, Rochester, MN, USA

Jennifer Busse, David Gottlieb and Krystal Ferreras
Anesthesiology, Morgan Stanley Children's Hospital of New York-Presbyterian at Columbia University Irving Medical Center, USA

Jennifer Bain
Neurology, Morgan Stanley Children's Hospital at Columbia University Irving Medical Center, USA

William Schechter
Anesthesiology and Pediatrics, Morgan Stanley Children's Hospital at Columbia University Irving Medical Center, New York, NY, USA

Frank Schuster, Stephan Johannsen and Norbert Roewer
Department of Anesthesia and Critical Care, University of Wuerzburg, Oberduerrbacher Street 6, 97080 Wuerzburg, Germany

Mehryar Taghavi Gilani and Majid Razavi
Anesthesia Department, Imam-Reza Hospital, School of Medicine, Mashhad University of Medical Sciences, Mashhad, Iran

Christine Vien and Brendan Ingram
Monash Health, 246 Clayton Road, Clayton, Melbourne, VIC 3168, Australia

Paul Marovic
Alfred Health, 55 Commercial Road, Melbourne, VIC 3004, Australia

Hao-Hu Chen, Li-Chuan Chen, Yu-Hui Hsieh and Mao-Kai Chen
Department of Anesthesiology, Kaohsiung Medical University Hospital, Kaohsiung 807, Taiwan

Kuang-I Cheng
Department of Anesthesiology, Kaohsiung Medical University Hospital, Kaohsiung 807, Taiwan
Faculty of Medicine, Department of Anesthesiology, College of Medicine, Kaohsiung Medical University, Kaohsiung 807, Taiwan

Chung-Ho Chen
Department of Oral and Maxillofacial Surgery, College of Dental Medicine, Kaohsiung Medical University, Kaohsiung 807, Taiwan

Enrico Giustiniano, Silvia Eleonora Malossini, Francesco Pellegrino and Franco Cancellieri
Department of Anesthesia and Intensive Care Unit, Humanitas Clinical and Research Center, Via Manzoni 56, 20089 Rozzano, Italy

Hiroe Yoshioka, Haruyuki Yamazaki, Rie Yasumura, Kosuke Wada and Yoshiro Kobayashi
Department of Anesthesiology, National Hospital Organization Tokyo Medical Center, 2-5-1 Higashigaoka, Meguro-ku, Tokyo 152-8902, Japan

Jose Soliz, Jeffrey Lim and Gang Zheng
Department of Anesthesiology and Perioperative Medicine, MD Anderson Cancer Center, Houston, TX 77030, USA

Yuki Sugiyama, Chiaki Kiuchi, Maiko Suzuki, Yuki Maruyama, Ryo Wakabayashi and Mikito Kawamata
Department of Anesthesiology and Resuscitology, Shinshu University School of Medicine, Japan

Yasunari Ohno and Shugo Takahata
Division of Pediatric Surgery, Department of Surgery, Shinshu University School of Medicine, Japan

Takumi Shibazaki
Department of Pediatrics, Shinshu University School of Medicine, Japan

Brian M. Osman
University of Miami, Miller School of Medicine, Department of Anesthesiology, 1400 NW12th Avenue, Suite 3075, Miami, FL 33136, USA

Isabela C. Saba
University of Miami, Miller School of Medicine, Department of Anesthesiology, 1801 NW9th Avenue, 5th Floor, Miami, FL 33136, USA

William A. Watson
University of Miami, Miller School of Medicine, Department of Anesthesiology, 1611 NW12th Avenue, Suite C-300, Miami, FL 33136, USA

Tobechi E. Okoronkwo, XueWei Zhang, Jessica Dworet and Matthew Wecksell
New York Medical College-Westchester Medical Center, USA

Suneel M. Agerwala, Divya Sundarapandiyan and Garret Weber
New York Medical College, Valhalla, NY, USA

Preeta George
St. Louis Children's Hospital, Washington University, 1 Children's Pl., St. Louis, MO 63108, USA

John E. Fiadjoe and Allan F. Simpao
Perelman School of Medicine at the University of Pennsylvania and the Children's Hospital of Philadelphia, 3401 Civic Center Blvd., Philadelphia, PA 19104, USA

Katherine L. Koniuch, Bradley Harris, Michael J. Buys and Adam W. Meier
University of Utah Department of Anesthesiology, USA

Michael Koeppen
Anesthesiology, Ludwig Maximilian University of Munich, Munich, Germany

Benjamin Scott, Joseph Morabito, Matthew Fiegel and Tobias Eckle
Anesthesiology, University of Denver School of Medicine, Aurora, CO, USA

Paolo Monticelli and Chiara Adami
Department of Clinical Sciences and Services, Royal Veterinary College, University of London, Hatfield, Hertfordshire AL97TA, UK

Luis Campoy
Department of Anesthesiology and Analgesia, College of Veterinary Medicine, Cornell University, Ithaca, NY 14853, USA

Tolga Totoz
Department of Anesthesiology and Reanimation, Nisantasi University, Istanbul Safak Hospital, Turkey

Kerem Erkalp, Ummahan Dalkilinc and Aysin Selcan
Department of Anesthesiology and Reanimation, Health Sciences University, Istanbul Bagcılar Training and Educational Hospital, Turkey

Sirin Taskin
Department of Anesthesiology and Reanimation, Health Sciences University, Istanbul Haydarpasa Sample Training and Research Hospital, Turkey

A. L. M. J. van der Knijff-van Dortmont, M. Dirckx, A. Gonzalez Candel, C. D. van derMarel, G. P. Scoones, V. F. R. Adriaens and I. J. J. Dons-Sinke
Department of Anesthesiology, Erasmus University Medical Centre, Rotterdam, Netherlands

J. J. Duvekot
Department of Obstetrics and Gynaecology, Erasmus University Medical Centre, Rotterdam, Netherlands

J. W. Roos-Hesselink
Department of Cardiology, Erasmus University Medical Centre, Rotterdam, Netherlands

Miyuki Niki, Yuka Sano, Hiroki Miyawaki, Yukari Okano, Nobutaka Kariya, Tsuneo Tatara and Munetaka Hirose
Department of Anesthesiology and Pain Medicine, Hyogo College of Medicine, Nishinomiya, Hyogo, Japan

Taihei Tachikawa
Department of Anesthesia, Meiwa Hospital, Nishinomiya, Hyogo, Japan

Aisa Matoi
Intensive Care Unit, Hyogo College of Medicine Hospital, Nishinomiya, Hyogo, Japan

Richard K. Patch III
Division of Critical Care Medicine, Department of Anesthesiology and Perioperative Medicine and Division of Pulmonary and Critical Care Medicine, Department of Medicine, Mayo Clinic, Rochester, MN, USA

Jason S. Eldrige and Susan M. Moeschler
Division of Pain Medicine, Department of Anesthesiology and Perioperative Medicine, Mayo Clinic, Rochester, MN, USA

Matthew J. Pingree
Department of Physical Medicine and Rehabilitation, Mayo Clinic, Rochester, MN, USA

M. D. Luca La Colla and R. M. D. Schroeder
Department of Anesthesiology, Duke University Medical Center, Durham, NC, USA

Hazem Kafrouni and Rami El Ojaimi
Saint George Hospital-University Medical Center, Beirut, Lebanon

Glenn van de Vossenberg, Selina van der Wal, Andrea Müller and Kris Vissers
Department of Anesthesiology, Pain and Palliative Medicine, Radboudumc, Nijmegen, Netherlands

Edward Tan
Department of Surgery, Radboudumc, Netherlands

Onur Balaban and Tayfun Aydın
Department of Anesthesiology and Pain Medicine, Dumlupinar University Hospital, Merkez, Kutahya, Turkey

Nitish Fokeerah, Xinwei Liu, Yonggang Hao and Lihua Peng
Department of Anesthesiology, The First Affiliated Hospital of Chongqing Medical University, No. 1, Youyi Road, Yuanjiagang, Yuzhong District, Chongqing 400016, China

Garret Weber, JuHan Yao, Shemeica Binns and Shinae Namkoong
Department of Anesthesiology, New York Medical College, Valhalla, NY, USA

Sangeeta Kumaraswami and Gabriel Farkas
Department of Anesthesiology, New York Medical College at Westchester Medical Center, Valhalla, NY, USA

William C. Fox
Department of Anesthesiology, Duke University Medical Center, Box 3823, Durham, NC 27710, USA

Matthew Read
Critical Care Medicine, Department of Anesthesiology, Duke University Medical Center, Box 3823, Durham, NC 27710, USA

Richard E. Moon, Eugene W. Moretti and Brian J. Colin
General, Vascular, Transplant Division, Department of Anesthesiology, Duke University Medical Center, Box 3823 Durham, NC 27710, USA

Index